HEALTH IN ACTION

series in physical education, health, and recreation
ROBERT N. SINGER, SERIES EDITOR

Warren R. Johnson
HEALTH IN ACTION

Ronald G. Marteniuk
INFORMATION PROCESSING IN MOTOR SKILLS

Robert N. Singer et al.
PHYSICAL EDUCATION: FOUNDATIONS

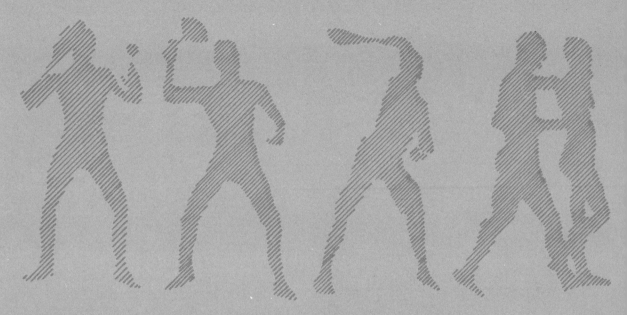

COLLABORATORS

Edwin G. Belzer, Jr.
Dalhousie University

Margaret W. Bridwell
University of Maryland

Michael S. Brock
Doctoral Candidate, University of Oregon

George W. Cox
San Diego State University

Johanna T. Dwyer
New England Medical Center

Albert Ellis
*Institute for Advanced Study
in Rational Psychotherapy*

Calvin J. Frederick
National Institute of Mental Health

Julia Ann Johnson
Consultant, University of Maryland

Warren R. Johnson
University of Maryland

Irving I. Kessler
Johns Hopkins University

Lester A. Kirkendall
Professor Emeritus, Oregon State University

Daniel Leviton
University of Maryland

E. James Lieberman
U.S. Public Health Service

Laurence E. Morehouse
University of California, Los Angeles

Ralph Nader
Public Citizen, Inc.

Elinor Jeanne Walker
*Graduate Student, University of California,
Los Angeles*

Holt, Rinehart and Winston

New York Chicago San Francisco Atlanta Dallas
Montreal Toronto London Sydney

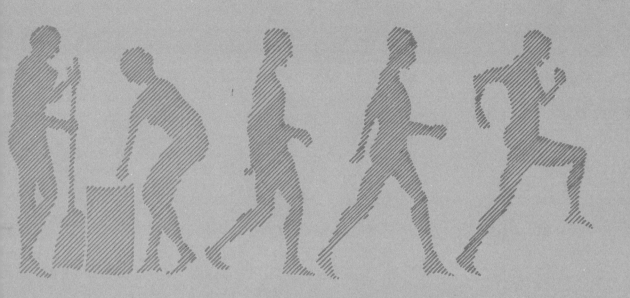

HEALTH IN ACTION

WARREN R. JOHNSON, Editor

Library of Congress Cataloging in Publication Data

Main entry under title:
HEALTH IN ACTION.
  1. Hygiene. I. Belzer, Edwin G.
II. Johnson, Warren Russell, 1921–
RA776.H448   613   76-26679
ISBN 0-03-014521-X

Printed in the United States of America
7 8 9 0   032   9 8 7 6 5 4 3 2 1

Credits and Acknowledgments

Chapter-opening photographs: 1, Leo de Wys, Inc.; *2*, Sybil Shackman/Monkmeyer; *3*, Mimi Forsyth/Monkmeyer; *4*, Laima Drushkis/Editorial Photocolor Archives; *5*, Marion Bernstein/Editorial Photocolor Archives; *6*, E. James Lieberman ("La Ronde" by Helen Phillips); *7*, Ian Berry/Magnum Photos; *8*, Michelle Stone/Editorial Photocolor Archives; *9*, Wide World Photos; *10*, Lida Moser—DPI; *11*, P. Rowntree—DPI; *12*, N.Y. Public Library Picture Collection; *13*, Mimi Forsyth/Monkmeyer.

Figure 5-2 on page 188 and the quotations on pages 186, 187, and 189 are taken from *Understanding Love* by L. A. Kirkendall and R. F. Osborne. Copyright © 1968, Science Research Associates, Inc. Reprinted by permission of the publisher.

EDITOR'S NOTE

In this book no effort has been made to conceal the fact that health is a controversial subject. Of course, there are a few areas of agreement: no one seems to find much good to say about cigarette smoking, air, water, or food pollution, or overpopulation. Even exercise has its critics, but no one recommends total inactivity or bed rest as a way of life for health reasons. Nutritionists have their differences, but they agree that the diet needs to include a variety of crucial nutrients. Beyond a short list of items such as these, however, health subjects are apt to provoke many conflicting opinions.

Health in Action was planned from the outset to take into account the crucial *what, where,* and *how* of health teaching. The following is a brief description of the basis for selecting what topics are included in this book, where highly authoritative information on these topics was located, and how the material was organized and presented to optimize learning.

Selection of subject matter. In every field there is a hierarchy of subjects ranging from what is most important to what is least important. To help me select the topics for this book, I found it convenient to visualize a bull's eye target. The bull's eye represents the crucial information relating to human health, and the rings moving away from the bull's eye represent progressively less crucial information. Thus the bull's eye might represent "urgent" information, the next ring, "very important," the next, "important," and finally at some distance, "nice to know." The problem, then, was to determine which of the numerous subject areas in the field of human health represent crucial information with respect to the intended audience, namely, first-year college students for the most part. The topics finally selected were the result of (1) studies conducted to determine areas of student interest and (2) what experts consider to be the most urgent health needs confronting individuals and society today.

Most of the chapters in this volume are tried and true in the sense that they deal with subject matter that has long been established as part of the college education curriculum. However, as a glance at the table of contents will show, some chapters deal with subjects that have not previously appeared in this particular literature. For example, crisis intervention and death education are not ordinarily included in health books, and the chapter discussing the role of language in relation to human health is entirely new. Including these chapters was a matter of judgment based upon broad experience not only with health educators but also with large numbers of students who found an introduction to these subjects of great value. These subjects may be like ecology, which was not recognized as a health problem by many people just a few years ago but is now a standard subject in virtually all health books.

Achieving balance in the types of subject matter included in a text of this type is important. Naturally specialists who prepare health books tend to see their own specialty as the most important, be it environment, mental health, biology, nutrition, disease, or something else. We have tried to make the coverage in *Health in Action* well balanced. The simple diagram shown here representing the various aspects of

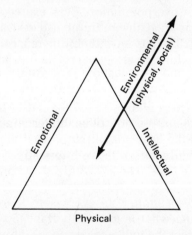

human personality functioning provided a guideline as to what categories of subjects should be considered to ensure balanced coverage of material.

The triangular representation suggests the essential oneness of the human personality and the interdependence of the physical, emotional, and intellectual aspects. The arrow, pointed at both ends and extending from the center of the triangle, suggests the interaction of the individual with his or her social (including language) and physical environment. The aim of this text is to present a balanced view of these individual-social factors in human health.

Part I is concerned with maintaining the basic physical self: tending medically to the common maladies of people, selecting foods which encourage feeling and being well, and maintaining a functional, adaptive body through judicious exercise. This is the base of our triangle which influences the status of the rest of the triangle. Part II shifts emphasis to the emotional and related social aspects of personality. Our emotions are determined to a large extent by our thinking and are sometimes channeled and expressed by means of a physical outlet. Part III focuses on matters of social importance—the part of the triangle where the two-way arrow reminds us of the interaction of our social-physical environment and human personality functioning. Here we broaden our experiences to include those outside our immediate sphere.

Source of valid information. The publisher and I agreed that the demands of a subject as broad and complex as human health would best be met by assembling a group of experts to write on their own specialties. Only those persons who are profoundly involved in a given area are in a position to make sensitive and informed judgments about what the status of the field is and what the most crucial factors involved in it are.

Presentation of material to assure learning through action. In order to distinguish our text from those currently in the marketplace, we decided to present our material in the following fashion. First, each chapter begins with an interest-arousing statement in the form of a brief abstract, or overview, of the subject. Second, we pose a challenge to our readers in the form of a few questions that will hopefully provoke them to read further into the chapter for answers. Third, the subject matter is then presented in a lucid and readable manner. Fourth, a general discussion concludes the chapter, pointing out highlights and commenting on implications for human welfare now and prospects for the future. Fifth, a short bibliography of outstanding sources is given with brief annotations to lure interested students into the available literature.

What about the action phase? How can we claim that this book encourages relevant action to a greater degree than most other texts? By interspersing action suggestions at strategic points in the major discussion sections where the subject is discussed in the greatest detail and the readers' interest has presumably been aroused. These suggestions were deliberately not placed at the end of the chapter, as is customa*
in other health books. This was done because by the time readers h*

reached the end of the chapter, their interest in what happened several pages back has generally declined, if not disappeared completely.

In a way it is artificial to distinguish between verbal and other activity suggestions because the ability to verbalize what is recalled and organized cognitively is certainly an important activity. However, the emphasis here is often physically going places and doing things. Of course, this action may have a prominent verbal element in it. Note that the activity suggestions given in the book are merely suggested *starting points* for action. The instructor and class can readily extend the list or replace it entirely with their own preferred activities.

All of us who have contributed to this book believe that this cooperative effort has resulted in a volume that is self-teaching to a surprising extent and in terms of its "systems" approach, a pioneer work in the field. This book does not pretend to tell the ultimate story of human health. But in every chapter there is information which, after careful consideration and testing, might lead to worthwhile modifications in health behavior. In evaluating this information with respect to making health decisions, real progress may be made in learning to utilize the scientific approach in practical day-to-day affairs. Perhaps this can also be a step in adopting a rational-action approach to health and life generally. We hope so.

We would like to thank those who have taken time to provide critiques for us in various stages of the manuscript. They are Mary K. Beyrer, Ohio State University; Verne G. Zellmer, American River College; James M. Pryde, American River College; Russel F. Whaley, Slippery Rock State College; Ellen Gillespie, Ohio University, Athens; Harriet Krantz, Queensboro Community College; Richard A. Windsor, Carl Shantzs, Syracuse University; Walter Lalor, Ithaca College; Willis R. Baker, Michigan State University; Patrick Earey, University of North Carolina-Chapel Hill; Marian K. Solleder, University of North Carolina-Greensboro; Robert N. Singer, Florida State University; Wesley Staton, New Mexico State University.

College Park, Maryland **Warren R. Johnson**

BIOGRAPHIES

Edwin G. Belzer, Jr., is a health educator at Dalhousie University in Nova Scotia. He is a member of the Nova Scotia Commission on Drug Dependency, which establishes volunteer committees and boards to initiate and oversee programs in the prevention and treatment of drug dependencies.

Margaret W. Bridwell is presently Director of the Health Center of the University of Maryland, College Park. She is also an assistant professor in the Department of Social Hygiene and Preventive Medicine at the University of Maryland Medical School and is on the faculty of the Family Planning Training Institute of Maryland Planned Parenthood. Her background is clinical, both as a general practioner and as an obstetrician-gynecologist. Human sexuality and health education are her particular interests.

Michael S. Brock is currently a doctoral candidate at the University of Oregon, Eugene. He wishes to concentrate in the areas of community health education, gerontology, and interpersonal relationships.

George W. Cox is Professor of Biology and a member of the ecology program at San Diego State University. He has taught and conducted research activities in the areas of basic and applied ecology, emphasizing avian ecology, conservation ecology, and recently the rapidly emerging field of agricultural ecology. He has authored numerous publications in the field of ecology.

Johanna T. Dwyer is Director of the Frances Stern Nutrition Center of the New England Medical Center Hospital, Boston, and is an associate professor in the Departments of Medicine and Community Health at Tufts University Medical School. She is also a lecturer in maternal and child nutrition at the Harvard School of Public Health. Her major research interests are child nutrition and obesity.

Albert Ellis is Executive Director of the Institute for Advanced Study in Rational Psychotherapy in New York City and Adjunct Professor of Clinical Psychology at Rutgers University. He has pioneered in the field of sex education and sex therapy for many years and in the field of psychotherapy as the originator of rational-emotive therapy (RET). He has written widely for professionals in the field of therapy and counseling as well as for general readers who want help with their sexual and emotional problems.

Calvin J. Frederick is Chief of the Disaster Assistance and Emergency Mental Health Section of the National Institute of Mental Health. He is also Associate Clinical Professor in the Department of Psychiatry and Behavioral Sciences at the George Washington University School of Medicine and Assistant Professor in the Department of Psychiatry and Behavioral Sciences at the Johns Hopkins University School of Medicine. As an advisor to the Pan American Health Organization, Dr. Frederick has developed initial studies into violent deaths in selected Latin American countries. Most recently he organized a new section dealing with mental health emergencies and problems of disaster relief within the Alcohol, Drug Abuse, and Mental Health Administration of HEW.

Julia Ann Johnson is Supervisor of the Children's Health and Developmental Clinic at the University of Maryland, College Park. Her particular interest is perceptual motor development, an area in which she has done consulting and presented workshops. She was a collaborator of *Human Sexual Behavior and Sex Education.*

Warren R. Johnson is Professor of Health Education and Director of the Children's Health and Developmental Clinic at the University of Maryland, College Park. He has written numerous books and articles on human health. For years he has been teaching parents and students alike about child health. Dr. Johnson is also a well-known authority on sex education and was president of the American Association of Sex Educators and Counselors.

Irving I. Kessler is Professor of Epidemiology at the Johns Hopkins University School of Hygiene and Public Health. He is also a consultant to the National Cancer Institute and the Uterine Cancer Task Force of the American Cancer Society, Maryland Division, and serves as Associate Editor of the *American Journal of Epidemiology*. Dr. Kessler has conducted a number of studies concerned with causal factors in Parkinson's disease, diabetes, and various kinds of cancer. He lectures and teaches on preventive medicine and disease detection at the University of Maryland School of Medicine.

Lester A. Kirkendall, Professor Emeritus of Family Life, Oregon State University, has been known for many years for his contributions to the fields of marriage, family life, and human sexuality. He was formerly Director of the Association for Family Living in Chicago. He has taught in various colleges and universities and was on the staff at Oregon State University from 1949 to 1968. He was cofounder of the Sex Information and Education Council of the United States and vice president and member of the Board of Directors of the American Association of Sex Educators and Counselors. He has recently published the booklet *A New Bill of Sexual Rights and Responsibilities.*

Daniel Leviton is Professor of Health Education and Director of the Adults' Health and Developmental Program, therapeutic program for older adults at the University of Maryland. He has pioneered in establishing and legitimatizing the study of death and dying, love and peace behaviors, and sexuality among older people.

E. James Lieberman is a psychiatrist in private practice. His particular interests are marriage, carefully planned parenthood, and sex education. He has actively worked toward the interaction of community mental health and social psychiatry. He has coauthored *Sex and Birth Control: A Control for the Young* and is editor of *Mental Health: The Public Health Challenge.*

Laurence E. Morehouse is Professor of Kinesiology at the University of California, Los Angeles. As National Research Council Senior Scientist at the Manned Spacecraft Center in Houston, he helped define the exercise needs of NASA astronauts. His work also includes physiological studies of astronauts and world class athletic champions. Dr. Morehouse is coauthor of the best seller *Total Fitness in Thirty Minutes a Week.* He believes that exercising need not be grueling to be effective, particularly in the case of nonathletic individuals.

Ralph Nader, a leading consumer advocate, is the managing trustee of the Washington-based Center for the Study of Responsive Law. From the time of his first major publication, *Unsafe at Any Speed* (1965), to the present, he has written, testified, and organized for improved safety and health legislation on the part of government, greater public accountability on the part of industry, and increased awareness on the part of consumers. Nader is the president of Public Citizen, Inc., which funds the Health Research Group, a group working in the areas of health care delivery, occupational safety and health, food and drugs, and product safety.

Elinor Jeanne Walker is a graduate student in kinesiology at the University of California, Los Angeles. Her goal is to apply the theoretical side of physical education and kinesiology to the practical side of movement activities.

CONTENTS

part three: **our health and society** *300*

HEALTH
IN
ACTION

part one

tending to
basic needs

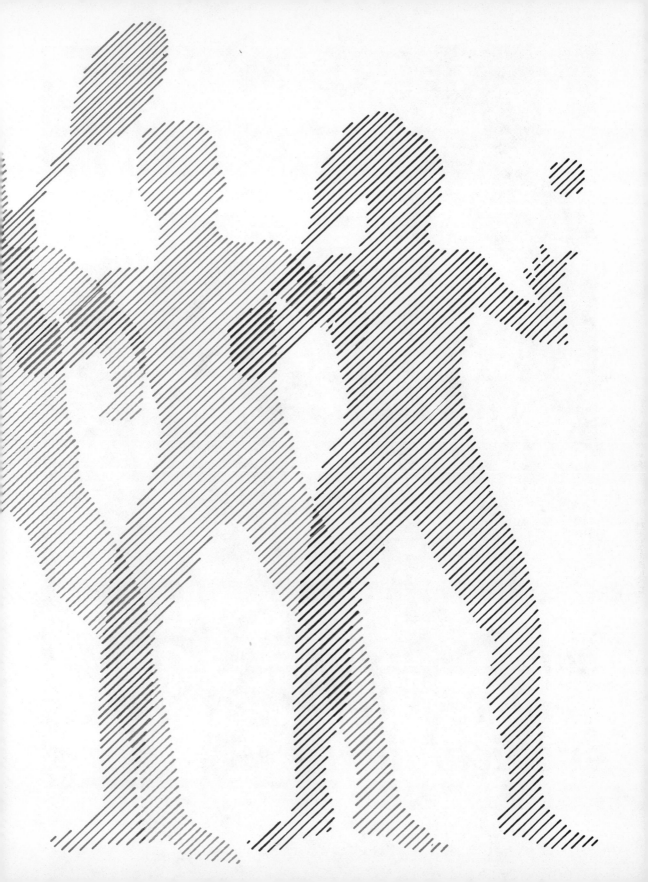

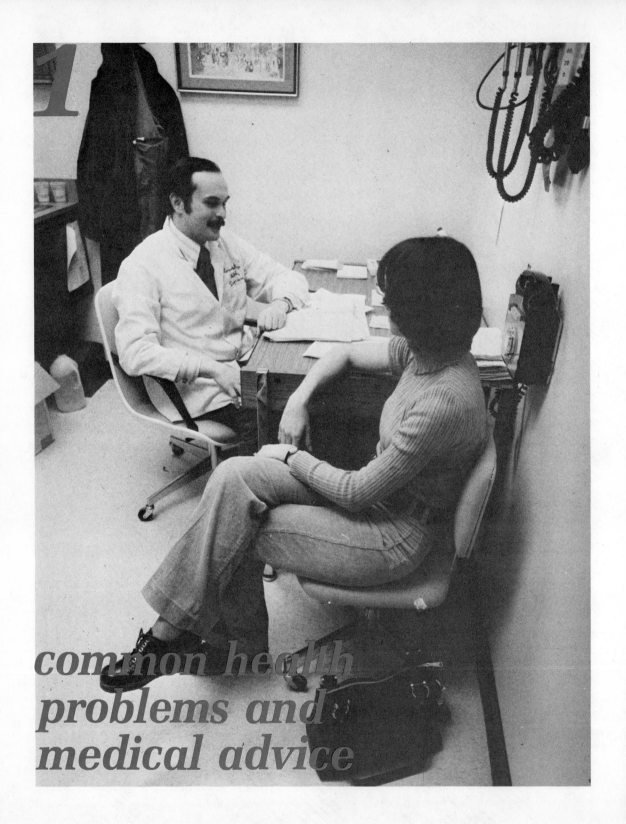

1

*common health
problems and
medical advice*

OVERVIEW

*In the final analysis, students are responsible for their own health.
Health education is concerned with helping them assume this
responsibility. However, virtually all campuses provide a health
service to take care of students in time of medical need. This
chapter is concerned with identifying what long experience has
shown to be the more common problems that lead students to
seek medical help. The general mode of medical treatment is also
described briefly. The approach used is to start with the head and
move downward, taking into account all parts of the body. Finally,
emotional health problems commonly seen by health service
doctors are outlined, with emphasis on how students may help
each other with such problems.*

INQUIRY

1. I've had a headache for two weeks. Could it be the tension I'm under,
   or is there a chance I could have a brain tumor?
2. I've heard that once you've had VD and been treated, you're immune
   for a while. Is that true?
3. There's been so much controversy first about the pill and then about
   the IUD that I'm confused. What is a safe and effective method of
   birth control?
4. Is it true that people my age can get ulcers? How do I know if I have
   one?
5. This morning during my shower I thought I felt a lump in my breast.
   Should I watch it for a while, or should I get it checked right away?
6. I have acne. Help! What do I do for it?

INTRODUCTION

Medical problems can be among the most anxiety-producing that we
can encounter. The very thought of illness conjures up all sorts of
questions: What do you do when you get sick? How do you know when
you are really sick? When should you seek medical attention? Is there
any truth to the stories you have heard about certain illnesses? All of
these questions are of valid concern, and some are not so easy to
answer. In this chapter we take a serious but nontechnical look at these
questions and apply them to the health problems that students most
frequently encounter.

Most of you, before you were even admitted to college, were required
to have a complete physical examination. An extremely important part
of that exam was a detailed history that the doctor or nurse took. You
were asked many questions about your body, and the questions were
usually grouped according to the parts of your body, such as the head
and neck, chest, abdomen, and so on. We will follow this same format
as we discuss the types of problems we see most frequently at a college
health center.

If you develop an understanding of your body, you can take better care of yourself. This is health in action. Today young people are insisting on being more involved in their own medical care; this too is health in action. The way you view your own body and take care of yourself will have an influence on others. You will find others asking you questions about your health and theirs and consulting with you about their health problems. Thus if you are informed, you may contribute to the health status of others as well as your own.

TAKING ACTION

1. Invite a physician from your college health service to visit class, describe just what services are provided, and answer your questions. Ask about such things as emergency procedures and when to and when not to seek medical help.
2. Pay a visit to your health service so that you will know just where it is and what its procedures are.
3. Form committees to discover and report on what off-campus medical and dental services are provided in the community.

HEAD AND NECK
Headaches

Headaches are a common complaint of young people. They can stem from a wide variety of problems and present themselves in various ways, but the most common types are tension headaches, migraine headaches, and sinus headaches.

Tension headaches are usually felt in the upper back part of the neck or lower part of the head. The pain can be dull and throbbing or very sharp. It is helpful to look back and determine what emotional tension may have contributed to your headache. This can either help relieve it or at least help you prevent a recurrence in the future. Measures to relieve your headache include massaging the shoulders and back of the neck to loosen tight muscles. Simple pain relievers such as aspirin or buffered aspirin are usually adequate for relieving a headache. Find out what medication works best for you, but don't be misled by the television ads that try to sell you special-strength tablets or headache medication "for women only." These products tend to be more expensive, and only you can best determine what is most effective for your tension headache. Do something about the situation that causes it, or at least try to learn to live with it. Chapter 4 on emotional health provides many useful suggestions in this regard.

Migraine headaches are commonly referred to but in actuality do not occur that often. They classically start with an "aura," such as seeing spots before your eyes or seeing colors. The aura soon progresses to pain. The pain formerly was considered to be only on one side of the head. The episode can also include nausea and vomiting. The medical profession thinks that migraine headaches may be caused by the constriction or tightening of the blood vessels in the brain. We do know that they seem to run in families. Moreover, they can be related to tension, and thus a migraine is sometimes difficult to differentiate from a tension headache. Treatment is most effective at the onset of the aura, but medication can also be effective during the actual headache. If you think you have had one or more migraine headaches, it is best to see a physician or nurse practitioner for evaluation.

Sinus headache is a broad term used to refer to head pain caused by congestion in or inflammation of the sinuses. Sinuses are pockets in the facial bones that help the voice sound resonate. They are small, and when inflamed, they do not drain as freely as the nose. This causes painful pressure to build up inside the sinus. The pain is usually in the forehead or cheekbones and may increase when you bend over.

Sinus congestion may be caused by a cold, an allergy, or a bacterial infection. Unlike tension headaches, which can usually be relieved by simple pain relievers, the sinus headache is best relieved by a decongestant to drain the sinuses and reduce the pressure. If sinus headaches persist and recur frequently, your physician should be consulted. You may be allergic to some substance, or you may have developed a sinus infection.

Brain tumors are most uncommon but are often feared when people have a headache for a prolonged period of time. Other symptoms that may be indicative are double vision, reduced peripheral range of vision to either side, difficulty keeping balance, and severe pain. Some tumors can be removed with relative ease and cause no further difficulty. Some are malignant and grow rapidly and are therefore very serious. Persistent headaches should be checked by a physician.

Headaches can also be caused by poorly fitted glasses, contact lenses, or the need for a change in your optical prescription. We will discuss contact lenses more in the section on eyes.

Eyes

Of all the senses, many people value their sight the most. They are remarkable receivers of information, and they deserve our most careful protection and attention. Problems with our eyes should not be taken lightly.

Conjunctivitis is an inflammation of the eyes. It may be caused by an allergy, eyestrain, an infection, chemical irritants, or a foreign body. If the inflammation is caused by an allergy, the source of the allergy should be removed. A change in shampoo, makeup, mascara, or soap is one possibility. Irritants in the air or clothing fibers also can cause it. If you cannot readily determine the cause and if the inflammation persists, you should seek medical attention.

The inflammation may be caused by an infection. You no doubt have seen people with red, irritated eyes having a yellowish discharge. This condition, called "pink eye," is caused by bacteria; it is contagious and should be treated with antibiotic ointments or drops.

If you get a foreign body in your eye, it is probably either a speck of dust or eyelash (even though it may feel much larger). Your eyes will

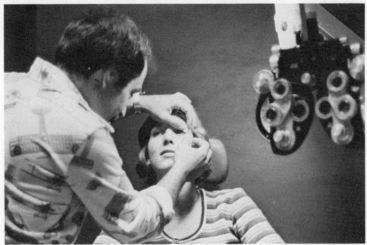

Robert de Villeneuve

tear and float the object away, but if the condition persists, you should seek medical attention.

Should you get any type of chemical solution (household cleaner, hair spray, makeup) in your eye, flush your eye *immediately* with large amounts of water. Do not hesistate to call your doctor or emergency room for advice whenever you get a chemical in your eye.

Contact lenses can be a marvelous solution for many people who need corrective lenses. They not only have cosmetic benefits but can improve your vision considerably. Contacts are small disks that cover the iris (the colored part of the eye). They do not actually touch the eye but float on a very thin layer of tears. Not everyone can wear them, and they must be properly fitted.

Contacts must have proper care. There are special solutions for cleansing, storing, and wetting the lenses. The wetting solution is the same as your tears, making it more comfortable for you to insert the contacts. When inserting them, *never* use saliva. Serious infections can result.

A few pointers to keep in mind:

Don't swim with contacts in (they may float away).
Don't sleep with your contacts in (you may get corneal abrasions).
Your eyes may be more sensitive to bright light with contacts. Tinted lenses can help reduce the glare, but sunglasses may be necessary.
Never wear your contacts for more than 10 to 12 hours. Corneal abrasions may result from overuse.

A corneal abrasion is a scratch on the cornea, which can be caused by contacts or a foreign body. The eye will tear, feel painful, often be sensitive to light, and feel as if something were in it. The eye should be examined by a medical person, who will usually treat it with drops and a tight patch for a day or so. Since the eye has a good supply of blood, it heals rapidly. If the abrasion was caused by contacts, you may need to go back to your original "breaking in" schedule when you start wearing the lenses again.

Ears

Ears are also highly sensitive organs. General care of your ears includes *not* putting anything in them. In medical school we were taught not to put anything smaller than our elbows in our ears, and it is still a pretty good rule. Unfortunately, some people use all sorts of objects to clean out their ears: hair pins, crochet hooks (shudder!), paper clips, and the like. Such objects can seriously damage the ear canal or, even worse, the eardrum. The damage can result in scarring and a reduction of hearing capacity. Actually, few people need to clean out their ears because nature has provided earwax to keep the skin from drying out and cracking, thus preventing infections from developing in these cracks. Some people, however, overproduce wax, and it becomes packed in the ear. This can easily be removed by having a nurse or doctor syringe it out with warm water. Using cotton swabs may only further impact the wax.

Reduction in hearing may be caused by several things, and it should never be neglected. If you suspect that you have a hearing loss, cover one ear with your hand and have someone whisper a word 5 feet away. Do the same with the other ear. If you still suspect a reduction, make an appointment with a physician. Often college campuses have a speech and hearing (audiology) department where you can have your hearing checked.

Infection in the ear can be either in the outer ear, middle ear, or inner ear. Infection in the outer ear, or ear canal, usually is evidenced by itching, pain, and the weeping of a clear fluid. It is most frequently caused by a fungus and is sometimes referred to as *swimmer's ear*. It should be treated by your doctor who may recommend the use of earplugs while swimming, at least temporarily.

Infections in the middle and inner ear are similar to each other, except that the inner ear infection may cause dizziness and nausea in addition to the other symptoms. Ear infection is usually characterized by severe pain, along with a feeling of fullness in the ear. This needs to be treated by a doctor who will prescribe antibiotics. Should the infection be allowed to progress without treatment, the pressure of the fluid may become so great that the eardrum will burst, which results in the drainage of bloody fluid from the ear. The eardrum might heal with scarring, thus reducing hearing capacity. There is the possibility that the infection may spread to the mastoid area and even the brain. Fortunately, antibiotic treatment of ear infections can arrest the problem before it leads to serious complications.

Ear piercing is often a topic of concern with young people. If you want to have your ears pierced, there is no reason not to have it done, so long as it is done carefully by someone trained in the correct technique. Avoid using any type of needle for piercing; it can lead to infection. A new instrument resembling a pistol now safely and antiseptically pierces the ear while threading the post of the earring at the same time. After the piercing, wipe the earlobe several times a day with alcohol for a week or so to keep it clean during healing. Incidentally, if you are the type of person whose skin develops rashes from rings and watchbands, you may develop a metal rash from the earring as well.

Nose

Your nose is used not only for smelling but also for filtering out bacteria and other substances that might enter your body and cause infection.

The *common cold* is the most frequent infection associated with the nose. Despite all of medicine's advanced technology we have not found a cure for the cold. Hence we have no choice but to let it take its natural course. Nevertheless, there are some measures that can help relieve the symptoms. Over-the-counter decongestants can break up the congestion, and aspirin can reduce the achiness and fever. Antihistamines help only if an allergy is involved, which is rare. Antibiotics are not effective against viruses (only against bacteria), and the cold is caused by a virus. So the all-too-common practice of taking an antibiotic for a cold is not only ineffective, it also may cause the user to develop a sensitivity to the antibiotic, thus making it impossible to be taken when it is really needed.

Nosebleeds are usually not serious, and the amount of blood lost usually appears to the victim to be far more than it really is. However, prolonged bleeding could be serious and may require medical attention. To stop most nosebleeds pinch your nose just below the bony part.

Teeth and Gums

Just brushing your teeth every day is not enough. Plaque-detecting tablets, available from your dentist or from your drugstore, demonstrate the problem. The tablets color the areas that need attention; the color goes away immediately, but the plaque that it shows does not.

Plaque is caused by bacteria and their film on the teeth, which can lead to tooth decay. Bacteria between the teeth or at the gum line can

Semiannual dental examinations help ensure the health of teeth and gums.

Blair Seitz/Editorial Photocolor Archives

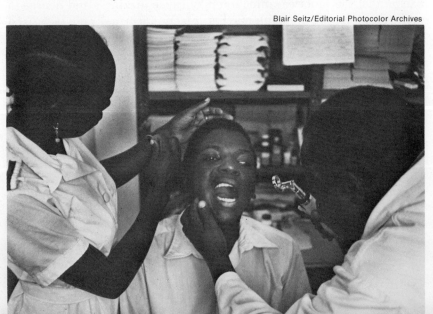

cause gum disease. If the bacteria are not cleared away, a hard deposit called *tartar* will be formed. Careful brushing and the use of dental floss to get to the hard-to-clean places can reduce the formation of plaque and thus cut down on decay and gum disease.

Bleeding from the gums can be due to poor care of the teeth and can be much more serious. Infection may be the cause; it can be treated by your dentist but can be serious enough to require surgical treatment. Bleeding gums can also be a symptom of medical problems. If your dentist finds no cause, you should have a complete medical checkup.

Throat

Sore throats are both common and painful, and their treatment varies significantly with their cause. The two most common causes are viruses and bacteria.

Viral sore throats are usually associated with the symptoms of a cold, have a slow onset, and generally are accompanied by only a low fever, if any. You may also notice swollen glands in your neck that are very tender to touch. A viral throat infection can be every bit as painful as a bacterial sore throat, but the treatment is different. The best way to determine the cause is to have a throat culture done by a nurse or physician. The results are usually available in 24 hours. If no bacteria are present on the culture, the sore throat is probably viral. Treatment is rest, fluids, hard candies or lozenges to soothe the dry, scratchy feeling, and aspirin for fever and pain. Again, antibiotics should not be used, since they would be ineffective.

Bacterial sore throats may have the same symptoms as the viral, but the fever may go up to as high as 103° F to 104°F. If you still have your tonsils, they may be enlarged with patches of whitish pus on them. Again, the only way to know for sure the cause of the sore throat is a culture. If it is bacterial, the organism is most often streptococcus, which responds readily to antibiotics. With strep throat it is most important to obtain adequate medical treatment because such complications as kidney and heart disease can occur.

TAKING ACTION

1. *Invite a medical specialist to visit class to discuss any of the foregoing symptoms that are of special interest. As an alternative, prepare questions to ask a specialist and report back to the class.*
2. *Invite a dental hygienist to talk with the class about preventive dental hygiene and common dental problems.*
3. *Form a committee to evaluate over-the-counter headache and cold medicines. Talk with the pharmacist about the actual value of each, their safety, and strength versus cost. Evaluate and discuss your own medication on the basis of what you learn.*
4. *Form a committee to visit a medical laboratory and observe demonstrations of actual tests such as throat culture, positive strep culture plate, and drug sensitivity.*

THORAX   Your thorax is the upper part of your body, not including your arms. Among college students two health problems are most significant: upper respiratory infections and breast masses.

Upper Respiratory Tract   *Upper respiratory infections* are infections of the nose, throat, and chest. They can be mild, like a cold, or severe, like pneumonia. We will discuss some of the most common ones.

Flu is an upper respiratory infection. Sometimes it has the same symptoms as the common cold, but it is usually accompanied by a fever, chills, and body aches and pains. Occasionally you may have some nausea and vomiting, but this is infrequent. The flu, like the common cold, will make you feel miserable, but it must take its own course since it too is caused by viruses, and antibiotics can't cure it. There is considerable discussion about flu vaccines. Some doctors strongly advise them, whereas others feel they should be given only to the high-risk populations such as the elderly and the chronically ill. One problem is that the flu virus with which you are inoculated may well not be the virus you encounter.

Pneumonia is an infection of the lungs that can be caused either by a virus or bacteria. Its frequency and severity these days has been greatly diminished by antibiotics, but we still see some cases among young people. It is most commonly a complication of another upper respiratory infection such as flu or bronchitis. When diagnosing pneumonia, a chest X ray is important to help rule out the possibility of tuberculosis.

Tuberculosis (TB) is still present; medical science has not conquered the problem. People must still be tested, diagnosed, and treated. However, there are very effective medications that people who have been exposed to TB can take to keep them from developing the disease. It is usually a long-term medication, up to several years, but the

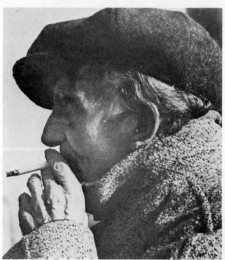

SMOKING IS
VERY DEBONAIR

American Cancer Society

12

treatment is most effective. If you think you have been exposed to TB, don't hesitate to get a skin test done by a nurse or doctor.

Asthma is another respiratory problem. This condition usually involves difficulty in breathing. Wheezing is caused by the tightening of the small air sacs in the lungs, making it difficult for the air to pass in and out of the lungs. Asthma usually is characterized by attacks rather than a continuous condition. It can be caused by external factors such as particles in the air to which a person is allergic or by internal factors such as respiratory infection. Asthma attacks are usually considered a medical emergency but are generally quite responsive to a shot of adrenalin given just under the skin.

Smoking is a matter about which you have probably learned a great deal already. It is well established that smoking is linked to cancer and heart disease, and millions of people have quit as a result. Our general word of advice to you is: if you don't smoke, don't start; if you smoke, quit; and if you can't quit, at least cut down.

Heart

Heart disease usually affects a considerably older age group; nevertheless, young people can sometimes also have problems. One example is the person who was born with a heart defect. Often this can be corrected by surgery soon after birth or even later in life. Following surgery, the person can usually live a completely normal life.

You may have been told you have a heart murmur. This is a sound made as the blood passes through the valves of the heart. It might be a normal condition and thus impose no restrictions on your living habits, or it could necessitate a change in your activities. Your doctor will advise you.

Another phenomenon related to your heart, not uncommon in young people, is an occasional short period of fast and hard heart beating. This is usually normal and should not alarm you. However, it's wise to have such symptoms checked by a physician.

Breasts

Breast lumps can frighten any woman; they should not be taken lightly. Your first thought is apt to be "Is it cancer?" If you discover a lump, have it checked by a physician immediately. *Do not wait.* All lumps do not have to be removed surgically. Medical opinion must determine what is "normal" for you, especially during menstruation. Removal may or may not be indicated. The most common lump is a tumor called *fibroadenoma,* which is a small, fluid-filled cyst. Some women have a tendency toward what is referred to as lumpy breasts. This is called *chronic cystic mastitis,* and it should be observed carefully. The cysts in chronic cystic mastitis may be very small and are often tender. If there is a change in the cysts, they should be further checked. Hopefully, all women will learn to check their own breasts. This way they become familiar with them and can quickly note any changes that take place. Self-breast exams should be done monthly after the menstrual period. This is the time when breasts are the least tender. Before

13

the menstrual period a woman's breasts prepare for pregnancy, that is, prepare to start producing milk. This makes them more tender and full and disappears with the period. Self-breast examinations should start at least by the age of 18 and should be done regularly.

The American Cancer Society recommends that women examine their breasts monthly for early detection of breast cancer. A simple three-step procedure is shown here.

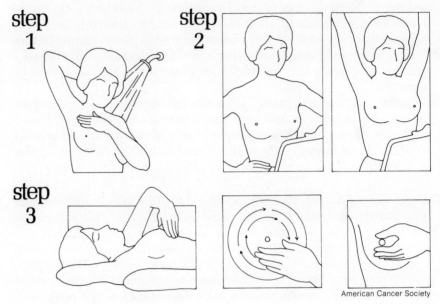

American Cancer Society

Men sometimes have an enlargement of their breasts. This condition, called *gynecomestia,* is seen most often in adolescent males. It generally disappears gradually. The enlargement can be caused by some hormonal imbalance in a man's system, but it should be checked by a physician to rule out the very small possibility of cancer.

ABDOMEN *The abdominal cavity* is the area of the body between the diaphragm or ribs and the pelvic area. It contains the stomach and all its related digestive organs: the liver, spleen, pancreas, and appendix, among other organs. Most problems in this area either are related to the digestive system or involve infection or inflammation of the other organs. Almost all of the problems cause some form of abdominal pain.

If severe abdominal pain continues for more than a few hours, you should consult your doctor.

Appendicitis is not nearly as common as it used to be, but it still occurs. Appendicitis usually starts with pain near the navel and is accompanied by nausea and vomiting and/or diarrhea or loose bowel movements. Shortly after the pain starts, it usually moves to the lower right side of the abdomen and can be quite severe. The treatment is surgical removal of the appendix. Most young people are up walking the day of the surgery or at least the morning after. The scar from the surgery is usually very small.

Gastroenteritis, an inflammation of the stomach and intestines, is usually indicated by severe nausea, vomiting, and diarrhea. Many times it has been mistakenly referred to as the "stomach flu" or "24-hour bug." The onset of the nausea and vomiting can be very sudden and quite severe. Fortunately, the symptoms do not last more than a day or two. The best treatment is to rest in bed (near a bathroom) and not eat or drink anything except ice chips or sips of ginger ale or cola for 24 hours. Then you can start taking clear chicken or beef broth, jello, and clear juices. After you're sure your stomach can handle that, slowly go back to a normal diet. If the rest and abstinence from food don't clear up the symptoms, a doctor can give you something to stop the vomiting and diarrhea.

Peptic ulcers do occur in young people. Actually, they're seen more often than one would expect in this age group, although the number seen in any age group has mysteriously decreased. An ulcer is actually a loss of the first layer of tissue in some spot in your stomach. This is like an open sore, which is irritated by the stomach acid that helps to digest your food. This irritation often causes a burning, cramping, or gnawing feeling, usually just below the breastbone (the stomach itself is quite high up in the abdominal cavity). The pain is often associated with hunger and can occur quite severely in the middle of the night.

Treatment should usually be supervised by your doctor and will include a diet low in spices and often milk between meals to help neutralize the acid in the stomach. Certain medications such as aspirin can increase the symptoms and should be avoided.

If you have an ulcer and ever start vomiting blood, contact your doctor right away. Bleeding ulcers can be severe and require immediate treatment—possibly surgery. We think ulcers can be brought about by or aggravated by emotional stress or tension. The reduction of the tension can help relieve an ulcer. Tension and stress are dealt with more specifically in a later chapter.

Constipation seems to be a great American concern—if one may judge from TV commercials. Actually, constipation is often overdramatized but nevertheless can be quite uncomfortable when you're affected. Constipation is defined as the passage of dry, hard stools or the absence of a bowel movement for more than three days. It is quite normal for some people not to have bowel movements daily. Constipation is best treated by good dietary habits. Plenty of water, fruit (except bananas), and whole grain cereal such as bran flakes, and whole wheat bread (instead of white bread) are all beneficial in treating constipation. Over-the-counter laxatives and stool softeners are effective but should only be used when dietary measures don't relieve the symptoms. The frequent or regular use of laxatives is not a good practice because it actually causes the bowel to get "lazy" and fail to do its work unless further laxatives are used.

Hemorrhoids or *piles* are actually varicose veins at the opening of the rectum, or anus. The veins are thin walled, and, the pressure of straining at stool can cause them to swell and become clotted, which is very painful. The veins can be up inside the opening to the rectum (internal hemorrhoids) and are therefore hard to see, or they can be outside the opening to the rectum (external hemorrhoids). They are usually very tender and become more so as they become more swollen. They may be discovered because you see bright blood on the toilet tissue or because the passing of a stool is painful. Alternatively, you may just discover the hemorrhoid itself, which may appear to be like a small tag of skin or cyst.

Treatment is usually warm, moist heat (sitting in a clean, warm tub for 20 minutes or so), or rectal suppositories and medication to soften your stools. Hemorrhoids can be removed surgically, but that is usually a last measure.

To help prevent hemorrhoids, establish regular bowel habits. It is not wise to sit for long periods of time on the toilet or to use your abdominal muscles, straining hard, to help push during the evacuation of a stool.

A *hernia* is a bulge on the abdominal wall, either through the navel or on either side of the groin. It actually is a weakening in the muscle wall of the abdomen that causes the intestines to bulge through the wall under the skin. This occurs where the muscle attaches at the lower end in the groin area or through a defect or weakness in the navel itself. It may be noticed when lifting too heavy a load, thus putting an unusual strain on the abdominal wall. Hernias are more common in men, but women can get them also. Usually hernias have to be treated surgically, so contact your doctor if you have the symptoms of one. Moreover, a piece of bowel can get stuck in the opening and become very painful—a real emergency.

Rectal itching can be caused by several things. One of the most obvious causes is pinworms. These are tiny, threadlike, white worms that lay their eggs around the rectal opening, usually at night. This is when the itching is most severe and when you scratch the most. When you scratch, the eggs get under your fingernails, and if you put your fingers in your mouth, the eggs go back into your system, and the cycle starts over again. The eggs can live for long periods of time in dust or on books. To prevent the spreading of the eggs always wash your hands after going to the bathroom. There is medicine available that will cure you, provided that you do not become reinfected.

A woman with vaginitis, which causes itching, can also have itching around the rectum, and it will clear up when the basic infection is cleared up.

Any kind of dermatitis, or skin rash, can be present around this area, especially if kept moist and warm by synthetic underwear. Sometimes the dermatitis is caused by tension. Your doctor can give you an ointment that will help ease the symptoms, but the underlying problem still has to be solved.

Let us stress that the organs and functions of elimination and reproduction are just as important and respectable as any of our other organs and functions. It is wise to learn to know about, care for, discuss, and seek medical help for them when needed—just as with any other parts of our bodies.

TAKING ACTION

1. *Determine which of the symptoms we have discussed are of special interest to the class. Invite one or more medical specialists in for detailed discussion and questioning. As an alternative possibility, make appointments with and visit specialists for specific information. Be sure to prepare questions in advance.*
2. *Contact the local cancer society and request a teach-in on self-breast examination.*

URINARY SYSTEM

The urinary system is composed of the two kidneys, the ureters or tubes that connect the kidneys to the bladder, and the bladder itself. The kidneys filter all the blood that flows in the body and remove the waste products that continuously flow into the bladder. Here the fluid is collected until the pressure triggers the feeling of needing to urinate.

Bladder infection is the most common type of problem of the urinary system. A person with a bladder infection usually feels a burning or painful sensation when urinating, often has a feeling of needing to urinate very frequently, and an inability to hold the urine for any length of time at all. Sometimes the urine will become red with blood. This is not uncommon, but it can be quite alarming.

Bladder infections need prompt and thorough treatment. They are treated best with antibiotics, increased water intake, and often a mild anesthetic for removing the pain associated with urination. (The latter usually contains dyes, so it will probably turn the urine orange or some other color, depending on the type of medication.) An important point to remember is that even though the symptoms may subside in just a few days, the entire course of medication must be taken.

Bladder infections occur more frequently in women than in men. This is logical because the distance up the urethra to the bladder is very short in women, and thus it is relatively easy for bacteria to invade the bladder.

Kidney infection, or *pyelonephretis,* is more serious than a bladder infection. It is often a result of a bladder infection traveling up the ureter to the kidney. With this type of infection there is general systemic evidence of illness: fever, chills, pain in the back at the waistline, and body aches. Kidney infections must receive prompt treatment since serious damage to the infected kidney can result.

REPRODUCTIVE SYSTEM

Problems of the reproductive system, which usually are of greatest interest to college students, relate to infections, venereal diseases, and birth control. We will discuss all of these very briefly.

Veneral Diseases

Veneral disease, or VD,[1] gets its name from Venus, the love goddess, an indication that the diseases in this category are transferred through sexual intercourse. The most common form of VD in college students, is *gonorrhea* ("GC," "clap," "dose," or "runs" are other names you may hear). It is transferred *only* by sexual intercourse.

Of the women who have gonorrhea, only about 20 percent of them have the classical symptoms of large amounts of vaginal discharge, pain in the abdomen, pain with urination, swelling of the vaginal area, and perhaps an elevation of temperature. The other 80 percent may have very mild symptoms, if any, and therefore do not seek medical attention, often finding they have contracted the disease only when they go to a doctor for a routine examination. Of the men, 60 to 70 percent or less of them develop the classical symptoms—that of discharge from the penis and burning with urination.

When gonorrhea goes untreated, it can cause serious complications in both men and women. In men, scarring can develop in the urethra, leading to difficulty in passing urine. In women, scarring and blockage of the fallopian tubes can occur. Each month an egg travels down the fallopian tube to the uterus. If the egg is fertilized, it is usually fertilized partway down the tube. Scarring of the tube can prevent the sperm from reaching the egg, thereby preventing the woman from becoming pregnant. In some cases the sperm is small enough to get through the scarred area, but the fertilized egg, being larger, cannot. It therefore stays and develops in the tube. This is called a *tubal,* or *ectopic,* pregnancy. As the fertilized egg grows, the tube is not able to stretch enough to accommodate it; after 6 to 8 weeks of the pregnancy, the tube will rupture, causing severe bleeding. Immediate surgery is then required.

The gonorrhea organism can also cause blindness in the newborn baby of a mother who has the infection. The baby must pass through the infected vagina during birth and can pick up the organism in its eyes. For this reason, we carefully check and treat pregnant women and put special drops in the eyes of all newborn babies.

The most effective treatment for gonorrhea is penicillin. There are also effective substitute medications for people allergic to penicillin. Prevention of gonorrhea is the best method of combating it. A condom is most helpful for prevention since it eliminates skin-to-skin contact. Another important preventive measure is to inform any of your recent sexual partners if you should discover that you have the infection so that they can also be treated.

Syphilis is another type of venereal disease. It is even more serious than gonorrhea because it gets into the bloodstream and is carried throughout the body. Syphilis is caused by a spirochete, *Treponema pallidum,* which enters the body through either the mucous mem-

---

[1]For further perspective on VD, see Chapter 12.

branes or a broken area in the skin. It is contracted by having sexual intercourse with an infected person.

There are three stages of syphilis. The primary stage is manifested by a painless chancre or sore at the location where the organism entered the body. The chancre appears about 10 days after contact and then goes away in a few days with or without treatment. This disappearance of the chancre without treatment does not mean the disease is cured. It is contagious while the chancre is present.

The secondary stage is usually a skin rash on the body, which can look like almost any skin disease. Thus the name "the great imitator." This skin rash denotes that the infection has gone throughout the bloodstream and now can be detected by a blood test. Occasionally a person won't have a skin rash but will have a sore throat or lose some patches of hair. All these, except the hair loss, which disappears more gradually, will go away in a few days.

The third stage, which develops after years of no apparent activity, is the stage where the very serious problems appear. These days it is rare for someone to reach this stage without diagnosis. Brain damage, blindness, nerve damage, and heart trouble are among the possible late complications of syphilis. The important thing to remember is that syphilis can be cured and that these things do not need to happen. The pregnant mother can pass the disease on to her unborn child. The closer to the time of the pregnancy that the infection occurs the more chance there is for the baby to be infected. The unborn baby can be treated at the same time the mother is; the penicillin will pass from the mother's bloodstream into the baby's and treat it before it is born.

Detection of the disease is done by blood test. One of these tests is called a VDRL; another, the first test to be used, is called a Wassermann, named after the doctor who discovered it. Syphilis is treated with penicillin, or other antibiotics, given over a period of about two weeks.

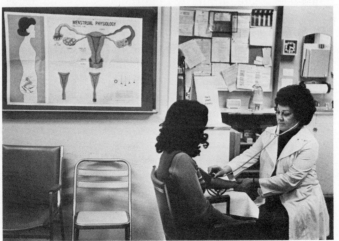

A young woman being examined by her gynecologist.

Sybil Shelton/Monkmeyer

19

There is another whole group of infections that are actually venereal, since they can be transferred by intercourse, although they can also develop without intercourse. These include moniliasis, trichomoniasis, hemophylis, herpes virus, and venereal warts.

Moniliasis is caused by a yeast and often is referred to as a vaginal yeast infection. The symptom is a whitish, sometimes curdy discharge that initially causes severe itching but when untreated can become quite painful. Yeast infections are very common, and are believed to be attributable to the use of nylon underwear and panty hose, which do not breathe and so trap warmth and moisture in the vaginal area, an ideal condition for the growth of the yeast. This problem can be helped by wearing cotton panties. Feminine hygiene deodorant sprays (which are most unnecessary) are irritating and can contribute to the infection. Yeast infection also tends to show up more frequently in women on the pill and can also follow a course of antibiotics. Monilia infection is treated by vaginal creams and tablets; there are no medications yet that can be taken by mouth.

Men, as a rule, do not catch the infection, but occasionally they can get it as an irritation of the groin area, where it is usually called "jock rot." It is treated with the same medications.

Trichomonas vaginalis is an infection caused by the trichomonas organism, a flagellated, pear-shaped organism that gives rise to considerable vaginal discharge, irritation, and itching. Men can also have the trichomonas infection, which is manifested by discharge from the penis and discomfort when urinating. For these reasons its sometimes confused with gonorrhea. There is a most effective medication, which is taken by mouth, but both partners must take it simultaneously or the infection can be passed back and forth.

Hemophylis is caused by rod-shaped bacteria and is most difficult to treat. It causes an irritating vaginal discharge which has a foul odor. Men may have discharge from the penis, but usually no other symptoms. It is treated either with antibiotics or sulfa drugs.

Venereal warts are similar to the warts found elsewhere on the body, but they appear around the vagina or on the penis. They are caused by a virus and can be passed back and forth between partners. Sometimes they go away by themselves, but often they have to be treated with a medication which makes them shrivel up and drop off. They grow well in high-moisture areas, so the use of cotton underwear is important.

Herpes is a serious disease that can occur in the vaginal area. It resembles the fever blisters people get on their lips, but it is usually caused by a different virus. It causes small blisterlike lesions, which are most painful. It can be found around the vagina, on the vaginal walls, or on the cervix. Sometimes the patient may ache all over, have a fever, and appear to have the flu. There is no definitive treatment at this time, but we do have some medications to put on the sores to help them clear up. Women who have herpes should have regular checkups and pap smears at least once a year. There is some concern for the possible relationship between herpes and cervical cancer.

1. *Invite a specialist to discuss and answer questions about VD, including its status locally and nationally.*
2. *Form a committee to visit and report back on the local health department's VD program.*
3. *List and discuss misconceptions about VD.*

Birth control is another topic of real concern to the college-age student. **Birth Control**
If you are sexually active but want to prevent pregnancy, you certainly need birth control information now. If you are not sexually active, you probably will be some day, and you need the information so you can make an informed decision at that time. You need to know something about all the methods of birth control so that your decision will be the proper one for you.

The most common questions are: What is the safest method? What is the best method? What about side effects? How do I obtain birth control information?

There are several types of birth control. The basic methods of action are:

1. Keeping the sperm cells from moving into the uterus, thus preventing their uniting with an egg.
2. Preventing the fertilized egg from becoming implanted in the uterus, where it would grow and be nourished.
3. Keeping the egg from being produced, so that pregnancy cannot occur whether sperm are present or not.
4. Abstaining from intercourse at the time when the egg may be present.

Condoms, foam, and *diaphragms* are three methods that keep the sperm cells from getting up into the uterus. A condom is a thin, rubber sheath that fits over the penis and is worn during intercourse. When the sperm cells are released from the penis at the climax of intercourse, they remain in the rubber sheath and do not move into the vagina. Condoms are available without a prescription from a pharmacy. They are a fairly reliable method of birth control but must be put on correctly prior to any skin-to-skin contact. They also have the advantage of reducing the chance of infection, as was mentioned earlier.

Vaginal foam is a medicine that kills sperm and therefore prevents them from traveling up into the uterus. Foam comes in an aerosol can and is put into an applicator. The applicator is placed in the vagina and the foam is deposited up near the cervix, or opening of the uterus (the means of insertion is similar to placing a tampon in position). Another application of foam should be used prior to each repeated intercourse. Foam used alone is about 80 percent effective, but when used in conjunction with a condom is about 100 percent effective. Foam is also available over the counter without a prescription.

Contraceptive devices. Shown here are birth control pills, condoms, intrauterine devices, a diaphragm, and foam with applicator.

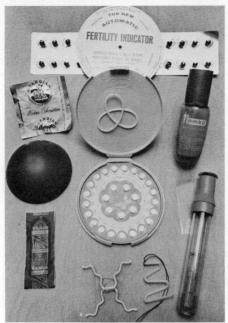

The *diaphragm* is a small rubber cup into which is placed a tablespoon or so of sperm-destroying medicine or jelly. Before intercourse, it is placed by the woman into her vagina so that it covers the cervix, thus leaving the jelly in place to destroy any sperm cells before they can enter the uterus. A diaphragm must be fitted, and its use supervised, by a medical person. Every woman should be carefully taught just how to use it correctly. When it is properly used, it is very effective as a method of birth control and has a low failure rate. Another advantage is that, with the exception of a possible allergic reaction to the jelly, there are no known complications or side effects.

The *IUD,* or *interuterine device,* is a small, plastic device that is placed inside the uterus by a physician or nurse. IUDs come in various sizes and shapes, and their method of action is not known, but it is believed that the foreign body in the uterus prevents the fertilized egg from becoming implanted. The IUD is about 90 to 99 percent effective, depending on the type used. The copper-coated type is the most effective but must be replaced every two years. Most other IUDs, which are not quite as effective, can be left in place for a longer time. When the IUD is first inserted, it often causes cramping and heavy bleeding. Once this stops, the only real evidence of its placement is heavier bleeding at the time of a woman's period. Not all women can wear them; sometimes the uterus will expel them, but this is rare. A woman is taught to feel the IUD's small string, which hangs from the cervix, to be sure that it is still in place and has not either come out or traveled farther up into the uterus. This should be done weekly. If she cannot feel the string, she should check with either her doctor or clinic.

Birth control pills are still the most commonly used method of birth control. They are tiny pills containing very small quantities of hormones that are regularly produced by the body. They are usually taken daily for three weeks, then stopped for a week. The cycle is then repeated. Sometimes there is a sugar pill to take during the week off the hormones, which means that the woman takes a pill each day and runs a lower risk of forgetting to restart. The pill acts on the ovaries to prevent an egg from being produced. With no egg, there can be no pregnancy. During the week a woman does not take the pill she will have light bleeding similar to her menstrual period. Cramps are usually reduced when a woman is on the pill.

There are still some complications related to the pill, so a woman must be under medical supervision when on it. The most common and serious complication is the development of blood clots in the calf of the leg. If a clot is released, it could go to the heart, the lungs, or the brain, causing a heart attack, lung problems, or a stroke. This of course is very serious, and although these complications are rare, any woman on the pill who feels pain in the calf of her leg, chest pain, or severe headaches should see her doctor right away.

If a woman has migraine headaches, if her periods are very irregular, or if she has had cancer, she should not take the pill. If she has liver trouble, diabetes, or epilepsy, her doctor would want to check her carefully before putting her on the pill.

It is a good idea for a woman to stop taking the pill once every two years. If her periods start up again normally, she may return to the pill. If they are not regular, she should not go back on it.

The pill comes in various hormone strengths. The smaller the amount the more careful you must be about taking the pill regularly. The mini-pill has only progesterone in it and occasionally may fail to prevent pregnancy. When determining the method of birth control or the pill you are to use, consult with your doctor.[2]

Diethylstilbestrol (or *DES*) is an important drug to know about. It is an artificial or synthetic form of the female hormone estrogen and has two important applications in relation to this discussion. It has recently been used as a morning-after form of contraception. It also was used 15 to 20 years ago to treat women whose pregnancies were threatened.

Its use as a morning-after pill has been stopped except in very unusual cases and has been discouraged by the Food and Drug Administration. What is of current concern is its use by pregnant women some years ago. Every young woman should find out whether her mother took this drug while she was pregnant with her. If she did, the daughter was exposed to DES and its potentially harmful effects. Moreover, the earlier the drug was given the greater the risk, because the tissues of the developing fetus were more likely to be harmed by medication before they fully developed. The daughters of women who

---

[2]For a discussion of the pill controversy, see Chapter 12.

were given DES are more likely to have cancer of the vagina and must be carefully checked at least from the time they start to menstruate or earlier if they have any vaginal bleeding. If cancer is detected in the early stages, it can be cured by surgery.

A serious question has also been raised with regard to possible effects on male offspring.

Withdrawal means withdrawing the penis just before ejaculation. This means that almost all the sperm cells are deposited outside the vagina, but there may be some leaking during intercourse. Some sperm cells may be about during intercourse and be placed near the cervix. For this reason withdrawal is not one of the best methods, but, like the rhythm method, it is more effective than nothing.

Rhythm is a method that takes advantage of the fact that an egg must be present for a pregnancy to occur. If intercourse takes place at a time before or after the eggs have been produced, then there is no pregnancy. Ovulation takes place about 14 days before the next period starts, so if your periods are quite regular, you could use this method. However, even with regular periods, the egg is sometimes present at a different time. Until we have better methods of determining ovulation, this is far from the best method. If you need to use it, consult with a specialist.

Sterilization. Some young people these days have already decided that they do not ever want to have children. They are not interested in preventing pregnancy just at the present time, but permanently. There are sterilization operations that can permanently prevent pregnancy both for men and women, but at this time the results are irreversible. Most physicians are reluctant to perform the procedures on men and women who are too young, feeling that they might later regret the decision.

Abortion. A planned pregnancy is a great thing, and medical care for the expectant mother is important and necessary. However, there is often the problem of an unwanted pregnancy. When diagnosed early enough, an abortion is available in most places now. This can be done safely and without great cost, and age is usually not a problem. The decision about continuing the pregnancy or having an abortion should be made carefully by the individual involved. After 10 to 12 weeks of the pregnancy most abortion clinics will not perform the abortion but will refer the patient to a hospital. After this time the procedure is not as easy, and there is more risk involved. The best solution is to plan ahead and not become pregnant until you choose to.

TAKING ACTION

1. *Visit a medical laboratory for information about most recent techniques of pregnancy testing.*
2. *Make a list of common misconceptions concerning birth control techniques, including vasectomy. Discuss them with the class.*
3. *Role-play some situations with another individual or with a small group.*

Choose situations in which personal problems come up and you work together in an effort to arrive at reasonable solutions. (For example, talk with a man who wants a vasectomy but is afraid that it will rob him of his sex drive or manhood.)

SKIN

Skin, of course, is the wrapping, or integument, of the body. It also includes a person's hair and nails. Healthy hair, skin, and nails usually reflect general health. So "skin" problems may be "more than skin deep."

Acne is a condition in which the oil-producing glands become plugged, inflammation and infection can occur, and blackheads are formed. The areas most affected are the face, neck, chest, and back. Acne that is not treated properly can cause permanent scarring, which will remain for life (unless cosmetic surgery is done). Squeezing or manipulating of the acne contributes most significantly to scarring. This worsens the infection and can cause serious, permanent markings on the skin.

A good routine to follow in treatment and prevention of acne is a regular schedule of cleansing the skin several times daily. Many people with acne also have dandruff, which compounds the acne problem, so regular shampooing with a dandruff shampoo is helpful.

Foods are thought to contribute to your acne problem but are probably not the chief cause of it. Chocolates, nuts, milk products, spicy foods, and excessive sweets or fats are evidently contributing factors.

Some women find that their acne problem develops or worsens just before their period. This is not unusual. Also, some women have noted an improvement of their condition when on the pill.

Emotional tension and the degree to which your acne upsets your general outlook can directly influence your actual problem. Keep this

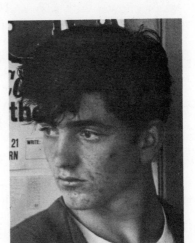

Youth with acne.

George W. Gardner

25

in mind as we discuss emotional health in a later chapter in the book.

Warts are growths caused by viruses. Although they appear most anywhere on the body, they have a tendency to develop on the hands or feet. There is some thought that they are contagious. They also can develop in the genital area, as already discussed. Warts often spontaneously disappear, but if they do not and are a source of concern for you, your physician can usually remove them for you.

Moles are dark spots of pigmentation on the skin. Some people have a few, but often fair-skinned or freckled people have a significant number of them. Usually, they are quite harmless. However, if you have a mole that is darkening, changing in size, or bleeding, it should be checked right away by a doctor. In most cases this is no problem, but moles can become a very serious type of cancer.

Sunburn is like any other burn to the skin, only it usually covers a large area and can be quite serious. It's nice to have a good tan, but a tan must be obtained sensibly with limited times of exposure to the sun. Fair-skinned people usually burn more readily and should be especially careful about the amount of time they are exposed to the sun. There are now some reasonably effective sunscreen products on the market that should be used by people who burn easily. There is clear evidence that prolonged exposure to the sun and skin cancer are linked.

Another problem with excessive exposure to the sun is the aging and drying process it causes in your skin. Think of the areas of your body never exposed to the sun and how much softer and younger feeling the skin is there.

Itchy skin rashes include poison ivy, scabies, crabs, and allergy. Poison ivy is a rash caused by exposure to the three-leaved poison ivy plant. It is more prevalent in some parts of the country than in others, and in some areas it can flourish into full vines growing up trees. To avoid contracting it, wear clothes covering your arms and legs when walking in the woods. Immediately after returning from the woods, take a shower with soap and water to remove any poison ivy oil (the cause of the rash) you may have on your body. The only way you can get it is from the oil itself. You can get the oil from the fur of a pet that has brushed up against the plant, or you can transfer the oil to parts of your body if it is on your hands. However, once you have washed the oil away with soap and water, the poison ivy will not spread.

There is no sure-fire treatment if you do catch poison ivy. A drying lotion like calamine can help, but if you get a really bad case of poison ivy, you may need to see your doctor.

Scabies are itchy lesions caused by microscopic mites or spiders that burrow under the skin, especially where the clothing fits tightly, such as at the waistline. It is possible to get scabies from using hairbrushes, clothes, or sheets of another infected person. They are contagious, but not nearly so much as lice or crabs. There is a specific medication for scabies, but it appears that mites may be developing a resistance to it.

Lice (or crab lice) are tiny parasitic insects that cause severe itching. An infestation (sometimes called *crabs* or *Pediculosis*) can be quite contagious, but fortunately there are specific medications that are very effective. Lice usually will settle in scalp hair or pubic hair, and occasionally you can see both the insect and the eggs. If you have them, see your doctor. Treatment is quite successful.

Allergy rash is hard to diagnose. It can look like any other rash and can be caused, for example, by some ingredient in soap, shampoo, makeup, or certain foods (especially seafoods). If the rash persists, you may want to see a doctor.

Dandruff and *psoriasis* are the most common hair problems. *Dandruff* is not contagious or infectious nor does it usually cause permanent hair loss. Contrary to some TV commercials, its cause is not known. It is best treated by regular shampooing with a dandruff shampoo. *Psoriasis* is a skin disease manifested by scaly whitish or reddish spots, especially on the elbows or knees or in the scalp. When the scalp is involved, psoriasis is difficult to tell from dandruff. Its cause is also unknown, and at this point there is no real cure, but sunlight and special ointments seem to help.

Perspiration can be a problem, especially in young people. There are two types of glands related to perspiration. One produces the moisture, and the other causes odor. That is why it is possible to have a wetness problem without an odor problem and vice versa. The human body is not designed to smell like a rose, and efforts to smell like one can be silly. In fact studies have shown that normal body smell is attractive if reasonable washing is practiced. However, when there is a problem, the best treatment is thorough, regular cleansing of the body with deodorant soaps and the regular use of deodorants or antiperspirants. The use of both the soap and deodorants builds up a residual protection against the microorganisms that cause odor. Contrary to popular opinion, you do not build up a resistance to the effective use of a given deodorant or antiperspirant. Sprays tend to be far less effective than creams or roll-ons. To minimize the danger of infections, avoid using a deodorant immediately after shaving under the arms. People with very sensitive skin are advised to use hypoallergenic deodorants.

Healthy nails are the result of a healthy body. Adequate protein in the diet helps to improve your nails. Try to protect them from dishwater and when you are working in the yard.

Hangnails are tags of skin along the side of the nail. They should never be pulled. They can become very tender and even severely infected if not left alone or carefully clipped. If they are infected, you should see your doctor.

Toenails should be clipped regularly and always straight across. Shaping or rounding of the sides can cause ingrown toenails, which are most painful and sometimes require surgery.

EXTREMITIES

Your extremities—your arms and legs including fingers and toes—can, of course, become infected or injured in some way. It's a good idea to know how to care for an injury if one should occur.

Sprains, especially to the ankle, are very common. Sometimes it is difficult to tell the difference between a sprain, which is damage to the soft tissues such as muscles, and a fracture, which is a break in a bone. Once you are sure it is a sprain, much can be done to help the pain. If there is a question about whether it might be a fracture, you will probably need an X ray. If the injury is a sprain, remember I.C.E.—that is, "I" for ice, "C" for compression, and "E" for elevation. Ice in a plastic bag placed on the injured ankle will help reduce swelling and pain. Never use heat on an injury immediately. Compression of the injured part can be done with an elastic bandage that will keep the swelling down with pressure. However, you must be very careful not to have the bandage too tight; if the toes feel numb, look blue, or feel cold, the wrap is too tight and must be loosened. Elevation is most important because it keeps the blood from pooling in the injured area and thus reduces swelling and also the pain. Keep the leg elevated, preferably on pillows, so that it is at or above body level. A serious sprain may need a cast on it to allow it to heal, but usually after a day or so some motion is helpful. Walking is permissible so long as no weight is put on the ankle, which is apt to become reinjured. Other joints in the body—wrists, fingers, knees, and so on—are also subject to sprains.

Knee injuries, which can be very tricky, require the care of a physician. The twisting type of injury so common in football or skiing can be both painful and serious.

Fractures are less common. However, with most painful injuries to an extremity, your doctor will order X rays to rule out the possibilities of a fracture. Casts are used with most, but not all, fractures. When the cast is removed, you will find the part to be weak because it has been inactive for some time. If your doctor recommends any exercises to do after your cast is removed, follow his instructions carefully.

Varicose veins appear in both men and women. These are large, lumpy, sometimes blue spots on the legs. They are not the spidery lines that look like someone took a fine pen and wrote on the skin. Those are quite harmless. Varicose veins are caused by weakness in the valves in the veins that support the column of blood and keep it from flowing backward down to the feet. These can be painful, can occasionally be snagged by something and bleed, or just look unattractive. Occasionally a clot can develop around an injured valve. This condition is serious because it can cut down on the circulation and also can cause more trouble if a piece of the clot breaks loose and proceeds to the heart, brain, or lungs.

Tight garters or any constriction above or below the knee can contribute to the development of varicosities. During pregnancy the weight of the baby in the uterus pressing against the pelvic veins can slow circulation and cause varicosities. Good support hose can help relieve some of the symptoms such as aching in the legs. If varicose veins become severe, surgery can be done. Young people do not often have varicose veins, but with so many women on the pill, there seem to be more and more questions about them.

TAKING ACTION

1. *Determine which symptoms or conditions discussed in the sections on skin and extremities are of special interest to the class. Invite one or more medical specialists in for detailed discussion and questioning. As an alternative, form committees to make appointments with and visit specialists for information. Be sure to prepare specific questions to ask the specialists in advance.*
2. *Have small group discussions on the foregoing topics of special interest.*
3. *Role-play the handling of likely, relevant situations. For example, three friends are hiking and one sprains an ankle. (If you create emergency situations for role playing, you may decide that you would benefit from an entire course in emergency first aid.)*

EMOTIONAL PROBLEMS

Sometimes students experience physical symptoms that stem from emotional problems. Adjusting to college life is no simple matter and may be emotionally stressful. Frequent headaches, stomach upset, or chronic fatigue often are such symptoms. In other cases there may be no physical symptoms, but instead such other symptoms as sleeplessness, nervousness, mood swings, depression, sleeping for long periods of time, avoiding contact with other people, not eating, or compulsive overeating. Doctors deal with these problems every day. However, you may have an important role to play in aiding others, both directly and by getting them to appropriate specialists. The following suggestions may prove helpful.

First, find out whether the person has seen a doctor. If so, find out whether the doctor has determined and explained a cause for the problem. This is always a good place to start, but one cannot always be sure that the physician has perceived the emotional part of the problem. Next, try to find out how the person is dealing with his or her problems. Is he or she trying to sort out the difficulties in a rational way, or is the person oblivious to them or being quite irrational about them? Try to do more listening than talking. Just speaking openly about problems may bring a great deal of relief and clearer perception of the situation. Solutions may emerge as problems are verbalized. You may be being most helpful just by listening.

Another good idea is to be stingy with your advice. Although you may suggest alternative solutions to problems, decisions for action cannot come from you but the person you are trying to help.

If you feel that the person is having difficulty working the problem through alone and needs professional help, there are resources. One already mentioned is the medical doctor. Residence hall directors can often be helpful. It never hurts to directly but gently approach the subject of emotional health counseling. People are beginning to realize that emotional problems are just as real as physical symptoms, and that seeking professional help for emotional problems makes as much sense as going to a dentist when you have a toothache. Ask if the person has

29

considered talking with someone who can help sort out his or her problems. The person's response may indicate openness to counseling. Most campuses have mental health facilities, counseling centers, or departments of psychology that provide either counseling or referrals. A local community hot line may also be helpful. These are often used to help people make the decision to obtain further counseling. If the person is actively affiliated with a religious organization, there may be someone there who can provide help through counseling.

There is a category of *unnecessary* stress symptoms, often not severe enough to be treated medically but a very real problem to many students. Only the student can treat it satisfactorily. It is that condition of chronic or frequent fatigue or anxiety brought about by trying to do too much and/or by scheduling time poorly—usually at the expense of sleep. Typically, individuals who suffer such stress fail to set priorities for their time, the not-so-important things getting as much attention as, or more than, the important ones. They let work pile up so that reasonable assignments become all but unmanageable, the only hope being sleepless nights of desperate effort. They do not set themselves a reasonable bedtime. They let recreational activities spread beyond sensible limits, perhaps endlessly bouncing a basketball as an escape from their work.

In other words, they goof off (which everyone does sometimes, but not habitually). Then they have to pay the price in frantic effort, emotional upset, sleeplessness, and fatigue. Often they make others pay the price for their goofing off by subjecting them to constant whining and complaining.

For your own good—and to save us doctors *unnecessary* work—consider how your way of life in college affects your health as well as your academic success. Take a look at your priorities and budgeting of time. Perhaps you need help with note-taking, study, or reading skills. If so, resources are available to help you. These things have a lot to do with your health status as well as what you'll get out of college. Reasonable health, play, and work habits formed now will serve you well for the rest of your life.

TAKING ACTION

1. *Discuss as a class or in small groups what you know of the tie-in of emotional stress and physical and psychological symptoms. Provide examples from observation or personal experience.*
2. *Role-play situations in which roommates or family members give evidence of emotionally based symptoms and you try to help them.*
3. *As a class or in small groups list some common examples of "goofing off" that you've seen or practiced yourself. Since this is obviously self-defeating behavior if practiced regularly, what courses of action might be taken against it? Role-play examples of the problem and possible solutions.*

Hopefully you are now better able to take care of your health. But even more important, you may be beginning to have a feeling for a broader scope of responsibility for both yourself and other people. These days it is difficult to separate one individual from the total mass of humanity when it comes to responsibility for health and well-being. A visit to your local health department, hospital clinic, or planned parenthood association could be a good starting point. This should give you an idea of the breadth of health care and even of some places where you could be of service. There are many opportunities to make a contribution that might be especially needed.

Staying well is important, and you can take care of yourself to the point of avoiding certain illnesses. If you know which symptoms are serious and which ones are not, you can save a lot of worry time.

Everyone has a responsibility for his or her own health and well-being, as well as a responsibility to others. Just as you try to avoid spreading a cold to others, if you think you have been exposed to VD, you had better get treated and see to it that anyone with whom you have had sexual contact is also treated. The point is, if you're at all health educated, you know that you can treat the cold yourself but not the VD. This is the kind of discrimination that can help you to handle many, if not most, personal health problems. But there is far more to health than the avoiding and treating of symptoms. Let us turn now to chapters aimed at the achieving of optimal health—where you, not the physician, play the major role.

FOR FURTHER READING

Asimov, Isaac, 1963. *The Human Body.* New York: Signet Science Library Books.

A concise, complete, easy-to-use book on anatomy and function.

Beeson, Paul, and Walsh, McDermott, eds., 1963. *Cecil-Loeb Textbook of Medicine.* Philadelphia: Saunders.

A medical textbook.

Boston Women's Health Book Collective, 1973. *Our Bodies, Ourselves.* New York: Simon & Schuster.

This presents the health issue from the liberated woman's point of view, using both opinion and fact.

Cherniak, Donna, et al., eds., 1972. *VD Handbook.* Montreal: Montreal Health Press.

Explicit factual information on venereal disease for college-age students.

———, 1974. *Birth Control Handbook.* Montreal: Montreal Health Press.

Explicit factual birth control information for the college-age population.

**tending to basic
needs**

Greenblatt, Augusta, 1974. *Why Do I Feel This Way?* New York: Pyramid Books.

Good general book on health written especially for young people.

Holvey, David, ed., 1972. *The Merck Manual.* Rahway, N.J.: Merck Sharp & Dohme Research Laboratories.

Concise reference book used by physicians for quick referral. Understandable to students.

Samuels, Mike, and Bennet, Hal, 1973. *The Well Body Book.* New York: Random House.

A popular, fairly comprehensive health manual.

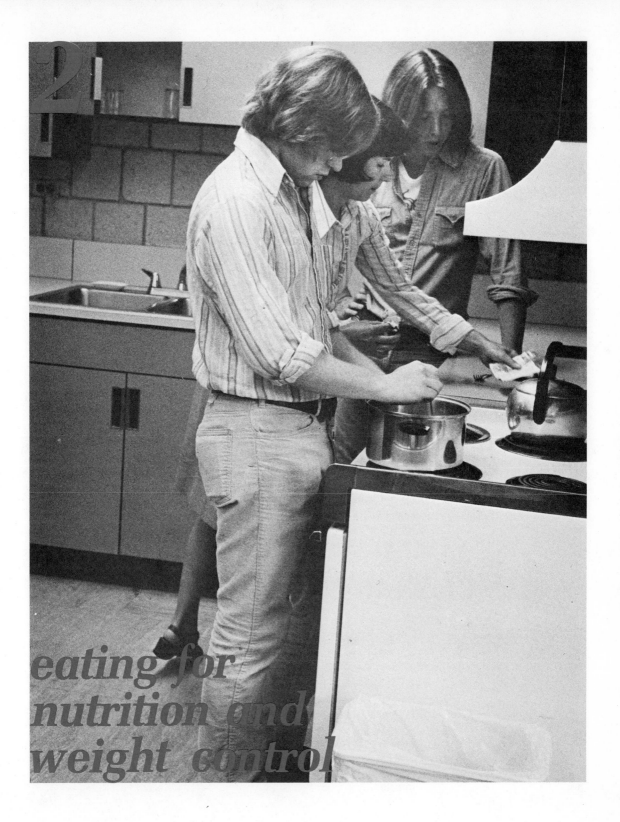

2

eating for
nutrition and
weight control

OVERVIEW

*Nutrition helps in health maintenance as well as in the prevention,
treatment, or cure of some diseases. Nutritional needs vary,
depending on the health status and physical characteristics of
individuals, but the same general principles apply to everyone.*

*Some nutritional problems are basically energy-related: either
too much (as in obesity) or too little (as in undernutrition). The
most common dietary problem in the United States is obesity.
Since many obese persons expend less energy than persons of
normal body fatness, the same number of dietary calories can be
excessive for them. Thus it is necessary to decrease calories eaten
(diet) as well as to increase energy expenditure (exercise) to bring
the level of fat down to normal. "Miracle cures" either do not
work or are not safe.*

*Heart disease rates may be increased by diets that are high in
calories, saturated fat and cholesterol, and low in polyunsaturated
fat. Changes in food intake that alter the type of fat and reduce
cholesterol in the diet are important for the control of this
condition.*

*Insufficient intake of the protective nutrients (protein, vitamins,
and minerals) rather than dietary excess is the problem in
iron-deficiency anemia. Some obese people have insufficient iron
intakes, and thus they suffer from both overnutrition and
malnutrition.*

*Some nutritional problems, such as diabetes mellitus, stem from
an underlying disease process or metabolic problem. Many
diabetics with mild desease can be treated with diet and exercise
alone. Obesity is extremely common in such persons, and it is
important to reduce their weight and thereby lessen their demand
for insulin.*

*Individual dietary change, altered food production and
processing techniques, more effective education, and protective
legislation and its enforcement are needed to further improve the
healthfulness of American diets.*

INQUIRY

1. How does the American diet measure up from the standpoint of
   environmental and ecological concerns?
2. Are food additives dangerous?
3. What are the major dietary problems in this country?
4. What steps can be taken to avoid obesity? If already present, how is
   it best to treat obesity?
5. Is obesity just a cosmetic problem, or are real health risks associated
   with it?
6. Where can you turn for expert help in matters related to nutrition and
   diet?
7. Are organic and health foods superior to other foods? Are they
   inferior?

We eat primarily because food tastes good and gives us pleasure. But concerns about eating also reflect our efforts to preserve our health, looks, and food budgets—and perhaps our ecology and environment.

Many Americans have the nagging suspicion that life was better and eating was more healthful in "the good old days." This is unlikely, but certainly food ways are different. Food production, processing, marketing, and the availability of foods, as well as eating habits, have changed a great deal.

Let's take a quick backward look over the past 50 years at the American diet. Fat intakes have so increased in the diet that now 35 to 40 percent of most of the energy intake of Americans comes from fat. This is due to increased intake of fat itself and animal foods as well (which in the case of such products as milk and red meat contain a good deal of fat as well as protein). In contrast to fat intake, which seems to have risen, the intake of carbohydrates has fallen, particularly that from fruits and vegetables and whole grains. Similarly the amount of dietary fiber in the diet coming from such undigested residues as pectins, cellulose, and other structural materials in plants has declined. Intake of simple sugars (such as sucrose) may have risen, while that of complex carbohydrates (such as starches, whole-grain cereals, and fiber) has fallen. In this chapter we will explore the effects of these alterations on human health.

The thrust of nutrition today is to find ways of preventing rather than simply curing nutrition-related health problems. This is a big step from 50 years ago, when little was known about either.

Preventive medicine focuses on the risks or warning signs of disease. These warnings, which may exist in seemingly healthy people, have been found to be associated with increased risk of later illness. Such risks include obesity, hypercholesterolemia or hyperlipemia, "pre-

NUTRITION, HEALTH, AND DISEASE

William B. Finch/Editorial Photocolor Archives

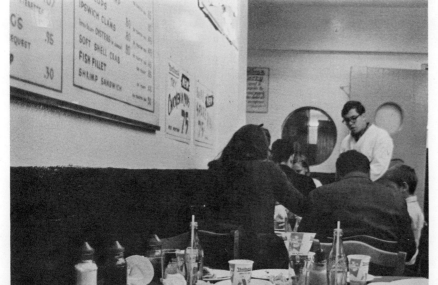

The American diet is often ample but not as nutritious as it should be.

diabetes" or abnormally high blood sugar, smoking, and excessive alcohol consumption. By acting early to avoid these risks we can often interfere with the process by which people become patients who need curative medicine. (Curative medicine is concerned with people who have developed clear-cut disease and tries to rescue these patients.) Nutrition has a place in prevention and treatment of disease, but since this is a book on health rather than disease treatment, we will concentrate on steps that can be taken to foster the optimal health of ourselves and others.

Nutrition and Health Maintenance: Finding Needs for Nutrients

Many a parent at one time or another says to his child, "Eat your spinach and drink your milk if you want to grow up big and strong." There is some truth to the statement that if nothing is eaten, no growth will occur. However, from the scientific standpoint no *specific* food is necessary for good nutritional health. The body does not require specific foods; it requires specific nutrients.

When foods are separated into their chemical components, the diets of healthy people have much more in common than they do if all the many foods that they eat were listed. Most diets supply at least certain minimal amounts of more than 50 nutrients, as well as many other substances. These nutrients are the chemical mixtures needed by the body for growth, maintenance, repair, or energy. It does not seem to matter when during the day foods are eaten, but certain patterns of eating may help ensure satisfactory intake.

Scientists have determined human needs for many different nutrients and can tell us with a fair degree of accuracy what these are. These requirements, with additional amounts to allow for a margin of safety and individual variation, are the basis of dietary standards or recommendations. The so-called "recommended dietary allowances" are estimates of the amounts of nutrients needed daily by the "average" person. They are intended to maintain a good nutritional state in most healthy persons and are set high enough to cover those with relatively high requirements for nutrients. (See the very valuable references, *Recommended Dietary Allowances* and *Composition of Foods,* at the end of this chapter.)

Although the kinds of nutrients we need to stay healthy are similar at all ages, the amounts necessary vary a good deal among healthy people because of differing amounts of body tissue, metabolic rate (including activity level), and whether growth is in process.

Surprisingly, infants eat *more* on a pound-for-pound basis than do adults. They use a great deal of energy for growth and must build up body tissue out of the materials supplied in the diet. Again at adolescence, when teenagers are shooting up in weight and height, a great deal of food is needed. Pregnancy involves producing an infant weighing about 8 pounds plus additional growth of the uterus, placenta, and other organs to support this burden. It also involves increased nutrient needs and a good deal of weight gain (usually 20 to 25 pounds), which is lost soon after delivery. Lactation means increased nutrient needs since the mother must produce daily about a quart of breast milk, high in nutrients, to feed the baby.

When parts of the body have been damaged, as by burns or surgery, growth must take place to restore the body to normal, so again nutrient needs are high.

Sex differences in nutrient needs are due partly to the fact that male and female adults (and, to a lesser extent, children) vary in their body composition. Males tend to be larger in bone and muscle and in other tissues that are actively using up energy. They tend to have higher needs for energy-providing nutrients simply because of this fact. Females have more body fat than males, and on the average they are smaller in height and weight. Fat is a storage tissue and does not use up large amounts of calories; thus females usually have lower energy needs than males. This sex difference is not true for all nutrients, however. The monthly process of menstruation, which involves blood loss, and the period of pregnancy, in which the maternal stores of nutrients must be drawn upon to supply the fetus' needs, mean extra drains on calcium, iron, and protein.

Physical activity is another factor that varies among healthy people and is particularly important in determining energy needs. In fact differences in physical activity are the major reason why calorie needs are often so different between people. Children and adolescents are generally much more physically active than adults and therefore have increased energy needs per pound. Adults are heavier and require more energy to move their bodies around than do children, but they may not move about a great deal. Thus 10-year-old children and 30-year-old adults may need the same amounts of energy a day.

Finally, of course, there is the state of health. As we will see later on, in certain disease conditions the needs for nutrients and the way they are handled by the body may be altered or changed. Dietitians and nutritionists work with physicians to help patients alter their diets to prevent, alleviate, or cure these various diet-related conditions.

FOOD AND FOOD GUIDES

Finding Nutrients in Foods

To find out what a food contains in terms of nutrients, a table of food composition is used. It is similar to a telephone book; you look up the name of the food, and numbers that represent the amounts of various nutrients in certain portion sizes of food are given. If this were done for every food eaten, it would be possible to get a fairly good idea of the intakes of different nutrients over the course of a day or a week.

Since many people who look up the nutrient values of foods are interested in doing so for reasons of weight control, short tables that state only the calories supplied by the energy-yielding nutrients in foods have also been published. These "calorie counters" may be helpful to some people, but it is important to remember that the calorie values apply *only* to the portion size given in the booklet.

TAKING ACTION

1. *The yardstick used for judging the nutrients provided by diets versus nutritional needs is the* Recommended Dietary Allowances. *Using the table in that book, find your own nutrient needs, taking into account your sex, activity level, and so on.*
2. *Identify and discuss four factors that may account for differences in the needs for nutrients among healthy people in your family.*
3. *Using a table of food composition, look up the nutrient content of a glass of milk and a glass of beer. Which supplies more protein, which supplies more calcium, phosphorus, vitamin D? How many calories are there in each?*
4. *Keep a day's record of your food intake, and using a table of food composition, look up your daily iron intake and compare it to your need as stated in the* Recommended Dietary Allowances. *How does it stack up?*

Food Guides Because we have both food composition tables that state each food's content of nutrients and the *Recommended Dietary Allowances,* it is possible to plan diets completely by matching the nutrient content of various foods against nutrient needs. But outside of scientific studies or medical situations, few have the time to plan daily diets by referring constantly to tables of food composition stating nutrient contents for each food eaten.

Fortunately, there is an easier way to choose foods over the course of the day that are in line with recommendations for levels of nutrients. Since many foods are similar in the kinds and amounts of nutrients they provide, foods can be grouped together into those high or low in particular nutrients by utilizing knowledge of their nutrient composition. For example, meat, fish and poultry all contain fairly high amounts of protein, varying amounts of fat, and roughly similar amounts of various vitamins. Therefore one food can be substituted for another within each group with very little effect on the nutrient composition of the diet. For example, it would not make much difference whether a person ate grapefruit or oranges since they are both citrus fruits high in ascorbic acid (vitamin C) and sugar and low in most other nutrients.

The "Basic Four" food group system is perhaps the most popular layman's food guide. These four groups of food are claimed to be "basic" for assuring adequacy of intakes of the "protective" foods, which are protein, vitamins, and minerals.

1. Meat groups: foods high in protein, including meat, fish, poultry, eggs, and legumes (beans and peas).
2. Dairy group: foods high in calcium and riboflavin.
3. Fruit and vegetables group: foods high in either carotene or vitamin C and other vitamins and minerals.
4. Bread and cereals group: foods high in carbohydrates and vegetable protein, B vitamins, and iron.

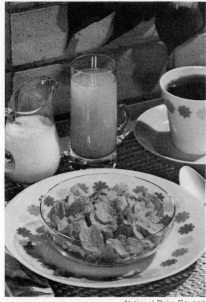 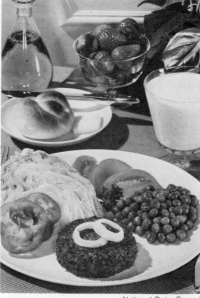

Two meals that contain necessary nutrients for a balanced diet.

Eating several servings of food from each of these groups each day is good insurance for meeting nutrient needs. Obviously the portion size selected is important, and it is assumed that a fairly wide variety of foods within the groups will be chosen.

There are certain problems in using such food guides if their purpose and limitations are not clearly understood. For example, eating the basic four food groups does not guarantee that obesity will be avoided. Eating excess calories from *any* combination of foods can result in obesity. Some people forget that the Basic Four do not include all of the various types of foods that are eaten each day. For example, butter, margarines, and oils are not included, nor are soft drinks, alcohol, and so on. These latter foods are high in calories and low in most other nutrients per serving. They are thus not considered "protective" foods, but they still "count" in terms of calories. Obviously the answer is to tailor the total diet—Basic Four and non–Basic Four foods—to be in line with energy needs.

Another problem with the Basic Four food guide is the difficulty of knowing how to classify many of the combination foods we eat so frequently. Pizza, beef stew, and various casseroles are examples of these. What is necessary here is some knowledge of the recipe composition of these foods.

Most food guides are also not very helpful to those whose favorite foods are very different from the typical American diet. For example, Chinese-Americans do not drink much milk, but they consume fairly large amounts of other foods that supply calcium and riboflavin. Thus the fact that a diet does not fit the "Basic Four" pattern does not necessarily mean that it is inadequate. More careful analysis of food sources of nutrients is necessary before judgments as to adequacy can be made. However, it is a good idea to get expert advice on how to meet nutrient needs if none of one or more of the Basic Four groups is usually eaten.

Nutritionists use other food guides for helping people with special dietary problems. Among the most common guides are the exchange lists for diabetics of the American Diabetics Association and the American Dietetics Association. These lists of similar foods that can be "exchanged" for each other are based not only on nutrient divisions but also on the calorie and carbohydrate content of the foods. Seven such food groups emerge in these listings. This type of food guide is helpful for counseling diabetic patients who must balance the amount, type, and timing of the food they eat against their insulin injections.

What happens if one of the Basic Four food groups is not eaten? The answer to this question depends on how often this is the case. If it happens only rarely, no harmful effects would be expected. However, if such a pattern continues for several weeks or months, the risk of nutritional deficiency problems is high. In such a case the diet may become poorly balanced in terms of nutrients. Proper balance is particularly important since little is known about the distribution of some micronutrients (such as copper and other trace minerals) in foods or the best relationships between levels of different nutrients.

TAKING ACTION

1. Using the Basic Four, examine your food intake over the past 24 hours. Did you meet recommendations? What are your plans to correct deficiencies or imbalance?
2. Someone in your family or a friend is probably a diabetic. Ask to see his or her diet prescription, and observe the various lists of foods that can be exchanged with each other (all having nearly the same protective nutrient content and carbohydrate values).

ALTERNATIVE EATING STYLES AND SPECIAL PROBLEMS

The food supply as a whole in this country meets human needs quite well *if* particular types of foods are properly selected. But this big "if" has worried many thoughtful persons who have wondered whether, for various reasons, it might not be safer or better for the diet to include "health," "organic," "natural" foods, to take large doses of vitamin-mineral supplements, and/or to adopt a vegetarian approach as preventive insurance.

Such dietary adjustments seem innocent enough, but for many years a controversy has raged as to their benefit. The very words "health," "organic," and "natural" suggest that these foods are these good things and other foods are obviously the reverse: nonhealth, nonorganic, and unnatural. The battle tends to be joined at this point, the alternative diet eater considering the traditional eater somewhat uninformed and perhaps irresponsible, and the traditional diet eater considering the other to be nuts or worse to question the majority way. Sometimes there is more than a little arrogance on both sides considering the scarcity of solid, scientific data on either side.

The effort here is to present a brief and hopefully objective view of the subject that may help the reader decide the merits of the case.

Health Foods

Health food stores usually carry all of the foods under consideration here, namely, health, organic, and natural. However, "health foods" usually refer specifically to protein supplements, mixtures such as Tiger's Milk, made of foods high in protein, and vitamins and minerals. So what can be controversial about such obviously "good" foods as proteins, vitamins, and minerals? The answer to this question is: the claims that are often made for them and their usually inflated prices.

Advertisements of health foods often suggest that eating ordinary foods is bound to result in crucial omissions that only health foods can correct. Moreover, it is sometimes suggested that certain diseases can be avoided, or even treated, by health foods. In the first place, a well-balanced diet can be selected in the ordinary market (which, these days, often stocks health and organic foods) at a considerably lower cost. This is a point of importance, especially to those on a low, fixed income. Deficiency dietary diseases can usually be avoided in the grocery store as well as in the health food store, and for less money. In the second place, it is dangerous to attempt to treat these diseases without medical care. If vitamin or mineral treatment is needed, self-treatment by health foods is likely to be inadequate since prescription quantities are probably required.

As to high protein intake, protein is, of course, needed throughout life, especially during the growth years and pregnancy. However, some people such as athletes practice a kind of "training-table magic" by consuming very large amounts of meat and other proteins made of various products including soybeans. They think that strength and thus performance in general will be enhanced. Unfortunately, there is no evidence that increasing protein in the diet *above adequate levels* improves performance. An adequate level for the healthy person consists of the well-balanced diet described earlier. (There is evidence that increasing carbohydrates may be helpful to endurance performance such as distance running and tournament wrestling.)[1]

Both vitamins and minerals are necessities throughout life; however, *assuming adequate levels* from a well-balanced diet, there is no evidence that supplements of either improves athletic or other physical performance. Physicians may prescribe vitamins or minerals for deficiency conditions, but these are medical matters, and the doctor is unlikely to send the patient to a health food store for the needed supplement. Moreover, some vitamins, especially A and D, may have ill effects if taken in excess.

---

[1]See J. Mayer and B. A. Bullen, 1974, *Science and Medicine of Exercise and Sport,* 2d ed., W. R. Johnson and E. R. Buskirk, eds. New York: Harper & Row.

Dr. Linus Pauling.

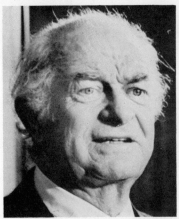

Wide World Photos

How are we to evaluate the controversy concerning the benefits to health (for example, avoidance of the common cold) and longevity of vitamin C? Linus Pauling, a most highly respected scientist, believed that the available evidence supports his view that "megavitamins"—in his case at least 2 grams of vitamin C daily and heavy vitamin B complex supplements—will prevent certain diseases and very significantly extend life. On the other hand, some respected nutritionists believe that such supplementation is not only unnecessary but potentially dangerous; for example, excess vitamin C evidently gives rise in some people to bladder stones.

Dr. Pauling, in his enthusiasm, seems to be arguing ahead of his data. He is aware of this and is calling for millions for research to determine *optimal* vitamin levels. On the other hand, some of his critics would seem more anxious to discredit him than to dig for the facts. From both sides we have heard assertions but few facts. Perhaps the best course at the present time for the nonspecialist is to withhold judgment and avoid either extreme position until more definite information is available.

Organic Foods

Foods grown without the use of pesticides or chemicals, chemical fertilizers, and usually marketed without food additives may be referred to as "organic foods." Such foods tend to become especially popular when publicity is given to some pesticide, fertilizer, or additive that is found to be, or is suspect of being, contributory to cancer or some other ill effect. Moreover, the word "organic" is attractive and tends to convey the impression that foods so labeled have special qualities that are beneficial to health.

All foods are organic, chemically speaking. Those so labeled tend to be high-quality foods, but no more so than their counterparts in the market. However, they do tend to be more expensive. Therefore people on a tight budget may need to think twice about the extent to which they can indulge this taste.

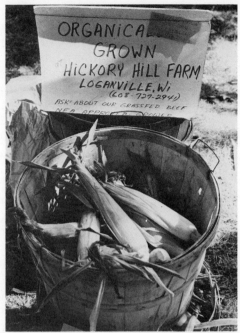

Daniel S. Brody/Editorial Photocolor Archives

Organic foods tend to offer protection from the occasional harmful pesticides and additives; however, Food and Drug Administration requirements have been tightening in recent years, and the chances of being hurt by "nonorganic" foods is small indeed. It is important to realize that given the present state of technology, as well as the necessity for producing huge amounts of food for great numbers of people and for getting this food to the table without spoilage, chemical fertilizers, pesticides, and additives would seem to be essential. The point for most people who cannot grow their own food is to wash fruit and vegetables carefully and try to insist on constant and close surveillance of all such substances by appropriate governmental agencies.[2]

Natural Foods

"Natural foods" are food products marketed without preservatives, emulsifiers, or artificial ingredients. Most of what was said about organic foods applies equally to them. On the one hand, certain preservatives and artificial coloring materials (for example, the notorious Red Dye #2 and suspect preservatives in bacon and frankfurters) have been withdrawn from the market or are being challenged as potentially dangerous to health. But, on the other hand, most people do not damn shoes or automobiles because they are "unnatural" in the sense of being man-made. The point is that we need a food-educated

---

[2]For a well-balanced discussion of the merits of organic farming, see Joan D. Gussow, March/April, 1974, *Nutrition Today,* p. 31.

public who will insist that our governmental agencies scrutinize carefully all such substances deemed important. (See Chapter 13.)

A note on the practices of enrichment, fortification, and supplementation seems in order at this point. Enrichment involves the addition of nutrients, vitamins, and minerals to foods that lost these ingredients in processing. Thus B vitamins (riboflavin and niacin) and iron are added to processed flour for the making of bread and dry cereals. Fortification refers to adding nutrients to foods that have not previously contained them. For example, baby foods are commonly fortified with iron, milk is often fortified with vitamin D, salt may be iodized, and vitamin A is added to margarine. Supplementation means adding nutrients to foods ordinarily eaten to meet a specific health need, as in giving iron and folic acid supplements to pregnant women.

By means of these techniques ordinary, relatively inexpensive foods usually reach consumers prepared to meet their nutritional requirements. Still consumers do need to exercise caution in selecting foods advertised to be so treated. For example, according to such groups as the Consumers Union, although some dry cereals are indeed quite nutritious, others actually contain virtually insignificant amounts of the enrichment claimed. Similarly, it would be necessary to eat very large amounts of some breads to get adequate amounts of the B vitamins with which they are enriched.

Vegetarianism

Vegetarians are people who eliminate meats from their diets; partial vegetarians eliminate specific meats; and "vegans" eliminate all animal products, including milk and cheese. Many groups avoid meat for religious reasons or because of some other conviction against killing. Some, like the Seventh-Day Adventists, have demonstrated the ability to maintain a high level of health by using suitable vegetable substances, and others are convinced that meat in particular and perhaps meat products as well are essentially poisonous and are therefore to be avoided for health reasons.

People thinking of changing over to a vegetarian-type diet owe it to themselves to plan their diet with a health professional who is competent to help identify satisfactory substitutes for meat. Radical changes, such as dropping meat products or going all out for "organic" foods and foods without additives or preservatives can lead to serious health problems if done on a hit-or-miss, uninformed basis.

TAKING ACTION

1. *Compare the prices of vitamins sold in health food stores, drug stores, and supermarkets and the potencies of the preparations with the* Recommended Dietary Allowances *for these nutrients. Which is the best buy?*
2. *What are several points you might make to an elderly person who is buying large amounts of health food supplements to cure his or her ills without medical advice?*

3. Compare natural or organic foods and their counterparts on the grocery shelf with respect to prices and ingredients.
4. As committees or individuals, interview health food store (a) advocates and (b) critics. Analyze their statements, comparing numbers of assertions versus facts. Do the same with regard to the vitamin C controversy.

In our society "obesity" (and "fat") is a dirty word when applied to people. Obese people are therefore discriminated against in various ways and are often led to believe that they are inferior—just as are certain other minority groups. In this discussion some disadvantages to health of being obese are presented, but in no way is a put-down of fat people intended.

The problem of being overweight is not a simple one. People are not always fat because they overeat, nor are they necessarily as fat (or thin) as they think they are. Teenage girls often think that they are obese when they are not because of their strivings to look like Twiggy. On the other hand, middle-aged men often think of themselves as lean and athletic although they may be fat and sedentary, their mind's eye still fixing on the way they may have looked when they were in their early twenties. Therefore people's own observations of their fatness are often inaccurate.

OBESITY

Obesity and Diet

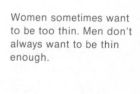

Women sometimes want to be too thin. Men don't always want to be thin enough.

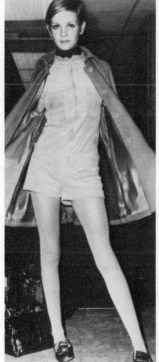

Wide World Photos

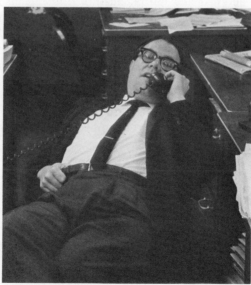
George W. Gardner

Early assessment makes possible early screening of those who need treatment before they become so obese that it is virtually impossible to reverse the condition. It also furnishes benchmarks against which progress in fatness reduction and fitness improvement can be measured.

Weight reduction is no easy matter for most people. A number of decisions are necessary. First, potential reducers must admit that they are too fat. Second, these people must then decide to do something about it; that is, lose weight. Next they must decide how to go about getting advice; shall they rely on their own ideas, go to a physician or other health professional, or go to a lay weight-control practitioner, such as a group leader in a commercial dieting concern or health club? The source chosen for treatment may help to make the next decision: how to go about losing the weight. There are several options: dietary modification, increased physical activity, medication, or schemes involving special equipment or devices.

Causes of Obesity and How to Avoid Becoming Fat

People usually get fat the same way they get thin: altered diet and exercise. Although it is true that a small percentage of overfat persons actually suffer from a disease or condition that leads to fatness, for most this is not the case.

There are three general rules for those who are lean but want to stay that way.

First, if you are physically active, keep it up. If you are not, learn to make some forms of activity a part of your life. (See Chapter 3 for details.)

Second, most people as they grow older become less physically active, although many young people are amazingly inactive. Their energy needs fall because of this and also because their metabolism, even when resting, slows down. Therefore food intake (especially of the energy-providing nutrients) must be adjusted downward or energy output increased as you grow older.

Third, watch your intake of foods that are high in calories and low in bulk (such as alcohol, fats and oils, butter, gravy, large portions of meat high in fat, most desserts, and snack foods high in carbohydrate and fat). They frequently are high in calories but provide few of the other protective nutrients you need. As time goes by they may cause you to gain extra pounds.

Reasons for Losing Weight: Handicaps of Being Obese

From the standpoint of *physical health* the handicaps of being obese are many and include greater risk of chronic diseases, more severe or prolonged courses of illness, declines in fitness, and poorer pregnancy outcomes.

The following are the most obvious handicaps to health. Angina pectoris (pain in the chest caused by heart disease) is more common to the obese. High blood pressure (hypertension) occurs more often among the obese. Complications after surgery are also higher in this group. Insufficient respiration (hypoventilation) is more frequent among the obese. In obese females failure to menstruate (amenorrhea) or irregular menstrual periods are more frequent. Obese females also suffer from increased frequency of toxemia (a kidney disease) during pregnancy.

For children, teenagers, and young adults these health problems are often many years away; it is the other handicaps of obesity that plague them more. Among other things, they are made to feel this society's intense prejudice against fatness.

Obese persons often have extremely negative feelings not only about the way their bodies look (that is, *body image*) but also about their *worthiness in other areas of life,* which are not related directly to their obesity. Unfortunately, even after losing weight, the formerly obese may still feel inadequate. They also may actually find themselves at a disadvantage from the standpoint of *social status* and *future social mobility.* Obese girls may find that the most eligible partners for marriage from the standpoint of physical appearance are not available to them. For adolescents their fatness may put them at a decided disadvantage for *college admissions* and *opportunities in other vocations* (such as work for the airlines or in sales jobs, where attractive appearance is important). *Parent-child* and *child-parent* relationships may also be stressful due to the issue of obesity: a formerly fat parent may nag her obese daughter about eating; a male parent may ridicule the unmanly look of his obese son. Obese adolescents and young adults are also at a disadvantage, for they have to restrain their eating because of their *low energy needs,* since they are usually less physically active than their peers. Being less likely to be successful in sports, they tend to avoid them and are deprived of a major recreational outlet. In addition to being less active, obese adolescents tend to mature earlier and thus the need for additional calories for growth is long past. Meanwhile their later-maturing and leaner peers are still growing and "chowing down" at every opportunity without getting fat.

A final handicap, which affects the obese at all ages, is the risk of being exposed to the adverse effects of worthless treatments. There is no field of nutrition that is so full of nonsense cures and charlatans as is the field of obesity. Unfortunately, these persons include a few unethical or unknowledgeable "health professionals" who charge high fees and use untried remedies such as dieting pills. But there are also thousands of commercial diet clubs and health spas, as well as mail order houses that dispense belts, exercise machines, sweating garments, diet candies, and special girdles that are supposed to do away with fat.

Treatment of Obesity

In the relatively rare cases of obesity caused by hormonal imbalance or other disease processes, curing the disease usually cures the obesity. But most cases of obesity are not in fact due to such disorders. The basic defect usually involves an inability to regulate food intake.

Treatment is a matter of increasing energy outputs and/or decreasing energy intake.

Sources of Dietary Advice

Everyone seems to have advice for losing weight. The suggestions range from the sensible to the silly. Since obesity sometimes is due to some other underlying health condition, it makes good sense before attempting to lose more than 5 pounds to consult a physician to make sure that a disease-related condition is not involved. After gathering information from a physical examination, history of past health, weight and other measurements, and clinical tests, the physician often calls in a dietitian or nutritionist who gets a dietary history and list of patient food preferences. Working together with the patient they can not only design a weight reduction diet and exercise program but also deal with other health-related dietary problems that may be present.

If the fatness problem is simple, that is, not connected or associated with some other type of health condition, many patients are able to lose weight with a sensible diet and exercise program on their own without much more advice. They may choose to enroll in a weight reduction group of one sort or another for motivation and reinforcement.

Other people attempt to treat themselves or rely on some friendly advice. Others pin their hopes on some advertised "guaranteed to work" miracle treatment. As we shall see, if the treatment they fix upon is essentially unsound, they may lose a great deal of money, subject themselves to unnecessary health risks, and fail to accomplish their objective.

Sensible Weight Reduction through Diets

Dieting is by far the most popular way most people in this country choose to lose weight. There are endless numbers of diets. They involve these principles if they make sense from the medical and scientific standpoint:

1. *If fat is to be lost, the calories taken in must be fewer than those needed for the body's energy requirements.* This is *always* true. Diets that do not involve caloric reduction decrease weight by loss of water (such as a low-carbohydrate diet) and fail to accomplish their real objective. Total fasts and very-low-carbohydrate diets involve loss of lean tissue as well as fat. Unless they are carefully monitored by a physician, these diets may be harmful to health if continued for any length of time. Some diet schemes (such as the "eat all you want but eliminate one certain type of food" diet) claim not to limit calories. On further examination, they do limit calories because people eat less than they would normally eat.

2. *The diet, though low in calories, is adequate in all other nutrients* so that intakes for these do not become dangerously low. Daily intakes of 500 to 1000 calories less than present intakes usually allow the patient to lose 1 to 2 pounds a week, while supplying enough food to furnish other nutrients. Diets below 1000 calories total per day can rarely do this.

3. The fact that *obesity cannot be cured for good but only controlled* is recognized. A diet establishes good food habits for permanent control. Some provision is made for helping the patient to maintain his weight after reduction and to watch his diet. If the patient is very obese (that is, more than 100 pounds too fat), he may have to watch what he eats for the rest of his life. Otherwise, once the patient reaches his lowered weight and goes back to his previous eating habits, weight will be regained rapidly. Such seesawing of weight may be harmful to health.

4. The *diet is something the patient can live with* for a long time. It should not set him apart as a freak; that is, it should have long-term possibilities. This is especially important if the patient is expected to stay on the diet for many months; otherwise the dieter may lose heart and give up the whole effort. There are some exceptions to this rule, such as total fasting, which is sometimes employed for patients whose health is such that they must lose weight very rapidly, but such diets should be undertaken only under close medical supervision.

5. The *advisability of getting a physician's advice* is emphasized.

6. It *recognizes that losing weight is not easy,* and that in addition to diet the person needs social support and help as well as rewards from himself and others for sticking to it.

7. It *doesn't forbid foods but emphasizes portion control.*

8. *Foods are used instead of vitamin-mineral supplements* or diet pills.

9. It has a *sensible balance of energy-providing nutrients.* This usually means that protein supplies 20 to 25 percent of total calories, fat 30 to 35 percent, and carbohydrates 45 to 50 percent. Since this is near the usual American pattern, it allows people to choose usual foods but in smaller amounts. When carbohydrates in the diet are cut to extremely low levels, the body is unable to obtain energy from all the body fat that is broken down, and compounds called *ketone bodies* are formed. In small amounts these can be eliminated through the breath and urine but in large amounts the body cannot cope with them, and the condition called *ketosis* results. This may be dangerous (especially for those with undiagnosed diabetes or kidney problems). The person may also become dehydrated and weak. Some people cannot eat even the foods in low-carbohydrate diets because they lose their appetites. Their weight loss is partly fat, partly water, and partly lean tissue. While there is no "recommended daily allowance" (RDA) for carbohydrate, it is wise to allow 5 g/100 calories or not less than 60 g in a day unless the person is under a physician's constant direction.

10. It is *realistic and does not call for superhuman effort.* The food should be readily available and come as close as possible to personal tastes and ways of eating. The diet should not require abandoning all social life or other activities to keep to it.

11. *Exercise* at the same time is recommended.

12. The *behaviors and emotions that lead to eating are examined, and advice is given to help the dieter control these.*

The behavioral approach to obesity treatment concentrates on reducing food intake and increasing energy output, but diets may not always be prescribed. This approach starts with the realization that starting, stopping, and selection of food are *not* due to biology alone but to a variety of deep-seated as well as more immediate factors. Long-standing and deep-seated factors that influence food intake include heredity and childhood experiences. These are hard to alter, although they are clearly important. More immediate factors surrounding the eating situation are somewhat more accessible to change. They include time of day, time available for eating, the place of eating, availability of food in the environment, cues that the person may pick up at the time of eating, and social aspects that surround food and mealtime situations. Instead of giving the patient a low-calorie diet, he is given help in cutting down his food intake by concentrating on those behaviors that lead to the eating of food. Obviously if the behaviors are changed, less food will be eaten, and the person will in effect be on a low-calorie diet.

Obese people often respond better to the modification of their food habits if they are taught to pay attention to these various environmental factors. Even though they may be attempting to stay on a diet that specifies exactly how much they are to eat, they may find that they eat very rapidly and simply do not stop until everything on their plates (or worse, on the table) is finished. Other obese people may discover that whenever they sit down to watch TV late in the evening they have an uncontrollable urge to eat, and before they know it they have polished off a large snack, again violating their diets.

It is often much easier to remove the cues to eat that these people get from their environments than it is to try to suggest what they should not eat in the very same situations in which they have always overeaten in the past. For example, teaching a person to always eat only in one specific room may help him more than telling him to cut out the late evening snack. The former advice is positive, the latter negative. Encouraging him to eat slowly may prevent him from needing to take "seconds" to keep eating while others are still on "firsts."

Each individual is unique; a situation that may cause one person to overeat may do nothing to another. Therefore it is necessary to collect information on the food intake (and exercise) patterns of individuals by having them keep careful records and to identify the most maladaptive behaviors within these. Then each maladaptive behavior is attacked and records kept of success in reducing the behaviors as well as the ultimate effects on decreasing fatness and weight of such changes.

Group Therapy and Dietary Clubs

Many of the group methods for treating obesity make use of the potential of the group for teaching each other, furnishing group support and a spirit of friendly competition and social outlets that are not food connected to help the obese person. Usually dieting clubs or commercial concerns employ a single reducing diet of roughly 1200 calories for women and 1800 calories for men, which is sufficiently low in calories to make most people lose 1 to 2 pounds a week, depending on what they were eating before. Group meetings give a chance to check up on weight reduction and to reward success, as well as to teach cooking techniques and habits that are helpful to the dieter. Since many people can be treated at one time, the costs of treatment are less than one-to-one dieting instruction by health professionals.

The group regimes suggested by the most common commercial weight-reducing companies have helped many, but they also have their problems. The reducing diets are usually adequate in nutrients other than calories, but they may not involve the special adjustments that those who are suffering from diabetes or possible early coronary artery disease may need. Emphasis is usually placed on weight loss, not fat loss or other changes (such as decreases in serum cholesterol), which might be more important for some persons. Obviously, in growing children or pregnant women sensible reducing diets do not necessarily aim for weight loss but rather fat loss since other tissues need to grow. Physical inactivity is usually given very little attention by these groups, and most of the advice is geared to diet alone: yet we know that the problems of the obese are often more related to inactivity than to overeating. It makes good sense to encourage greater physical activity, not only to burn up calories and improve fitness but also to provide a substitute for all the food-related life activities that are often so important to the obese. When commercial dieting groups are conducted by lay people, the nutrition information taught in the classes is sometimes incorrect. Also, especially if the club or company produces low-calorie foods or owns a health spa, these may be heavily promoted and the false impression given that it is these special foods or special exercises (and not simply a low-calorie diet or greater physical activity) that is necessary for weight loss.

Crash Diets

These diets usually promise that weight will be lost very quickly (faster than 1 to 2 pounds a week) and in a more or less miraculous manner. Very often a person who has supposedly been "cured" promotes it by personal testimonial or reference to complicated metabolic processes.

In the past few years a number of physicians and hundreds of nonphysicians have written books on various crash diets such as the Stillman diet, the Atkins diet revolution, the banana and skimmed milk diet, the total-fast diet, and so on. The major problem with most of these diets is that they do not supply the nutrients other than calories that humans (including fat people) need. Although weight loss may occur, it will not be any faster than it would be on a diet more sensible from the standpoint of other nutrients. Many "diet books" contain false or misleading information and claim that one or more foods (grapefruit, bananas, cider, honey, vinegar, and so on) have especially good properties that will allow the dieter to shed pounds simply by eating them, while at the same time the person's beauty, strength, sexual prowess, or other characteristics will miraculously change for the better. Such claims are false. Since the calorie levels of these diets are usually low and the diets are made up of only a few foods, the combination of low calories and boredom (which may lead to loss of appetite) may in fact lead to weight loss. It is just not necessary for a diet to be that unpleasant.

Most of the crash diets fall into two general categories. The first group suggests low-calorie diets that are higher in protein and fat and lower in carbohydrate than most Americans' usual food habits. While many of these diets are harmless, they can cause real health problems, including ketosis and elevated serum cholesterol levels when carried to extremes. Changes in the proportions of carbohydrate, protein, and fat do not have any particular positive effect in stimulating fat loss. In the first week of weight reduction more weight may be lost, due to the fact that on low-carbohydrate diets water loss is faster.

The second group of diets often has special appeal because they claim that the dieter can eat all he wants of a particular group of foods and thus seem to promise "something for nothing," that is, weight loss without limiting calories. Unfortunately, the gimmick is that only a few foods are allowed on the diet, and the dieter quickly becomes so bored that he is unable to eat enough of these items to amount to a high caloric intake.

If these diets "work," they work by getting the dieter to take in fewer calories than he needs so that body stores of fat are burned up.

Fasting Total fasts are of course the ultimate crash diet. They have their place *only* if done under the supervision of a physician, since they may cause or heighten disorders such as gout, liver damage, and ketosis and lead to a substantial loss of body protein and minerals along with the fat. Very often people who have fasted on their own go back to their old ways as soon as the fast is over, and as a result they rapidly regain the weight they lost. Under a physician's care such diets may be quite useful in bringing about very rapid weight losses, for example, in patients who need surgery, but the risks of operating on very heavy patients are great.

Drugs The most appealing way to solve an obesity problem would be to do away with it by taking a pill. While there are many pills to swallow, none has yet proved to be the answer to reducing fatness. Perhaps the most popular and widely used medications for obesity are drugs that can be bought over the counter in drugstores. These are sometimes in the form of diet candies, sometimes pills. The most active ingredient they contain is the sheet of directions for a low-calorie diet that usually accompanies them; the expensive pills or "special candies" that are supposed to cut appetite do little good.

The next most widely used are appetite-suppressing agents, which are only sold by prescription from a physician. Probably the best known of these are the amphetamines and related compounds such as diethylproprion, phenmetrazine, and fenfluoramine. These substances act on the central nervous system to inhibit food intake and may help to curb appetite for a few weeks. Their main problem is that most people develop "tolerance" for the drugs; that is, larger and larger amounts of the drug must be given to get the same effect after a few weeks of treatment. Even then, over the long term they do not make much difference in weight loss; after six months the difference is only a few pounds between those who use these pills and those who do not. Since high doses of some of these drugs may have effects on the emotions or mental health, they are by no means without risk.

Diuretics are also sometimes prescribed by physicians. These assist in water loss but not fat loss. These are not usually necessary because in most people body-fluid balance readjusts to a lower level as fat is lost.

Thyroid preparations have sometimes been used to treat obesity. They are not called for unless thyroid function is abnormal to begin with, which it is not in most obese patients. If they are given to obese persons in moderate amounts similar to the levels found in normal persons, they have little effect on weight, since the hormone that is taken merely decreases hormone secretion within the body. If very high doses are given, weight loss increases. However, the weight lost is not fat tissue but lean body tissue, and very high doses may cause heart failure. Then there are the "rainbow diet pills" regimes, so called because each of the many pills is a different color, which have from time to time been prescribed by unethical or unwise medical practitioners. These pills sometimes combined a regime of appetite depressant, thyroid hormone, a diuretic, and tranquilizers for reducers. The use of a combination of these drugs plus a very low-calorie diet has in some cases led to its own health problems, since under certain circumstances this may cause a potassium deficiency and resulting heart problems.

Another useless treatment that has been advertised for obesity is a hormone called human chorionic gonadotropin (HCG). A Swiss physician first popularized this "injectable" pseudo-cure, and it became very popular in some "fat clinics" to employ injections of the hormone with a 500-calorie reducing diet for spot reducing. The diet works, but the hormone does not. The Food and Drug Administration and the Federal Trade Commission recently evaluated the claims for this hormone treatment and found them false.

Exercise

As most Americans have become more affluent, their activities, jobs, and daily living patterns have tended to demand less and less energy. The objective in obesity treatment is to reverse this trend. Exercise helps not only by raising outputs but by controlling appetite, decreasing numbers of tempting situations for eating, and lessening the strictness of the reducing diet, since it too contributes to the calorie deficit. In treating obesity with exercise the first principle that must be grasped by the fat person is that *exercise must become a way of life*—an everyday event, not a special weekend task.

The amount of energy expended in physical activity depends on the number of muscles used, the size of these muscles, and how long, hard, and fast they are used. Thus it is not how vigorous and exhausting exercise efforts are, but how often calorie outputs are increased above the resting level and for how long that are important. (See Chapter 3.)

Reducing and Body-shaping Devices

We have all read those ads that say, "Take 2 inches off your hips, and add 2 inches to your bust overnight." Personal testimonials from so-called "satisfied" users and claims by promoters of reducing devices about doing away with lumpy hips, double chins, and spare tires around the middle would lead you to think that the old-fashioned diet and exercise approach to obesity control was sadly out of date. Unfortunately, all they really illustrate is that their promoters have discovered loopholes in the law that allow them, at least temporarily, to make totally false statements and claims.

The most popular of these devices claim that they can "spot-reduce" various parts of the body; others claim that by body wraps of various parts or all of the body, fat will be removed by inducing perspiration, or that body fat can be shaped by mechanical vibrators. Such claims are false. The only way to remove fat from the chin, neck, thighs or other parts of the body is through loss in total body weight.

The manufacturers and promoters of these devices get away with making false claims since there is no law that covers reducing devices and makes the promoters test their safety and effectiveness before they are put on the market. Court proceedings are necessary to show that advertising is false or misleading or that the product is dangerous to health, and very few complaints against these devices reach the courts. Since there are so many being sold, the enforcement agencies concentrate on the devices that are harmful and tend to ignore the ones that are simply worthless.

Dennis Stock/Magnum Photos

Weight-reducing machines—an exercise in salesmanship.

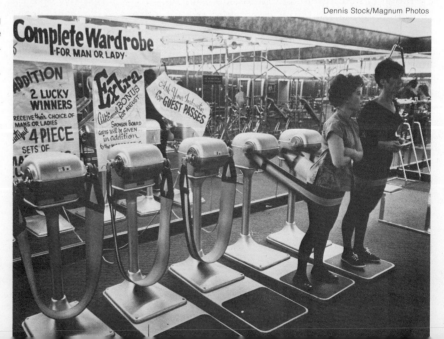

1. *Judge your own fatness both subjectively (by what you think) and objectively (by use of a table of ideal weights for heights or even measurements by experts). Were you right or wrong?*
2. *Give examples of times during the day when you could do extra vigorous walking or other exercise, and estimate the extra energy output this would involve.*
3. *Keep a weekly account of your physical activities and the time spent in each, then calculate your daily calorie output. Does it match your intake?*
4. *Examine sugar-snack and soft-drink consumption in your own diet and that of friends, and compare to the national averages.*
5. *Discuss environmental considerations that encourage you or others to eat excessively. How might these be modified?*

Diseases have very different effects on nutritional needs. Therefore if we wish to talk about diets for disease, we must talk about diets for specific diseases. The fact that a person is "on a diet" does not always mean that his illness was caused by a nutritional disorder, nor does it mean that it can be cured by food. Diets may be used to prevent, treat, control, cure the disease, or, if this is impossible, simply to make the patient more comfortable.

DISEASES AND NUTRITIONAL NEEDS

Every year about a million persons in the United States either have a heart attack or die suddenly of coronary artery disease. Unfortunately, many young people have signs and symptoms of precoronary artery disease. One of the early signs of this disease is thought to be hyperlipemia, or high levels of certain fatty substances or lipids (cholesterol and triglycerides) in the blood. Certainly, these substances are found to clog the medium and large arteries of heart attack victims. This discussion will make reference to hypercholesterolemia (high cholesterol in the blood) and hypertriglyceridemia (high fat in the blood) since both can be influenced by diet.

Hyperlipemia and Heart Disease

Even with good care at least a third of the persons experiencing their first heart attack in middle age will die within a few hours or weeks after the attack. Those who survive are still much more likely to die than other people. Therefore medical science is now looking for ways of finding cases earlier and preventing people from getting the severe form of the disease in the first place.

The "big three" things related to the way we live which can be changed to help prevent atherosclerosis are diet (which affects cholesterol and triglyceride levels in the blood), blood pressure, and cigarette smoking. Persons who are free from abnormally high serum cholesterol values and high blood pressure and who do not smoke are very much less likely to have heart attacks than others.

Prevention of Atherosclerosis

55

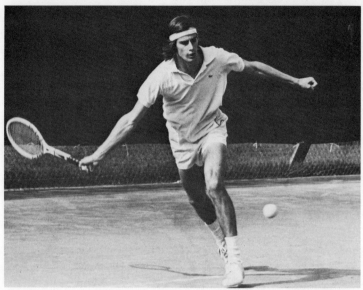

Exercise, whether moderate or strenuous, is essential to our health.

John T. Lewis/Editorial Photocolor Archives

Diet and Serum Cholesterol

When diets high in cholesterol and fat are fed over a long time to experimental animals in scientific laboratories, a condition similar to coronary artery disease in humans can be produced. Also, with very few exceptions, human populations with diets like our own, which are high in saturated fat and cholesterol (such as the diets of the British Isles and the Scandinavian countries), have high cholesterol levels in their blood and often suffer coronary artery disease early in life. On the other hand, people in countries in which the diets are low in cholesterol and saturated fat (such as Greece, Guatemala, or Japan) have lower cholesterol levels and a lower rate of heart disease. Even among people in this country whose diet is rich in these components, the risk of developing coronary artery disease early in life increases as the serum cholesterol level rises. Therefore while diet alone is not enough to either cause or cure the disease, it is evidently related to prevention.

Other disease processes and factors may also aggravate atherosclerosis. One is diabetes mellitus. Diabetics have atherosclerotic disease more often, more severely, and earlier in life than nondiabetics. Control of diabetes is related in part to diet, as we shall see later.

Another is obesity. The obese also suffer heart attacks more often than the nonobese. This is largely due to the fact that overweight persons, especially men, are more likely to have high blood pressure, hyperlipidemia, and diabetes. Weight reduction may help on this score, since it may lessen some of these symptoms.

Sedentary living also seems to elevate the risk of heart disease, as do psychosocial tensions—either related to personal life situations or simply built into the lifestyle of the culture. Exercise not only helps to keep body weight in line but also may be helpful in other ways such as in reducing tension.

It seems that the best way to prevent atherosclerosis is to decrease hyperlipemia, obesity, hypertension, cigarette smoking, and sedentary living—all at the same time.

In terms of benefits for both now and the future, there is a great payoff in adopting living patterns early in life that encourage low blood lipids, nonfatness, normal blood pressure, and good physical fitness.

Diets for Better Heart Health

The following diet recommendations are extremely important for those who have some of the warning signals of early atherosclerosis such as hypertension and elevated serum cholesterol. The general public would also benefit from adopting them.

1. *Reduction of obesity.* Obesity should be avoided and weight should be reduced or maintained at near "ideal" levels. This helps to lower blood pressure in some hypertensive patients, decreases blood glucose levels in some patients with maturity-onset diabetes, and lowers elevated serum triglyceride levels.

2. *Reduce dietary cholesterol intake to less than 300 mg per day.* Since the average daily diet in the United States contains about twice this much cholesterol, foods high in cholesterol must be eaten less frequently. These include eggs, organ meats (such as liver), and shellfish. Chicken, fish, and lean red meat are lower in cholesterol and saturated fat than these foods and are useful substitutes.

3. *Reduce saturated fat.* When saturated fat in the diet is lowered, serum cholesterol levels usually fall. Less than 35 percent of total calories should be obtained from fats of all sorts and less than 10 percent of total calories from saturated fats. Unsaturated fats may be used to replace a portion of the saturated fats in the diet, so that 10 percent of the fat comes from polyunsaturated fat and 10 percent from monounsaturated fat. To make this possible, Americans need to modify their practice of eating the five major sources of fat: meats, dairy products, baked goods, eggs, and table spreads or cooking fats. This can be done on the practical level by following these suggestions:

a. Use lean cuts of beef, lamb, pork, and veal cooked in ways to get rid of saturated fat. Eat moderate amounts.

b. Eat poultry and fish more often.

c. Use products that are fat-modified (that is, made with reduced saturated fat and cholesterol content). These include fat-modified processed meats (such as hot dogs, sausage, salami, luncheon meats). Check labels to determine which are fat-modified.

d. Use low-fat and fat-modified dairy products (such as skim milk and low-fat cheese) and avoid high-saturated-fat dairy products (such as whole milk and high-fat cheese).

e. Use fat-modified baked goods (pies, cookies, cakes, sweet rolls, doughnuts, and so on) and avoid baked goods high in saturated fat and cholesterol. Watch portion sizes.

f. Use more grains, fruits, vegetables, and legumes, which are low in

57

cholesterol and saturated fat as well as in calories.

g. Avoid butter, margarine, and shortenings high in saturated fat.

h. Minimize consumption of candies such as chocolate that are high in fat, as well as egg yolk, bacon, lard, and suet.

TAKING ACTION

1. *When you have your next checkup, ask the doctor what your serum cholesterol and blood pressure are. Discuss them with him and plan your diet accordingly.*

2. *Analyze your own diet for a day, and plan ways to eat that encourage good heart health.*

3. *Record your diet for several days, and find the saturated, unsaturated, and monounsaturated fat content of your diet from the tables of food composition. Does it meet the guidelines for percent of total calories from each of these substances?*

Iron-Deficiency Anemia

Lack of dietary iron is perhaps the most widespread nutritional deficiency in the United States. Iron-deficiency anemia is a common condition, especially among infants and children and women in the childbearing years. The reasons why this condition is distributed mostly among the young and among childbearing females are interesting examples of how diets that are adequate for some are inadequate for others.

Iron is an important nutrient, since it forms parts of the hemoglobin and myoglobin molecules (which transfer oxygen and carbon dioxide to, from, and within various tissues) as well as many enzymes. Because it is so important, the body is careful to retain what it has, and in healthy people very little iron is lost from the body once it is absorbed from the gastrointestinal tract.

Iron needs in the first years of life are high since infants must grow and increase their body tissue and blood volume. Although infants are normally born with some iron stores, they are not sufficient unless iron is supplied in the diet. This is particularly true for premature infants, who are born before their iron stores are built up.

Women of childbearing age also have greater needs to make up for losses of iron in the blood during menstruation, transfer to the fetus during pregnancy, and blood loss during lactation due to milk production. Thus, an intake that might be perfectly satisfactory for an adult man would be inadequate especially for a pregnant woman or rapidly growing baby.

When we examine the iron content of foods, it is easy to see where problems of inadequate intake arise. Small amounts of iron are present in nearly all foods. Especially good sources are meat, liver, peas, and beans. These foods may not be enough to meet the high iron needs of pregnant women, and so it is usually recommended that they take an iron supplement in addition to increasing their consumption of iron-

58

rich foods during pregnancy. Infants consume large amounts of milk, but it is low in iron. For this reason commercial infant formulas are fortified with iron. Iron drops may be added to homemade milk-based formulas or the other foods eaten by breast-fed infants. Infant cereals are enriched with extra iron. Wheat flour and cornmeal are sometimes also enriched, but at lower levels.

Preventing iron-deficiency anemia in babies is not very difficult today since a variety of foods enriched with iron are available to supplement milk. Preventing the problem in older infants, toddlers (who no longer eat infant cereals, drink formula, or receive iron supplements) and older children and youth, particularly female adolescents, is much harder. It involves the careful selection of foods, and in some special cases use of iron supplements.

TAKING ACTION

1. *Check your own food intake for its iron content. Are you in need of more than you're getting?*
2. *Check ten foods with nutrient labels for their iron content.*

High Blood Sugar and Diabetes Mellitus

Diabetes mellitus usually involves high blood sugar and a disorder in fat and protein metabolism, which lead to such effects as excessive thirst, urination, and eating (polydipsia, polyuria, and polyphagia) and even coma in persons who are acutely ill with the disease. We do not know what "causes" diabetes. The likelihood of developing it is at least in part inherited, but it is not due only to heredity. Among the contributing factors that may be related to nutrition are obesity, diet, exercise, and ethnic eating habits. You will note that diet is not a sole cause, nor can it cure the condition, although as we shall see it may affect the likelihood of getting the disease, and it certainly may help to control it.

Maturity-Onset Diabetes

Noninsulin-dependent persons with mild diabetes mellitus make up the greatest portion of the diabetic population. At least 50 percent of these persons are overweight and underexercised. These patients apparently make enough insulin to do well in the fasting state but not quite enough insulin to handle the loads of nutrients that must be disposed of after feeding. They may also have trouble producing enough insulin to support normal metabolism if they are obese. In a genetically susceptible person obesity may further enhance the possibility that this type of diabetes will develop. When you eat, the passage of food through the gut and the absorption of the glucose and amino acids into the blood all stimulate insulin secretion. However, noninsulin-dependent diabetics' bodies seem to resist the action of insulin on both muscle and fat tissue, so fuels become trapped in the blood and cannot be stored or used by many tissues. Thus while insulin

59

in the blood may be increased, it may still be inadequate for the normal metabolism of food.

In order to eliminate the symptoms of diabetics who are not insulin-dependent, diet or a combination of diet and drugs usually will prevent polyuria, polydipsia, and polyphagia. Since insulin and some oral hypoglycemic agents make them fatter by increasing insulin secretion or bringing about other undesirable side effects, the best ways of treatment at present include diet and exercise reeducation. However, although the symptoms disappear, the underlying problems of abnormal metabolism such as higher-than-normal blood sugar levels remain; the disease is simply controlled but not cured.

Again, factors which influence control include obesity, diet, and physical activity. The most important of these would seem to be obesity, since more than 60 percent of maturity-onset-type mild or moderate diabetics are obese. Obesity evidently increases demands on the beta cells of the pancreas because the lipid-loaded, large fat cells packed with fat resist the action of insulin, and it therefore takes more insulin to do the same amount of work and to maintain normal blood sugar in the fat diabetic. If normal healthy volunteers deliberately gain weight and become obese, their insulin secretion also becomes inadequate to preserve normal metabolism. If these patients lose weight, they improve their control over blood sugar with lesser amounts of insulin. Therefore it is very important for obese diabetics of this type to reduce their weight to normal levels if they are to adjust to their bodies' inability to produce insulin.

Drugs other than insulin may be used if diet alone and weight reduction are insufficient to achieve satisfactory blood sugar levels and remission of symptoms. However, since these drugs (called oral hypoglycemic agents) have certain undesirable side effects, it is preferable to stay with diet alone if this is sufficient. Changes in diet and physical exercise may frequently reverse the diabetic state, while prolonged use of oral hypoglycemic agents or insulin may not. The importance of increased levels of physical activity are means of prevention and treatment that should not be ignored.

Lifestyle changes in eating and physical activity are essential components in the management of this condition, as they are in simple obesity. Started early they may provide effective prevention. Started later they may still restore near-normal function both in maturity-onset diabetes and (as we shall see later) in the hyperlipidemias, which are early warnings of cardiovascular disease and often are also present in those who suffer from diabetes.

"Juvenile" or Insulin-dependent Diabetes

The other, more severe form of diabetes requires entirely different treatment. Its characteristics include insulin dependence, an age of onset early in childhood or adolescence, and a tendency for the end products of fat metabolism to accumulate and spill into the urine, as well as other signs of ketoacidosis.

Insulin-requiring diabetics lack insulin altogether and must have insulin to control their blood sugar. They generally have a more severe form of the disease, which tends to be more ketosis-prone. Again, diet and exercise as well as insulin are important in treatment. The goal of therapy is to match food intake and physical activity with insulin activity. Since these patients are thin, it is not necessary to use reducing diets to bring about weight reduction. Rather, what is strived for is adequate nutrition, maintenance of ideal body weight, and timing of food intake to correspond to the time of insulin action. Since the pattern or daily rhythm of insulin secretion cannot be maintained like that of normal persons by any known pattern of insulin injections at present, diet must help to maintain blood sugar levels. This is done by controlling the amount of carbohydrate and protein in the diet as well as the calories and the timing of when they are given.

However, even in insulin-dependent diabetes, exercise is important since it lowers the requirement for insulin. Thus diet therapy, insulin, and exercise all carefully keyed to each other are life-saving measures.

TAKING ACTION

1. *Discuss dietary and activity regimes of some heart and diabetes patients with some individuals who have these conditions.*
2. *Find an insulin-dependent diabetic among your friends or acquaintances. Discuss how they handle diet and insulin.*

DISCUSSION: IMPROVEMENTS NEEDED

If the battle to modify dietary lifestyles for better health, economy, and ecology is to be won, agricultural production, the food industry, food advertising, the alcohol products industry, and most of all consumers are going to have to make some changes. In many ways these very same institutions can be effective comrades in helping to get the American consumer out of destructive lifestyle habits and the diseases and disorders they produce. The real challenge is to do this by eliminating bad practices and enhancing good practices through education.

For example, in the areas of agricultural production and the food industry, what kinds of changes are needed to do a better job of preventing atherosclerosis? If we are to have a diet that is better for the health of our hearts, American agriculture and the American food industry should be encouraged to make available leaner meats as well as processed meats, dairy products, frozen desserts, and baked goods that are reduced in saturated fats, cholesterol, and calories. Visible fats and oils such as margarines, shortenings, mayonnaises, salad dressings, and cooking oils of low saturated fat and cholesterol content are already available and helpful to those on such diets.

The cattle industry should be involved in making changes in meats so that they are low in saturated fats. To produce red meat lower in saturated fats, many changes in cattle breeding and feeding practices

61

will be needed. In this country beef cattle are kept in yards and heavily fed before slaughter so as to increase weight by fattening. Changes in feeding practices as well as in the breed of the animal are needed to lower the fat content of the beef and produce more protein and a leaner cut of meat. For processed meat products the problem is easier since it is possible in production to add vegetable oils and other foods low rather than high in saturated fat. We also need an intensive educational program to teach people how to cook the leaner cuts of meats, since they must be cooked slightly differently to taste their best.

It is also important to find ways to reduce the saturated fat and cholesterol content of dairy products. The farmer receives the most money for dairy products containing the highest amount of butterfat, because years ago this was deemed to be a good thing. This is now obviously incorrect, and the dairy industry and government need to establish policies that encourage the development of low-fat, low-cholesterol milk and milk products, and the breeding of cows that produce large amounts of high-protein, low-fat milk. The manufacturing of cheeses also needs to be changed so that saturated fat and cholesterol in them are reduced.

Creamers (powdered creams) need to be developed that are low in total fats, saturated fats, and cholesterol. At present these products are very high in saturated fat.

The baking industry needs to start using more fat-modified products to reduce the saturated fat, cholesterol, and calorie content of baked goods.

The oil industry should continue to produce and promote fats and oils low in saturated fats and cholesterol for table spreads, shortenings, and cooking and salad dressings. Butter substitutes should be widely available in restaurants as well as elsewhere.

Since egg yolks are the single highest source of cholesterol in the American diet, the food industry must continue to develop acceptable substitutes (such as low-cholesterol, low-saturated-fat egg substitutes), and the use of egg yolks in commercially prepared foods should be avoided by industry whenever possible. They should use the substitutes instead.

Food labeling needs to be changed so people will know how much fat products contain and how much saturated fat is a part of this. Consumers need to be able to identify the amount and type of fat and cholesterol as well as other nutrients in foods, including commercially prepared mixed dishes. The advertising, production, and sale of products low in saturated fats and cholesterol should be allowed.

Government feeding programs such as school lunch programs and meals for the U.S. Armed Forces, veteran's hospitals, and so on should pay more heed to these sorts of preventive habits since they feed millions of persons each day.

A second example of the kinds of changes that need to be made is the matter of food advertising to children and the unfortunate effects that

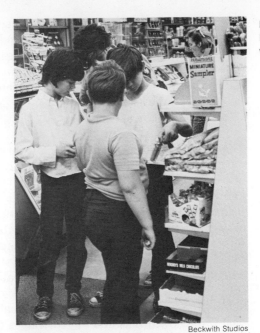

Bad—and good—eating habits are developed when we are young.

Beckwith Studios

this may have on their dietary habits. By school age, children have had a heavy dose of indoctrination, other than that which their parents provide, about which foods are good to eat on the basis of television. TV commercials may promote overconsumption of certain food groups such as sweets, desserts, or convenience foods, which may be extremely costly and relatively low in nutrition. Only some food products are advertised, and these only by brand. Thus, children may get a very distorted view of what is good food, since "good" depends largely on advertising exposure.

Since most of the food products advertised on television push the sensory qualities of food, particularly sweetness, the child may learn to believe that only these foods are good foods. He may fail to understand that many nourishing foods not advertised on television can also be enjoyable. Finally, sweetness may become linked in the child's mind with being the taste of "reward food." Children, on their own, do not necessarily choose an adequate diet unless the foods from which they are allowed to choose are adequate. If children themselves are allowed to decide what will be on the pantry shelf, they are likely to overload it with large numbers of low-nutrient reward foods at the expense of the necessary nutritious foods. Clearly changes and countereducation are needed here to teach children more sensible eating habits.

Where to Turn for Expert Help

Whenever people decide that something is radically wrong with them and it is due to what they are eating, it is wise to consult an expert, just as they would do if their cars were acting peculiarly. Physicians are prepared to deal with serious dietary deficiency conditions. The

tending to basic needs
dietitian or nutritionist, whose first concern is food and its relationship to health, is able to assess the food-related aspects of problems and help with their solution. There are also other experts who may be helpful in answering questions concerning food and diet. These persons include nutritional biochemists, health educators, home economists, and hospital-based dietitians.

CONCLUSION

The food consumption patterns of every culture, including our own, have elements that may be detrimental from the standpoint of nutrition and health. Malnutrition is *not* confined to the poor, nor is lack of knowledge about nutrition and wasteful use of food budgets or food resources. It is easy for us to overlook the negative aspects of our own eating habits on health. The diet of most Americans—with its high saturated-fat and cholesterol content and its superabundance of calories, high sugar (sucrose) content, and (at least until recently) low iron content—may also lead to health problems of various kinds. Our lifestyles, which favor little physical exercise, excessive smoking, obesity, and stress, may also exert threats on health. There is a great deal in our own diets and our own lives that we need to set right if we are to optimize our eating from the standpoint of health, appearance, budget, environment, and, of course, enjoyment.

FOR FURTHER READING

Hafen, Brent Q., ed., 1975. *Weight and Obesity: Causes, Fallacies, Treatment.* Provo, Utah: Brigham Young University Press.

An excellent source of readable articles on the topic of weight control.

Margolius, Sidney, 1975. *Health Foods: Facts and Fakes.* New York: Walker and Co.

A fair and thoughtful examination of the health, natural, and organic foods movement.

Mayer, Jean, 1968. *Overweight: Causes, Costs and Control.* Englewood Cliffs, N.J.: Prentice-Hall.

Answers most of the scientific as well as practical questions people have on obesity.

———, 1973. *Human Nutrition: Historic and Scientific.* Springfield, Ill.: Charles C. Thomas.

A wide-ranging series of short articles on nutrition-related health problems.

National Academy of Sciences, 1974. *Recommended Dietary Allowances.* 8th ed. Washington, D.C.: U.S. Government Printing Office.

For a copy write to Printing and Publishing Office, 2101 Constitution Ave., N.W., Washington, D.C. 20418.

Pyke, Magnus, 1971. *Man and Food.* New York: World University Library.

Discusses many different questions on food technology, poverty and nutrition, the science of nutrition, and related topics in a popular and easy-to-read style.

Trager, James, 1970. *The Food Book.* New York: Grossman Publishers.

A fascinating collection of short, readable pieces on various topics concerned with food.

Watts, B. K., and Merrill, A. L., 1973. *Composition of Foods.*

A 190-page handbook, which can be obtained by writing to the U.S. Department of Agriculture or to Composition of Foods, P.O. Box 17873, Tucson, Ariz. 85731.

3

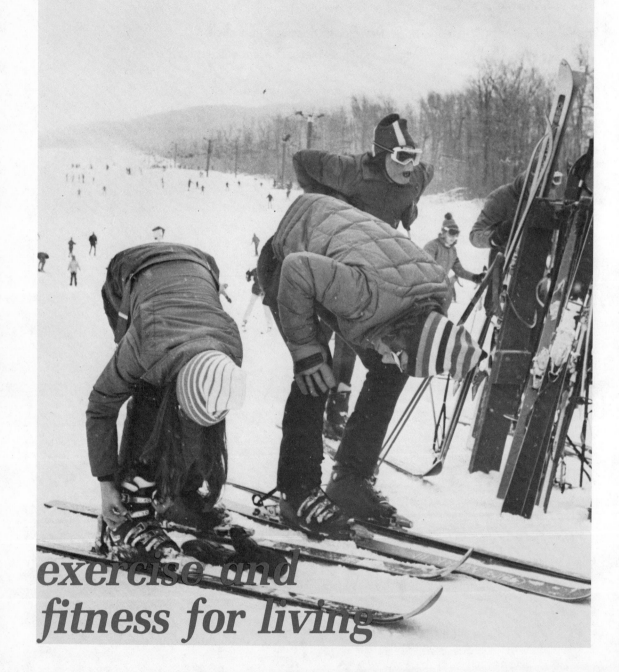

exercise and
fitness for living

To put it as simply as possible, exercise is a voluntary increase in physical activity for the purpose of enhancing or improving body functions. Therefore we cannot consider as exercise those ordinary physical activities you do in carrying out your routine daily life. Just performing these regular functions on a day-to-day basis without additional exercise or physical activity leaves you only marginally fit. To improve your body, you must add some form of "overload."

Perhaps the best way to understand what exercise does is to look at what happens when you do not exercise. The common symptoms of inactivity are easily recognizable: exhaustion after slight or moderate exertion, fatigue that comes late in the day, and the inability to carry out those little extra demands or common emergencies that happen in everyone's life.

From what has just been said, or perhaps from what you already know about exercise, you can see that even if you are playing two sets of tennis on a daily basis, you still need additional exercise or activity in order to place that all-important overload on the body's systems. If this is not done, your body will become adapted to that one level of activity, and in a sense your body systems will reach a plateau, showing no further improvements without the added stress of extra activity.

If you are a moderately active individual, this degree of exertion may be sufficient to prevent deterioration of your structure and function. However, you will probably experience, or have experienced already, some of the symptoms mentioned above as a result of insufficient activity.

If you are an extremely sedentary individual, one who spends your days sitting and/or lying around, worse things can happen to you in addition to experiencing the signs of lack of exercise already mentioned. Your body's systems will begin to deteriorate. Your bones will start to disintegrate. You will become weak and feeble because you will be literally wasting away. The bright spot about these symptoms of deterioration is that they are all easily reversible at any age and at any time of your life. All you need to do is increase your level of physical activity.

INQUIRY

1. How do you feel about your present state of physical fitness and the amount and type of activity in which you regularly participate?
2. What kind of a lifestyle do you see yourself having 10 years from now? 20 years from now?
3. What are some of the physical activities you've always wanted to try but never got around to? What are your reasons for not trying some new activities?
4. Do you know what happens to your body systems when you exercise? When you don't exercise?
5. Do you have to "kill yourself" to get into shape?

HOW FIT DO YOU WANT TO BE?

Good physical fitness rarely "just happens." More often than not it is the result of knowing what to do. Students at the college level have an excellent opportunity to learn the skills and the sources of motivation that will help them maintain good physical fitness throughout their lives.

What Do You Want to Be Fit for?

People should never look upon physical fitness through the eyes and lifestyle of another person. You must decide for yourself what kind of person you are or would like to be and the kind of lifestyle you have or would like to have. From the answers to these questions you can choose the types of sports, games, and exercises you wish to pursue or avoid. For example, do you have aspirations of becoming a champion, world-class athlete? Or is your goal to become a professional dancer? Does your choice of a career involve a moderate amount of physical activity?

A person's needs and activity preferences are an extremely personal matter. Not everyone needs or even wants to be skilled in some sport. Some people enjoy games and others do not. For many people sports provide an effective and enjoyable means of meeting activity needs; others may choose such nonsport activities as walking, bicycle riding, or hiking. A few people, for whatever their reasons, choose to reject any kind of vigorous physical activity. But whatever the choice of involvement may be, the important question to be answered is: "Does your present attitude and practice of exercise reflect choices based on thought-out decisions about you, your lifestyle, and your health, or did they 'just happen'?"

Review of the Possible Levels of Fitness   To make responsible decisions regarding fitness and exercise, people should have a good background of precise information concerning their own activity needs along with the limitations, possible detriments, and potential benefits of the numerous varieties of physical activity.

Traditionally exercise has been viewed from two extremes of the continuum; at one end are the athletes who are in excellent condition, and at the other end are the hospital patients whose activity needs fall along the lines of therapeutic exercise. In the middle of the continuum lie the overwhelming majority of Americans who are neither athletes nor hospital patients but are still capable of varying degrees of physical activity. Yet it is this category of persons that engages in almost no regular exercise at all!

A more realistic view of the human condition is the continuum shown in Figure 3-1.

Figure 3-1
A scale of physical fitness levels.

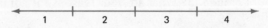

Level 1 is characterized by the person who is totally dependent upon the help of others and on motorized devices. This level also contains

the activity of therapeutic exercise for patients on the mend. These patients recuperating from illness or injury tend to focus their fitness efforts on the injured or diseased parts of their bodies rather than on the whole. If you are at this level, you typically spend your day doing little more than sitting or lying around.

Level 2 is characterized by the person who does the minimum amount of activity necessary to reduce the risk of coronary heart disease, obesity, and other degenerative changes resulting from lack of exercise and activity. If you are at this level, you are merely meeting the five simple requirements to achieve minimum maintenance:

1. Turn and twist your body joints to their near-maximum range of motion.
2. Stand for a total of 2 hours a day.
3. Lift something unusually heavy for 5 seconds.
4. Get your heart rate up to 120 beats a minute for at least 3 minutes.
5. Burn up 300 calories a day in physical activity.

Level 3 is characterized by the individual who is totally fit for regular life plus possessing the necessary reserve for those extra demands and common emergencies of everyday life. This is the housewife who when asked by her husband to go out dancing at the end of the day doesn't have to decline because she's too tired. This is the man who eagerly looks forward to that extra tennis or golf game following a regular workday without the embarrassment of having to cancel the date due to fatigue. The individual at this level is not a fitness fanatic but instead is one who enjoys living life to its fullest and is always ready when friends suggest recreation activities.

Level 4 is characterized by the person who is maximally fit for peak levels of performance. This, then, is the level of the serious athlete. This individual has already made the decision that his or her sport is more than just a leisurely pursuit or recreational pastime. If you are at this level, you have committed yourself to a lifestyle that is different, both psychologically and physiologically, from the nonathlete's. You will be dedicated to your sport and training. You will sacrifice social pleasures, endure pain, discomfort, and even punishment in order to create the tolerances necessary for champion performances.

TAKING ACTION

1. *Determine your present fitness level. Compare with classmates.*
2. *At what level of fitness would you like to be? Specify why.*
3. *Have you ever tried altering your lifestyle to change your fitness level? (For example, have you tried jogging or taking up some new sport?)*
4. *How did you feel about the alteration(s)?*
5. *Discuss with others what exercise means to you.*
6. *Talk to someone whom you consider to be exceptionally fit and get his or her ideas on exercise and fitness. Can you use any of these ideas?*

In a very short time you will be graduating from college. Possibly at your commencement ceremony you will hear something to the effect that you are the hope of the future and the leaders of tomorrow. How many times do you suppose that has been said to people your age? Do you believe it? Do you really believe your actions could change the world? Or, on a smaller scale, could your actions and beliefs actually have an influence on those people around you—your family or friends?

If you are willing to believe that, you are placing a tremendous amount of responsibility upon yourselves. Are you up to handling this challenge? It has been said so many times before that "it's now up to you." And this was never more true than it is right now. You will have the knowledge to save America's health and fitness. Right now people's health and concepts of fitness are deteriorating simply because the information they need now was not available to them when they were in school or the information that they have now is inaccurate.

Try to pass on the knowledge you are acquiring now to help turn America from a nation of inactive, obese individuals into once again a nation of energetic, fit, and ready-for-anything people.

FITNESS IS A TEMPORARY THING

The word "fitness" suggests a relationship between a task to be performed and an individual's capacity to perform it. General fitness can be thought of as a person's ability to perform work, resist disease and infection, and resist the physical stresses imposed by the environment (cold, heat, atmospheric-pressure changes from water depth or altitude, and the velocity changes of jolts and vibrations). In other words, to be in a good state of physical fitness one must be able to dominate his ordinary environment. When you exercise, you actually are creating an artificial environment by increasing the stress placed on your systems in order to raise your level of adaptation. Each individual requires his own degree of general fitness that is related to the degree of stress he must be able to overcome in his environment. This degree of stress is highly specific to each individual and is easily subject to changes as the environment changes around him. Specific physical fitness, then, is the condition of the body's systems in readiness to meet special demands.

Adaptation and Deadaptation to the Environment

An individual's state of fitness for exercise relies upon three important factors: the suitability of the individual's body structure for the task to be performed, the ease and effectiveness with which the body's organs and systems support the effort, and the attitude that the individual takes toward the task as he approaches it and completes it.

The importance of the three factors just mentioned is their level or state at the present time. Because your body automatically adjusts to the daily demands you place upon it, you can see that what you have done in the past 4 weeks is far more important than what you have done in the past 4 years. This is the principle of adaptation.

The principle of adaptation also works in reverse. Since exercise results are transient, once you stop exercising at a certain level, you will slowly lose the results of that level. Your body will quickly adjust and react to the lack of demand placed upon it. If the demand diminishes, your body will register this fact. This is the problem one faces with patients requiring long periods of bed rest. Recall a time in your life when you had to stay in bed for an extended period of time due to an injury or an illness. Do you remember how weak and unsteady you felt when you first tried to walk? This is because you were experiencing hypokinetic deterioration (deadaptation to diminishing or reduced stress from the environment). It has been proved by experiments with subjects maintaining complete bed-rest conditions for long periods of time that the body loses approximately 5 percent of its strength for every 3 days of bed rest.

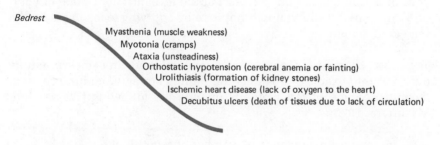

Figure 3-2
Conditions of
hypokinetic disease.

The sloping line in Figure 3-2 shows the steps of deterioration that take place in a period of 8 weeks of complete bed rest.

The following scale shows the adaptation-deadaptation phenomenon to environmental stress conditions.

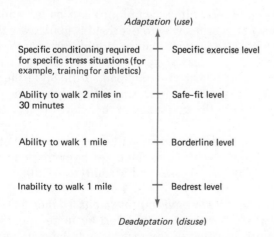

Figure 3-3
A scale showing physical
adaptation as it relates
to general health.

The area below the borderline level represents the condition of hypokinesis. The borderline level represents the minimum maintenance level referred to earlier. At this level we know that very slight amounts of activity every day will keep a person near the borderline. The safe-fit level is the level of total fitness for regular life plus fitness for the extra demands. And the specific exercise level is, of course, the level of the athlete.

Overload Overload is the foundation and the key to any fitness program. The overload principle is based on the biological law of adaptation-deadaptation just mentioned. This training principle (overload) must be used in all programs to achieve desired results. No matter how poor your physical condition and no matter what your age, you can improve your physical condition by using the principle of overload. Overload is any resistance greater than that which you typically encounter in daily living. For practical application what this means is that when you start your fitness program, you will start at the level just above that of your ordinary activity, and you will improve by applying loads in gradually increased amounts.

Types of Overload There are several methods for incorporating overload into exercise programs for gaining strength, endurance, and flexibility. Some of the methods include the following (Wessel and MacIntyre, 1970):

1. Increasing the distance or number of repetitions
2. Increasing the duration, or lengths of time, of the exercise
3. Increasing the intensity (strength) by increasing the resistance or load (weight to be lifted)
4. Increasing the speed of the exercise movement
5. Decreasing the rest interval between exercises

Some of these overloading techniques are better and safer than others. The most dangerous way to overload is to increase the intensity of the effort by lifting a heavier load or moving faster or moving against a heavier resistance. A less risky way to overload is to increase the duration of the effort by carrying the load a little bit farther or hanging on a little bit longer. The safest way of applying the principle of overload is to increase the frequency of the effort—that is, to do it more times a week.

The type of overload you choose will depend upon what you decide your specific fitness goals are, such as strength, endurance, and flexibility improvement (Wessel and MacIntyre, 1970):

1. *Overloading and strength improvement.* To increase strength you must increase the intensity of effort by increasing the weight of the object to be lifted or the resistance to be overcome.

2. *Overloading and endurance improvement.* To increase endurance you must increase the duration of the effort. Endurance overloading must be specific to the type of endurance you wish to improve (that is, muscular endurance or circulorespiratory endurance).
3. *Overloading and flexibility improvement.* To increase flexibility you must apply the overload principle by gradually and progressively forcing the muscles and the surrounding connective tissue to stretch through their full range of motion.

When applying the overload principle to any exercise it is important to keep in mind that a little overload will go a long way. Moderation is the key; therefore excessive overloading is not only undesirable but may also be dangerous as well. The symptoms of excessive overloading are easily recognizable (Wessel and MacIntyre, 1970):

1. Disturbed rest and sleep
2. Muscle soreness or stiffness occurring the next day that limits your activity
3. A feeling of tiredness or depression following the exercise or the next day
4. Failure of heart rate and respiration to return to normal within 15 to 20 minutes after a vigorous, strenuous workout

Elements of Fitness

Physical fitness from a layman's viewpoint is an individual's capacity to carry out reasonably vigorous physical activities along with the normal activities of daily life. The components of fitness are those qualities that relate to the individual's general health and well-being rather than those specific motor skill qualities that are vital for performance (speed, agility, power, balance, coordination, reaction time, and so on). There are only perhaps five or six qualities that are basic to physical fitness. They are circulorespiratory capacity, muscular endurance, strength, flexibility, body composition, and relaxation.

Circulorespiratory capacity (also referred to as circulorespiratory endurance or aerobic power) is the fitness quality that enables an individual to continue with reasonably vigorous activity for extended periods of time. In more physiological terms, circulorespiratory capacity is the ability of the body to supply oxygen-rich blood and food to active body tissues. This type of endurance is related to the strength and tone of the heart, lungs, and blood vessels, and the mobilization of energy reserves in the body to meet exercise stress (Wessel and MacIntyre, 1970). Circulorespiratory fitness is generally thought of as involving activities such as running, swimming, cycling, and other activities that require the use of much of the large musculature of the body. These type of activities force the respiratory system to operate at a much higher level of efficiency than usual.

Muscular endurance is the fitness quality that enables an individual to continue in localized muscle-group activities for extended periods of time. It is this local endurance of the muscles that is involved in specific activities such as pull-ups, pushups, sit-ups, and the like, as well as other typical test exercises involving primarily local muscle groups. This type of endurance is also dependent upon muscular strength in addition to an adequate blood supply to the individual muscle groups. Muscles possessing greater strength will also have greater muscular endurance—the ability to continue prolonged activity.

Strength in human movement is the ability to mobilize force to overcome resistance. In contrast to muscular endurance (sit-ups, push-ups, and so on), muscular strength is properly defined as the maximal force exerted at one time. The ability of an individual to mobilize muscular force is essential for nearly all human activities. Strength is specific to a given muscle or muscle group and is dependent upon the nature of the resistance (movable or stationary).

Two types of strength can be defined: *isometric strength* and *isotonic strength.* Isometric or static strength is the maximal amount of force you can apply against a fixed resistance during one all-out contraction or effort. Isotonic or dynamic strength refers to the amount of resistance you can overcome during one application of force through the full range of motion of a particular joint or joints (for example, a bench press or arm curl on a weight machine).

Flexibility is the fitness quality defined as the basic capacity to move a joint through its normal range of motion. Flexibility can be specific to a single joint (such as the shoulder joint), or it can be related to several joint actions involving bending, reaching, twisting, and turning in total body movements. Flexibility is actually far more dependent upon the connective tissues, ligaments, and musculature surrounding a joint than on the actual bony structure of the joint itself. Not using joints frequently and regularly through their full range of motion causes them to become limited in their range of possible movement. This again, is a good example of the principle of adaptation-deadaptation. In addition, flexibility is also an important requirement for the ability to exert muscular force through the full range of motion.

Body composition may tentatively be listed as one of the qualities of physical fitness because there seems to be increasingly strong evidence at the present time that excess fat stored in the body limits health and physical fitness.

It may be surprising to many people to consider the ability to relax as one of the basic components of physical fitness. Relaxation in human movement means the ability to release tension in the muscles. A state of slight tension is always present in our muscles. This is called *tonus,* and it is essential for free and easy movement and quick response to the stress of exercise. An excess of stress or stimulation results in the condition called neuromuscular hypertension. Emotional upsets, fatigue, lack of sleep, inadequate nutrition, problems with posture, hypertension, or excessive noise and other environmental conditions may cause neuromuscular hypertension.

Everyone needs some form of relaxation. Enjoyable and vigorous activities that will release the tensions and strains of everyday life are essential for everyone's well-being. If you find that your tension is stemming from boredom, you must seek activities that will be stimulating and refreshing for you. If you find, however, that you are constantly left with a feeling of fatigue or tiredness, you should take a look not only at your activities but also at your rest, sleep, and nutritional habits.

Relaxation, like physical fitness itself, is an individual matter. Each person has his or her own activity preferences. There are many methods and techniques that can improve a person's ability to relax. Exercise may work for one person, while meditation or special breathing exercises may be the key for another. Jacobson[1] has devised specific relaxation techniques based on the principle of contrast. The techniques are called *progressive muscular relaxation.* Essentially what these techniques involve are strong muscle contractions followed by voluntary relaxation, with an increased awareness of the decrease in muscular tension. For example, starting with the large muscles of the leg, completely contract and tense each muscle group for 3 seconds and then let go. Follow each complete contraction and relaxation with a "one-half" contraction and relaxation, "one-fourth" contraction and relaxation, and so forth. Many people have found Jacobson's methods and others similar to it to be quite effective for achieving states of relaxation during the day or just prior to sleep.

TAKING ACTION

1. *Explore the movement patterns you use in your daily routine activities. Which ones require strength? Circulorespiratory endurance? Muscular endurance? Flexibility? Compare your evaluations with those of others.*
2. *To check flexibility explore the range of motion possible in the various joints of your body. Experiment with total movements involving multiple joint actions.*
3. *Keep track of your work and recreational activities. Which ones do you feel contribute the most to helping you maintain your full range of motion in your joints?*
4. *What activities in daily living and playing contribute the most to muscular endurance? To circulorespiratory endurance?*
5. *Explore different methods of relaxation. Which ones work best for you?*
6. *List the leisure-time activities (activities done by choice) you enjoy the most and those you enjoy the least. Which activities provide you with feelings of tension release, refreshment, and relaxation?*

---

[1]Edmund Jacobson, 1957, *You Must Relax.* New York: McGraw-Hill.

75

Exercise is a natural part of our lives when we are young.

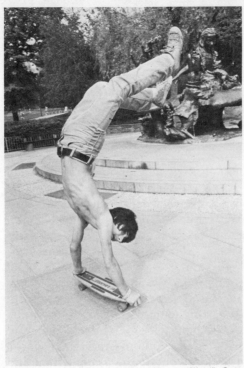

John Marmaras/Woodfin Camp

Discussion The title of this section, "Fitness Is a Temporary Thing," is the key to healthy living. Physical fitness, like a good relationship, must not be taken for granted. Both take planning, commitment, and work.

At this time in your life you're likely to assume that your health, your fitness, and your youth are things you will always have and never need be concerned about. But as you grow older, you'll begin to cherish these aspects of life more and more. Try to imagine, if you can, what you will be like when you reach the age of 35, 50, or even 65. Can you project yourself that far into the future? At 65 will you be a burden to your family and friends because you've let yourself become sedentary and bored with life? At 50 will you still be looking for new things to enjoy and exciting things to do? At 35 will you still have the enthusiasm and zest for living that you have now? A lot of what happens to you in the distant and the near future depends on what you are doing right now. You are laying the groundwork for some very important years ahead.

FORMULATION OF AN EXERCISE PROGRAM The most important consideration in forming your own exercise program is for you to act according to your own needs and desires. If you are not happy and satisfied with your program, you will not be likely to stick with it. Each individual must search for new ways to put physical activity back into his or her life. Here are the three common approaches to putting an optimal level of movement into daily living (Wessel and MacIntyre, 1970):

1. A prescribed exercise program regularly scheduled
2. Regular physically active leisure-recreational activities
3. Stepped-up physical activity in one's daily routine

Each person will have to decide which approach is the best, the most practical, and (of greatest importance) the most enjoyable.

In our world today modern living requires so little physical effort because technology and automation have all but replaced the demand for muscular work. If you find yourself caught in the trap of having succumbed to all the "modern conveniences" (always riding rather than walking, sitting rather than standing, or lying down rather than sitting), it's time to do something to change your sedentary habits. There are three steps involved in such a change (Morehouse and Gross, 1975):

1. The first step is simply to accept the importance and necessity of physical activity. You know you can always find time to do the things you really want to do.
2. The second step is to schedule the activity in spite of everything else you have to do. It then becomes one of the high-priority items of your day or week.
3. The third and probably the most difficult step is to work on your attitude toward exercise.

There are so many excuses for not exercising: no one else does it, we don't know enough about exercise, we don't have the skill, we'll look bad, we have other things to do that are more important, we don't have the time, we'll get tired and sore, we'll hurt ourselves, and the list could go on and on.

There are three important factors to consider when formulating an exercise program for yourself: frequency, persistence and adherence, and positive reinforcement. Once you have decided what you are going to do for your exercise program, whether prescribed exercises or recreational sports, you will need to determine how many times a week to engage in these activities. It is best to avoid the extremes of the "once in a while" or "always without fail" spurts and try to maintain a regular schedule of three to four times a week. It's also a good idea to work out on alternate days—Monday, Wednesday, and Friday, or Tuesday, Thursday, and Saturday. Sunday can then be used as a makeup day. The hour of the day doesn't matter. But remember, you have already decided that your fitness program is going to be number one on your priority list of things to do, so it shouldn't be hard to get into the habit of putting regular workouts into your weekly schedule.

Factors to Consider When Formulating an Exercise Program

77

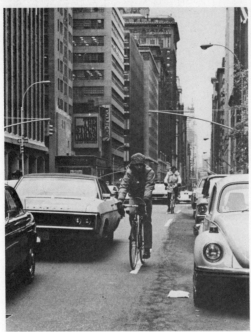

Mimi Forsyth/Monkmeyer

Persistence and adherence are as important to any exercise program as the activities or exercises themselves. You will obtain much better and much more lasting results from a program of three to four steady and regular workouts each week than a program where you go all out every day for one week and then do nothing at all the following two or three weeks. Once you commit yourself to your program, stick with it and don't let anything interfere with it. Your maintenance program, once you have reached your desired level of fitness, might be less strenuous and/or slightly less frequent, but you will lose whatever results you have built up or gained if your activity program ceases completely or becomes too sporadic.

Psychological research has discovered that a response that is reinforced by some means is more apt to be repeated than one that is not. When this kind of research was first being studied, it was thought that the reward of desired behavior and the punishment of undesired behavior created equal and opposite effects. It was quickly discovered that this was not the case. Punishment seems to have a less permanent effect than reward, and punishment may even bring about the opposite result from the intended one. Therefore it is positive reinforcement that we are seeking. Although there seems to be plenty of positive reinforcement built right into your fitness program (looking and feeling better are terrific payoffs), you will also need to be reassured that you will be receiving praise and encouragement from the people around you as you get started and continue in your fitness program. This also works both ways. If some member of your family or someone you know is attempting a change in his or her fitness condition, by all means offer encouragement and praise. Make them feel good about what they are doing or trying to do. Obviously it goes without saying that criticizing or belittling are the easiest ways to put a damper on, or even wipe out completely, a person's confidence in himself and his enthusiasm for his program.

Different Programs Develop Different Capacities (Specificity)

Specificity is a well-known principle used in conditioning programs. Briefly stated it means "adaptation to imposed demands." In other words, the closer your activity involves or simulates the exact fitness quality you wish to improve, the greater will be your improvement of that quality. Your body will respond to the way you place demand upon it. For example, you won't improve your circulorespiratory capacity by a program of lifting weights; likewise, you won't improve your muscular strength by a weight-lifting program involving many repetitions with very light weights as much as you would by working with greater resistance and fewer repetitions. And, of course, flexibility cannot be improved by a relaxation-improvement program.

Just as you can't improve one physical fitness component to its fullest by concentrating on another, you can't expect to get in shape for one sport (such as tennis) by working on another one (such as swimming). The point to remember here is that if you have chosen only one sport to comprise your fitness program, you will, with a few exceptions, have to schedule some different exercises or activities to cover all the components of being physically fit.

One of the exceptions mentioned above is swimming (Morehouse and Gross, 1975). At the fitness level, swimming is a terrific activity. People seeking an adequate degree of fitness could get all the strength, endurance, flexibility, and relaxation they needed using swimming alone as their exercise—as long as their swimming efforts were gradually intensified (overloaded).

TAKING ACTION

1. *Observe your activities for a week. Which approach to increasing your daily physical activity will best suit your lifestyle—a prescribed exercise program regularly scheduled, regular physically active leisure-recreational activities, or more physical activity in your daily routine?*
2. *Take a look at your typical week's schedule of activities and determine when would be the best times to schedule your workouts so that they would become a regular part of your week?*
3. *There are many excuses for not exercising. After discussing these in a group, make a list of all the reasons you can think of for exercising. Discuss rational responses in the event that you are belittled or teased.*
4. *The next time you see someone exercising or engaging in some physical activity, make it a point to compliment or offer encouragement (positive reinforcement).*

5. Suggest to a member of your family the possibility of starting a fitness program. Offer to share some of your new knowledge on the subject.

6. Design a fitness program to improve (a) circulorespiratory capacity, (b) muscular endurance, (c) muscular strength, (d) flexibility, (e) relaxation, (f) a specific sport that interests you.

Discussion

So many of us have grown up with a false concept of what it means to be fit. Images of a Mr. America–type physique or a dancer's figure crowd our imaginations. These are encouraged by the promoters of the fitness cults who spread the belief that *everyone* should attain an exalted degree of fitness, even if it's unattainable and undesirable for the majority of us.

Thank goodness we are now beginning to see the light. Now we have the chance to formulate our own fitness programs based on our individual goals, desires, and lifestyles. We no longer feel we have to attempt to reach someone else's goal or strive to compete on someone else's level. We can be ourselves.

Because we have the knowledge we can formulate a fitness program that fits our lifestyle right now. And we can also change our program without having to answer to anyone but ourselves. We realize that we will be changing our fitness concepts and programs many times as we grow older. We know that few things remain unchanged as time passes. So we are prepared to change with the times, always following what is right and good for us.

THE EFFICACY OF EXERCISE

Effects of Physical Condition

A program to improve your physical fitness state can actually be defined as a conditioning program. Conditioning or training is simply the use of regular exercise to enhance or improve one or more of the components of physical fitness. Training can also mean the attempt to improve one or more of the components of physical fitness. Training can also mean the attempt to improve performance or a specific skill.

Muscle building.

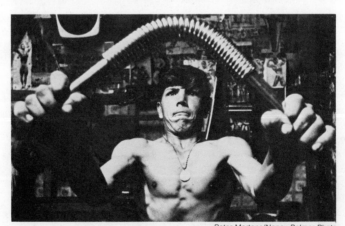

Peter Martens/Nancy Palmer Photo

The effect of a single exercise workout leaves an imprint that lasts for several days on almost every organ and system of the body. This is shown by improvements in subsequent workouts and performances and also by increased efficiency, that is, less effort to do the same work. The body quickly becomes "conditioned" to a new level of physical work, using fewer wasted motions and less tenseness during the effort and often through the acquisition of improved skill.

The Effects of Physical Conditioning on Muscular Development The most noticeable change in the body as a result of physical training is the increase in strength, hardness, and size of the exercised muscles. Part of the increase in muscular strength comes from an increase in muscle mass, but the majority of the increase comes from a better-organized system of nerve impulses that can reach the working muscles at a faster rate and result in a stronger contraction. Inhibitions of the degree of contraction caused by specific nervous system controls are thought to be safety mechanisms. An unconditioned body would not be able to handle a contraction of maximum strength. Training seems to lessen some of the inhibitions, which allows the muscles to contract to more nearly their full capacity. It is the degree of tension under which your

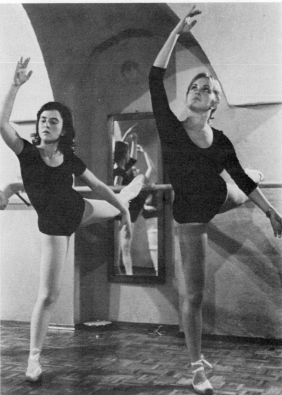

Roberto Borea/Editorial Photocolor Archives

Female dancers often wish to build up muscle strength without substantially increasing muscle size.

muscles contract that dictates the strengthening effect of the training program. The number of times the muscles are contracted has very little to do with pure strength development. A single strong contraction is far more effective toward the development of strength than 100 weak ones.

About 15 to 20 moderate heavy contractions repeated in a pumping motion will result in increased muscle size. If you desire to increase muscular strength without increasing muscle bulk, your program should include single repetitions of near-maximal effort. This fact is important to many persons whose particular activities require agility and speed and to whom heavy, bulky muscles would be disadvantageous. For those activities in which muscle mass is required or simply for the person who desires large muscles for appearance's sake, weight training with the pumping motion is the most effective means of achieving this goal.

Trained muscles are harder than nontrained muscles. This is due to the greater degree of contraction that is achievable by bringing more muscle fibers into action. The trained muscle is firm but supple in the relaxed state, possibly because the ratio of muscle fibers to fat cells is increased.

The Effects of Physical Conditioning on the Circulatory and Respiratory Systems The response to exercise training of heart muscle is similar to that of skeletal muscle. The heart can contract more strongly and in a more coordinated way after training so as to expel more blood with each contraction. In endurance training (circulorespiratory capacity) the musculature of the heart becomes larger, increasing the power potential of each beat. One of the prime benefits of endurance training is that the heart rate becomes slower at rest. This decrease in resting heart rate can be as much as 10 beats per minute with intensive endurance training.

The coronary circulation, which is the heart muscle's own blood supply (separate from that of the general blood supply of the rest of the body), increases as the result of endurance exercise training. This increase in the number of coronary vessels increases the endurance of the heart and may also aid in surviving a heart attack.

As a result of endurance training, new blood vessels appear in all active tissues. This aids in the delivery of supplies carried by the blood and in the removal of wastes. There is almost no increase in the volume of blood to fill these newly formed vessels, but the improvement comes from a better control of pressures that provide for a better shunting of blood to the active muscles used in exercise and away from the tissues and organs that tend to shut down during heavy exertion (for example the kidneys).

The lungs themselves are not affected to any great extent by exercise, since their capacity for ventilation is not reached even during a maximum effort. The muscles used in breathing, the rib musculature and the diaphragm, however, are worked very hard during heavy, strenuous exercise.

The Effects of Physical Conditioning on the Nervous System   It is the nervous system, more than any other system, that is the most affected by exercise training. Often the mere anticipation of an exercise bout can trigger an overwhelming response in an untrained person. As you become more accustomed to exercise, your body seems to acquire the ability to size up the precise amount of effort required for the exercise to be performed and then to adjust all its systems to the proper setting to accommodate it.

Exercise training improves the nervous control of body systems from the perception of the task difficulty to the setting of the response levels. This improvement is a result of a shift from voluntary control to a more conditioned involuntary reflex control. Overactive mental processes in the voluntary control of movement can cause "paralysis by analysis" (Morehouse, 1974). It is not until a movement or a task can be performed almost unconsciously that it can then be accomplished with the greatest ease and skill. This accounts for the apparent ease and casualness with which champion athletes achieve record performances.

How to Measure Exercise Responses: Pulse Rate

Your pulse is the heart-initiated wave that travels throughout your arterial system each time your heart beats. The wave is actually the change in the condition of your artery at the end of each heartbeat. For the majority of people this change (your pulse) can be felt in several places on the body, as shown in Figure 3-4.

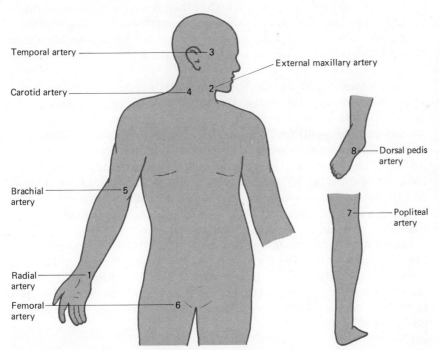

Temporal artery — 3

External maxillary artery

Carotid artery — 4   2

8 — Dorsal pedis artery

Brachial artery — 5

7 — Popliteal artery

Radial artery — 1

Femoral artery — 6

Figure 3-4
Pressure points. (1) Radial artery, on the thumb side of the wrist. (2) External maxillary (facial) artery, at the point crossing the jaw. (3) Temporal artery, at the temple above and to the side of the eye. (4) Carotid artery, on the side of the neck. (5) Brachial artery, on the inner side of the biceps. (6) Femoral artery, in the groin. (7) Popliteal artery, behind the knee. (8) Dorsal pedis artery, above the instep.

The rate of each person's pulse is as individual as his fingerprints. When you read your pulse, you are not reading the volume of blood that is flowing out of your heart into your body, nor are you reading the force or pressure of the blood flow. All your pulse does is give you an accurate index of how many times your heart is beating against the column of blood in your circulatory vessels.

This index is one of the most accurate and precise measures the body has to indicate changes that are taking place internally due to external forces. Your pulse can tell you if your body temperature goes up or down. It can tell you how fast you're using oxygen from the air and burning energy. It will tell you how effectively your body can handle the chemical wastes that are by-products of exercise. It will also tell you the degree of muscular work and involvement. Your pulse can even monitor your psychological state of emotions and attitudes. It combines and coordinates all these conditions together and ends up with a signal that can singularly report your overall condition. Your pulse is your body's single most important indicator of illness, stress, or well-being.

Not only is your pulse a reliable index and simple to measure, it is very easy to locate and count. After a light exercise bout, it's impossible to miss; after moderate or heavy exercise, you don't even need to search for it. You will be able to feel it beating if you simply sit quietly.

Your pulse rate will vary throughout the day. It will be at its lowest after you have been asleep about 6 hours. It will increase from 5 to 10 beats per minute upon awakening. As you go through the day your resting pulse rate gradually increases, and at bedtime it is likely to be another 5 to 10 beats per minute higher than it was when you got up in the morning. Any activity, no matter how slight, even eating, will raise your pulse rate. Your pulse rate can be elevated for the duration of a day and most of the night by a single hard bout of exercise.

Your Pulse and Fitness

There are four things you can feel when taking your pulse (Morehouse and Gross, 1975). The first is the force of your pulse against your fingers. As you become more fit, this force will become stronger. The second thing you will feel is the volume or the expansion of the artery. As your fitness level increases, this volume will increase and the artery will feel thicker, yet soft and elastic. The third is the regularity of the force and the rhythm. Your pulse beat will become stronger and more regular as you become more fit. The fourth and final feeling you will be able to sense is the frequency of your pulse. As you become more fit, the frequency of your pulse beats will diminish.

Lowering your pulse rate is an advantage and a goal of your fitness program because it indicates that the heart is taking a longer rest period between each beat, which means that it is filling more slowly and completely. Your supply of oxygen to the heart is increased by the improved coronary blood flow in addition to an increase in the heart's pumping efficiency.

An important source of information about your fitness and health is your resting pulse rate while seated. Men average 72 to 76 beats per minute, while women average 75 to 80 beats per minute. An average sitting pulse rate for boys is 80 to 84 beats per minute, and for girls the range is 82 to 89 beats per minute. It is not understood why the average beats per minute is higher in women and girls than in men and boys.

According to the American Heart Association, the range for "normal" is between 50 and 100 beats per minute, varying extremely between individuals. There are always exceptions, of course, but as a general rule the lower the resting heart rate the healthier you are. If you have a resting heart rate of higher than 80 beats per minute, this suggests a poor health and fitness condition and makes you an increased risk of coronary heart disease and death in middle age. If this is the case, you should see your physician and follow his advice in taking steps to improve this condition.

A fast pulse rate is not dangerous in itself, nor does it necessarily indicate that there's something wrong with you. What it does mean is that the body is being forced to work under a heavier load than necessary. The body's effectiveness and efficiency is measured by the amount of external work that can be accomplished at a moderate heart rate of 120 beats per minute. If your heart rate reaches 120 or above after only mild exertion, it means that you are not as efficient as you could be. Your system shows the signs of being deconditioned, probably due to a lack of, or insufficient, exercise.

Your exercise pulse rate is another important source of information about your state of health and fitness. Your exercise pulse rate will have little or no relationship to your resting heart rate. The intensity of your exertion will determine how high your pulse rate will go. No matter what your resting heart rate may be, moderate exercise will elevate it to about 120 beats per minute.

If upon taking your pulse you find that it exceeds 100 beats per minute, this could mean one of several things. It could indicate that you've had previous physical activity, that you're emotionally upset, that your body is not in a resting condition (even though you may be sitting), that you have a slight fever, or that your heart rate may have been stimulated by coffee or cigarettes (both caffeine and nicotine can raise your heart and pulse rates by as much as 10 beats per minute). If the cause of your accelerated heart rate is not any of these things, then you have a condition called *tachycardia,* which is an unusually high resting heart rate. If your resting heart rate reaches near 100 beats per minute or the upper limits of the scale of normal, then it is imperative that you attempt, again with your physician's help, to lower your rate. An unnecessarily high resting heart rate, indicative of a heart that is working harder than it should, is inefficient and tiring, and it may be dangerous.

Even if your resting heart is at the lower limits of the normal range, it is still beneficial to lower it even further. Again, a slow heart is beating more efficiently. So there's no danger in lowering your heart rate, no matter how low it is to begin with.

Physiological Responses to Various Degrees of Exercise   *Responses to light exercise.* Light exercise such as walking can be continued for hours without undue fatigue. Your rate of breathing will usually be less than 17 per minute, while your heart rate will rarely exceed 110 beats per minute. At this degree of exertion the blood constituents are undisturbed. Bowling, archery, housework, shopping, auto repair, baseball, and table tennis are only a few of the many examples of light physical exercise.

Responses to moderate exercise. Easy running or jogging on level surfaces are considered moderate exercises. A heart rate of around 120 beats per minute and a respiration rate of about 18 per minute would accompany this degree of exertion. Basketball and football, with bursts of additional strenuous exercise, are typical moderate physical activities. Also included in this group are boating (canoeing), skating, downhill skiing, and golf (where you walk the 18 holes and carry your own clubs).

Responses to strenuous exercise. Wrestling, running at maximum or near-maximum speeds, gymnastics, speed swimming, sprint skating, and fast snow shoveling are examples of activities involving heavy exertion. These types of activities can be endured for only a short while. Chemical waste products of muscle activity, acids, quickly accumulate in the blood. If you are not conditioned for this type of activity, you will become fatigued within minutes. During this activity

Bowling is a good form of light exercise as well as a social activity.

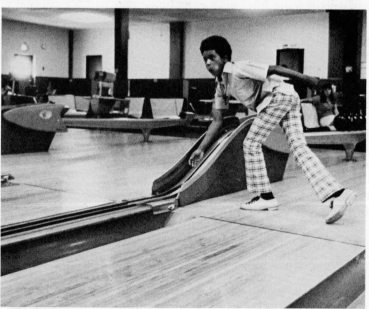

Sylvia Johnson/Woodfin Camp

your respiration will exceed 20 per minute, and your pulse rate will exceed 130 beats per minute.

Responses to static exercise. Weight lifting and other strenuous activities, including holding nonmoving endurance positions (that is, isometrics), involve fatigue of the localized musculature. The chemical processes and the heart and lungs are placed under severe stress if these activities are continued beyond 1 minute.

The following table (Morehouse and Gross, 1975) shows the approximate pulse rates as a result of continuous exercise at varying intensities.

Scale of Perceived Exertion	Pulse Rate (beats/minute)
Very, very light	Under 90
Very light	90
Light	100
Fairly light	110
Neither light nor heavy (moderate)	120
Somewhat heavy	130
Heavy	140
Very heavy	150
Very, very heavy	160

Exercise and a Lower Heart Rate   Surprisingly enough, the best way to lower your resting heart rate is to make it beat faster during short periods of exercise. This effort will make your heart stronger by enabling it to perform more efficiently at a lower rate. This lowered heart rate is a characteristic of many endurance athletes and is termed the *bradycardia* of training (as opposed to tachycardia).

When you exercise, you will be strengthening your heart in two ways: first, by changing and improving the quality of the myocardium (the heart muscle), and second, by improving the heart's coordination of beating. Through training, the fibers are able to contract more simultaneously and with better coordination. Without training and with lack of sufficient use, myocardial fibers will become uncoordinated and, like people themselves, lazy. This will require some of the fibers to work harder and more frequently to compensate for the "lazy" fibers in order to circulate the blood in the required amounts.

When you exercise or put some strain on your heart, you will be increasing the quantity of blood return from the veins. This return gives your heart the resistance to beat against. The resistance, sometimes called *loading,* is what causes your heart to develop. The formula is simple:

↑exercise→ ↑resistance (loading)→ ↑myocardial development

87

Just as the skeletal muscles need overload to become conditioned, the heart also requires overload. To achieve overload on your heart is simply a matter of engaging in some form of activity that pushes your heart rate to a higher level than you are accustomed to from your ordinary routine daily activities. Your goal eventually should be to raise your pulse to 120 beats per minute and sustain it at that level for a few minutes every day. A less strenuous activity that does not result in a 120-beat-per-minute heart rate is better than nothing, but it is not enough to improve your heart to the degree you would desire.

Your Pulse Test

Before you attempt anything, a fitness program or the pulse test, it's best to make sure that your present fitness condition is sufficient that you can undertake these activities without endangering your health. Your best assurance is from your physician. If it's been quite some time (over a year) since you've had a thorough medical checkup, it would be wise to schedule one now. If you've seen your doctor within the past 12 months, you should be able to start your program. If your doctor had found something wrong with you, some reason why it would be harmful to engage in moderate exercise, he most likely would have told you at that time. Just for safety's sake, however, it would be sensible to call your doctor now and tell him what you have in mind for your fitness program.

If in your recent past you've noticed any of the following symptoms after mild exertion (for example, running up a flight of stairs), you definitely should see your doctor as soon as possible and refrain from beginning your fitness program until you receive medical clearance.

Respiratory problems: difficulty in breathing
Gastrointestinal upsets: stomach aches or cramps
Dizziness or faintness
Chest pains
Flulike symptoms: nausea, vomiting, headaches, fevers, and so on

You should also obtain your physician's go-ahead before starting your fitness program if any of the following conditions apply to you.

History of heart disease in your immediate family
High blood pressure
Extreme tension or stress
Total lack of exercise
Heavy smoking habits
High cholesterol levels

One method of determining whether you are fit enough to engage in moderate exercise is your ability to walk 2 miles. If you are unable to do that, it's a clear warning, and your doctor should be informed.

One important further restriction against starting an exercise program is obesity. The medical definition of obesity is when the body is composed of 30 percent or more fat. You can easily tell if you're obese—you can see the fat hanging from your body in suspended folds. If that description fits you, then it is strongly suggested that you lose some weight before you begin any intensive activities program. What you can do if you are anxious to get started is to begin an easy walking program as the groundwork to the fitness program you'll be starting as soon as you've lost some weight.

Even if you've seen your doctor fairly recently and you've been cleared for your exercise program, there's one additional test you can take yourself before you begin your program. Because most physical examinations don't include the important exercise electrocardiogram on a bicycle ergometer, treadmill, or stepping bench, your physician almost always sees you in the resting state. Therefore when you first begin your program you will need to be on the lookout for any signs or symptoms of poor tolerance that would only show up when you exercise.

You will administer and evaluate this test yourself by counting your pulse rate in various conditions of rest, mild exercise, and recovery. Physical exercise should be fun and leave you with a good feeling; you should feel absolutely no discomfort or pain. This test will ensure that there won't be. The test will be as simple as climbing a few stairs. It involves taking your pulse as you sit, then stand, and ultimately step up and down for three 1-minute periods. And the results of these tests will give you an added reassurance that it is indeed safe for you to begin increasing your physical capacity. For your pulse test you will need a ruler to measure the exact height of the step you'll be using and a wristwatch or a clock with a sweep-second hand to count your pulse beats.

Counting Your Pulse Beats   First you should determine the best place to feel your pulse. Check back on the diagram of the pressure points. In order to amplify your pulse, be active in any manner you wish for a couple of minutes. Then explore the following places:

The radial artery in your wrist, which is located at the base of your thumb joint just inside your wrist bone

One of your carotid arteries on either side of your throat, located at the side of your jaw and directly above your collarbone

One of your temperal arteries, located at the side of your forehead just in front of your ear (the temple)

Most of you will prefer to take your pulse from the radial artery in your wrist. If that's the method you choose, then follow this simple procedure (Morehouse and Gross, 1975):

Place your wristwatch on your wrist so that you can see its face when the palm of your hand is up. Next, place the wrist on your other hand, so that the watch falls into the crotch between the thumb and forefinger. Let the tips of your fingers curl toward your thumb. Now your third and fourth fingers will rest over your pulse. The little pads at the ends of those fingers will fit right into the groove of the wrist. The pad on your middle fingers is the pulse "feeler." If you press slightly against the wrist with your fingertips feeler, you should be able to find your pulse. Don't panic if you can't find the pulse at first; it takes a few minutes of practice.

Remember that what you are feeling at each beat is not the blood flow, but the pulse wave that is moving along your arteries at a rate of about 12 to 18 feet per second.

There are several ways of calculating your pulse. Doctors and nurses may use any one of the many methods: counting pulse beats for 1 minute, counting pulse beats for 30 seconds, then multiplying by two, or counting pulse beats for 15 seconds, then multiplying by four. For our purposes, we will use still another method: counting pulse beats for 6 seconds and adding a zero. This is done for a specific reason. For a person at rest the longer count is ideal and is more accurate in general terms. But since we will be engaging in activity, a long count would not tell you about your exercise response as precisely as would a 6-second count taken instantly after the exercise. At that count the pulse (and the heart) will be beating at a rate that most accurately reflects the exertion you achieved during your exercise. Your pulse rate will diminish from its peak within 15 seconds, more within 30 seconds, and within 1 minute still more. The variation can be as great as 30 beats between your pulse rate immediately after exercise and the rate 1 minute later, depending upon your recovery.

So you will now determine your most accurate rate by counting the number of pulses in 6 seconds and adding a zero to obtain the per-minute rate. Before actually beginning the count, take a few seconds to catch the rhythm of the pulsations. Then when your pulse coincides with an easy time interval (a five-second mark), start counting. To avoid miscalculation it is important to begin counting with "zero" as the second hand crosses over the 5-second mark. Then, simply count the number of beats in 6 seconds. Practice and retest a few times to be sure you are getting consistent readings.

Your pulse test has six parts. Part 1 is to take, record, and interpret your pulse rate at rest. Part 2 involves the same procedure as Part 1, except it is performed while standing. Parts 3, 4, and 5 will depict your reaction under conditions of mild exertion. And finally, your rate of recovery will be tested in Part 6.

Your pulse test should be taken a couple of hours after any smoking, eating, or drinking, because all three will cause an increase in your pulse rate. Coffee, with its high caffeine content, should be especially avoided. It is important to avoid talking to anyone during your test since any conversation has the tendency to raise your pulse rate. If you have been physically active just prior to your test, you should rest for a few minutes to let your pulse return to a low level and become steady. If your body temperature is higher or lower than normal as a result of overheating or chilling, you will get a false reading because both conditions will accelerate your pulse rate.

Once you have sat down and calmed yourself, repeated counts of pulse rates should give you nearly the same scores. This score actually represents your average resting pulse rate during the day, which is different from your basal pulse rate. The only time you would be able to obtain a basal reading accurately would be upon awakening in the morning and before leaving your bed. Your resting pulse rate while seated comes closest to equaling your normal condition of wakefulness.

If you cough, yawn, sneeze, or even clear your throat during the test, stop and rest a few minutes until you're perfectly calm again and then start over. Keep in mind that you can raise and lower your pulse with deep and forceful breathing. Your pulse will follow the rhythm of your respiration. Therefore try to keep your breathing pattern calm, steady, and relaxed during your test. Your pulse will have a regular rhythm if you're quiet and breathing softly. (If you should notice any irregularity in the rhythm of your pulse—a missed beat or an extra out-of-rhythm beat—tell your doctor before you increase your physical activity.)

A method for deliberately slowing your pulse rate is through "biofeedback exercises." This technique can be very relaxing and a good way of getting rid of the excess tension in your body. After you have achieved a steady resting pulse rate, try some of these simple suggestions to put your mind in control of your body (Morehouse and Gross, 1975):

Instead of sitting on a chair, let yourself sit into the chair. Let all your weight go into the chair. Instead of holding your legs up off the floor, let the weight of your legs move into your feet so that your feet feel heavy on the floor. Now let your shoulders drop comfortably outward instead of holding them up. Let your face relax; feel that you are no longer furrowing your forehead, squinting your eyes, or clenching your teeth. Finally, let your belly relax. Put your hands on your belly. Do they rise or fall as you take a breath? In two out of every five cases I have examined, the belly is drawn in as a breath is drawn in. You're creating excess tension. Try to reverse the pattern. As you take in a breath, let your hands move outward.

After you have finished the biofeedback techniques, take your pulse once more. If you've really concentrated and done all of the above correctly, your pulse should be appreciably lower.

You should obtain your lowest seated pulse rate in this quiet, calm state. Your pulse rate should register less than 100 beats per minute. If you find your seated pulse rate near 10 counts in 6 seconds (100), you should remain seated and try a full 1-minute-count pulse rate. If, after the 1-minute count, your pulse is still higher than 100 beats a minute, try some more biofeedback exercises. Then if your pulse remains at 100 beats a minute or higher, you may have an infection or a fever. If this is true, you should definitely stop the pulse fitness test until your illness or infection has subsided.

If you discover that you don't have a fever and you have no explanation as to why your pulse is higher than 100 beats a minute, then it would be prudent to check with your physician to be sure that the rapid pulse is a normal condition for you and that there is no reason why you shouldn't have the green light for activity.

If your pulse rate is less than 10 beats in 6 seconds (100 beats/ minute), you may go on to Part 2.

Part 2 deals with *orthostatic tolerance,* which is another aspect of your response to exercise. Orthostatic tolerance tests your circulatory ability to adjust to the vertical position after having been seated for a while.

Stand quietly in an easy resting position for about 1 minute. You may wiggle your toes or shift your weight, but avoid moving around or standing rigidly at attention. Take your pulse at the end of 1 minute. The difference between your standing pulse rate and your sitting pulse rate is another good indication of your present fitness level. If your standing pulse rate is more than 20 beats higher than your seated pulse rate, you probably should again check with your doctor to be sure increased physical activity is not taboo. A pulse rate at that level is more than likely higher than it should be. If your pulse rate is near 110 beats per minute (11 or more beats in 6 seconds), or if you feel dizzy or faint, there may be a reason for this poor showing of orthostatic tolerance, and your doctor should know about it. Remember that neither athletic ability nor an exercise program will increase your ability or tolerance to quiet standing.

Your pulse rate should increase upon standing; up to 10 beats a minute is well within the range of safety. For our method of calcula- tion, if your sitting rate was eight beats in 6 seconds and your standing rate was nine beats in 6 seconds, then you're ready to advance to Part 3. Any change of one count in 6 seconds is fine, as long as you don't reach 11 counts in 6 seconds.

Part 3 is the first of three 1-minute tests on a step. First measure the height of your step. Now compare it with your body weight in Table 3-1 to determine your stepping rate (steps per minute). Locate your body weight, then move horizontally across the table until you intersect with the height step in the vertical column. For example, a man using a 9-inch step and weighing 200 pounds will step at a rate of 20 lifts or step-ups per minute.

The test itself is easy. Step up with your left foot, then your right foot. Step down with your left foot, and follow with your right foot. Repeat the lifts as many times as indicated on the table. Try to finish in exactly 1 minute—no more or less. You will be able to tell after about 15 seconds whether or not your rhythm is enough to achieve the required number of steps. Adjust accordingly if you're going too slowly or too fast.

Table 3-1

STEPPING RATE IN STEPS PER MINUTE

Body Weight (in pounds)	Height of the Step (in inches)					
	7	8	9	10	11	12
100	30	30	30	30	30	30
120	30	30	30	30	30	30
140	30	30	30	30	20	20
160	30	30	30	20	20	20
180	30	30	20	20	20	20
200	30	20	20	20	20	20
220	20	20	20	20	20	20

Source: Morehouse and Gross (1975).

Be sure to stop your test at the first symptom of poor tolerance. The signs of poor tolerance are many. Some physical symptoms would be a pounding heart that hurts, difficulty in breathing or shortness of breath, a tremor or twitching in the legs, aching legs, cramps, or profuse sweating. Another indication of poor tolerance is attitude: you ran out of gas, you wanted to slow down, you felt like quitting. Any of these symptoms, either physical or mental, in 1 minute of mild exercise is a warning to stop your test and seek medical advice. Remember to sit down when you stop. Never stand quietly after exercise.

Immediately upon finishing your test for Part 3, sit down and count your pulse. If your count is 12 or more in 6 seconds or if you feel strained, your test is over. You will have determined that you have a low tolerance to exercise. If such is the case, you are in a deconditioned state, and you are in need of a special exercise program. Talk it over with your doctor.

If you show none of the symptoms of poor tolerance and your pulse count is less than 12 in 6 seconds, you may go on to Part 4. Immediately repeat the 1-minute test exercise. Then sit down and count your pulse. Again, you must stop if it exceeds 12 counts in 6 seconds. If it's below 12, proceed to Part 5. Once more repeat the exercise test and take your pulse. The standards and the admonitions for Part 5 are the same as for Parts 3 and 4.

Part 6 is a test of your recovery. After taking your final pulse rate following exercise in Part 5, sit down and rest for 1 minute. Then take your pulse one more time. The difference between your pulse rate following exercise and your pulse rate 1 minute later should be no less than 10 beats, and your final pulse rate should be no more than 110 beats per minute.

You're in poor shape if it took only a small amount of activity to raise your pulse to 120 beats per minute. But if after taking the three stepping-exercise tests your heart rate remains under 120 and you were fairly comfortable during the whole series, you're in pretty good condition.

You must understand that this pulse test is not a diagnostic or medical test. But it has a purpose for us. What it does is reveal any signs or symptoms of poor tolerance that may have been hidden before. Also it designates your present level of fitness for exercise. It gives you an accurate guide as to where you should begin your program.

If your heart rate has not passed 120 after having gone through all six parts of the test and you recovered quickly at the end of your test, you've shown a sufficient degree of fitness, and you have two choices: you can either begin a maintenance program or a conditioning program to raise yourself to an even higher level of fitness.

If you've had to stop at any time before the end of the test, you haven't failed the test. You have simply established your present exercise tolerance level. From discovering this vital data point, you need a developmental program before you try a maintenance program. No matter what your level is, you will need a program geared to your own specific needs.

Exercise Prescription

From this point you will have decided the kind of fitness program you think would best fit into your desired lifestyle. You will have determined which of the components of fitness you would like to improve. You have learned the importance of frequency, adherence, and persistence in any self-improvement program. You are ready to apply the principle of positive reinforcement to your efforts. You have obtained a medical clearance, and you know at what level of physical fitness you stand. And, finally, you have gained the knowledge of carrying out your program in the safest, most effective way—pulse-rate monitoring.

A sample 1-week exercise program that can serve as a model for fitness maintenance and/or building is given on page 95. This is a brief program (Morehouse and Gross, 1975) that is easily accomplished and fits into anyone's schedule. *Every other day* (three times a week) you may choose any one of the three workouts depending upon what particular area you need to improve, such as strength or endurance.

To briefly explain the exercises in this program, let's start with the limbering warm-up. This is simply a stretching warm-up to improve flexibility. You twist, turn, reach, and stretch in a slow, easy manner. There should be no strain.

Push-aways are exercises that can be modified to help improve either strength or endurance of the arm-shoulder-chest region. The basic push-away is done in this manner: start by standing a little past arm's reach from a wall. Place your hands on the wall about shoulder height. Lean forward until your chest comes near the wall, then push away until you're back in your beginning position. You can adjust the difficulty of this exercise by placing your hands in a lower position on the wall or standing farther back. When this becomes too easy, move to an even lower level such as a chair or table until you eventually end up

Minutes	Exercise
	Workout A (for muscular strength and cardio-vascular conditioning)
0–1	Limbering warm-up
1–1½	5 strength push-aways
1½–2	Strength sit-back, held 5 seconds
2–10	Endurance lope
	Workout B (for muscular strength and endurance and cardiovascular conditioning)
0–1	Limbering warm-up
1–2	20 expansion push-aways
2–3	Expansion sit-backs, held 20 seconds each
3–10	Endurance intervals (30 seconds of rapid circulorespiratory exercise, alternated with 30 seconds of "active rest," such as walking or slow pedaling, for 7 minutes)
	Workout C (for muscular endurance and cardio-vascular conditioning)
0–1	Limbering warm-up
1–3	50 endurance push-aways
3–5	Endurance sit-backs held 50 seconds each
5–10	Sprint intervals (15 seconds of rapid circulo-respiratory exercise, alternated with 15 seconds of "active rest," for 5 minutes)

doing regular pushups on the floor. When these become too easy, you begin to reverse the process by raising the legs until you reach the level of handstand pushups. Now to apply this to the workouts, let's use workout A, for example. For the five strength push-aways, you find the level of difficulty at which you can do only five push-aways. This will be different for each person. The same principle applies to workouts B and C.

Sit-backs are also exercises that can be modified for strength or endurance improvement of the abdominal region. The basic sit-back exercise is as follows: sit on the floor with your knees fully bent, and hook your feet under a piece of furniture. To begin with, work your chest as close to your knees as possible. This is your starting position. Now lean back away from your knees until you feel your abdominal musculature coming into play. As with the push-aways, you will hold the sit-back for the required amount of time as stated in each workout. The sit-back can be adjusted for increased difficulty by leaning back farther and farther until your shoulder blades are almost touching the floor. Then you can increase difficulty even more by placing your hands across your chest or above your head or even adding weights.

The fourth part of each workout is the cardiovascular lope or conditioning exercise. These are activities that generally involve total body movement and are used for conditioning the heart. Good examples are brisk walking, running, swimming, bicycling, rowing, rope skipping, and dancing. The important thing for this part of your workout is to select an activity that you will enjoy doing.

The Importance of Internal Effects

Most physical fitness or exercise programs rely on performance. It is the external effects of these programs that are important. *How far* you can run, *how much* weight you can lift, *how many* sit-ups you can do, and *how long* you can continue at an activity are the measures of success. But the problem with these measures is that they actually tell you nothing about your body's response to the exercises. They can't tell you if you're working hard enough or not. They are only based on your perception of exertion, which could be totally inaccurate for any number of reasons. There is only one way of determining whether you're working at the right intensity, and that is by directly measuring the amount of effort.

In the laboratory this measuring can be accomplished in several ways. We can measure oxygen consumption, air ventilation, rising blood pressure, or increasing pulse rate. Of these, the pulse rate is the easiest to measure. And it has the added advantage of computing the relative effort expended by all the various body systems and coming up with a final score that is a reliable indication of the intensity of physiological effort.

Now, for the first time, we can separate physical activity as a sporting event and physical activity as a fitness event. This is important to your program to decide what you will be using your physical activity for.

TAKING ACTION

1. *In a group discuss the differences in the perception of exertion of activities of varying intensities.*
2. *Do research on some of the popular fitness programs that have been developed, such as the work of Dr. Dudley Sargent of Harvard, Walter Camp's Daily Dozen, Charles Atlas' dynamic tension method, the Royal Canadian Air Force Exercises, and Cooper's Aerobics.*

Discussion

You have learned how much more important it is to keep track of the internal measures of exercise and exertion rather than the secondary external measures, which are likely to be false measures due to the differences in perception of exertion. There are many ways of measuring internal exertion, and you have seen that the easiest way by far is by counting your pulse beats. In nonemotional states it is impossible to go wrong, and your pulse rate is a truly accurate measure of exertion. What's more, now that you know the value of this simple measure, you can easily get into the habit of checking your pulse regularly while participating in different activities of varying intensities.

Now that you are informed, it is important for you to pass the word along. It might be fun to administer the pulse test to your family or a group of friends. You might precede the tests with a good explanation of what you are doing and why. After giving the tests be sure to evaluate and explain the results to your subjects. Your final job would be to prescribe a fitness program geared specifically to each of your subjects.

GENERAL FITNESS FACTS AND FICTION

Most people have only a vague idea of what comprises fitness. We blindly accept "rules or principles" of fitness that are actually old wives' tales not based on scientific facts. Here are some of the commonly and erroneously accepted myths of physical fitness (Morehouse and Gross, 1975).

Myth: Never drink while exercising. This is absolutely false. If you know you are losing water, you should replace it immediately even if you are not thirsty. It is even a good idea to drink an extra glass of water before exercising the first thing in the morning.

The cells of your body are unable to function adequately if they lack fluid. They depend on the circulation in order to obtain their required energy and to dispose of their waste products. If you become dehydrated, the fluids bathing your cells diminish. When that happens, the strain on your heart increases, and your muscles are unable to keep up the work you are doing. The strain on your heart comes from the fact that some of the fluid you lost is blood fluid, and this means that the heart must pump more times to recirculate your decreased blood supply.

Myth: Avoid certain foods before activity. Extensive tests and research done at the Human Performance Laboratory at UCLA have not yet proved that the kind of food (not the amount) you eat makes any difference in your final performance or well-being. All the so-called forbidden foods (heavy foods, gas-producing foods, spicy foods, and so on) were given to athletes on campus. Neither in the laboratory nor on any playing field could any difference be determined in performance. Moreover, none of the athletes became ill from eating the forbidden foods.

Myth: Sugar taken before exercise raises the energy level. Extra sugar does not give extra energy. The only time you need to eat sugar to replace that which may have been depleted is after at least an hour and a half of steady, continuous exercise such as long-distance swimming.

Myth: Do not eat before swimming. There seems to be no history or science to support how this tale got started. The supposed "theory" behind this myth is that blood is drawn into the intestine for digestion; when you start exercising, the heart is placed under great strain because the muscles also need blood. What actually happens is that once you start exercising, the circulation to the intestine cuts off, and the blood is diverted to the working muscles, which have greater priority.

Cramps do not cause drowning. Heart attacks are typically the cause of supposed drowning from cramps. The most you may expect to get from exercising after eating is a stitch in the side. Cramps are not known to be related to food. This is not to suggest that a strenuous swim should follow a huge meal. Any vigorous activity following a meal will probably cause nausea. But certainly swimming leisurely around in a warm, heated pool won't hurt you.

Myth: Use salt tablets to prevent fatigue. It is a fact that you do lose salt when you sweat. So if strenuous exercise has caused you to sweat profusely, you will need to replace the salt to prevent muscle cramps. But salt should not be replaced by tablets. A salt tablet is a solid piece of brine, and brine resting on mucous membranes of the stomach can cause nausea and vomiting.

It is a good idea to add a little extra salt to your food before or after any activity if you know you are going to perspire heavily during your exercise bout. As always, avoid excess because your body cannot store salt as it can sugar. If you overdo salt intake by restoring more salt than you have lost by sweating, you could induce the muscle cramps and weakness you were hoping to avoid. In addition, body fluids from the cells will be drawn into the digestive tract and bloodstream to make excretion of the excess salt easier. So excess salt intake will dry out your body tissues.

Myth: Sleep extra hours before a contest or when you are very tired. Sleep cannot be stored. If you try to catch up on missed sleep by sleeping 12 hours, you will be worse off than if you got 8. Beyond 8 or 9 hours (individuals may vary greatly as to what they "need") bed rest will not give you extra energy. Based on the principle of adaptation-deadaptation, bed rest has a severe deconditioning effect. All body processes slow down with sleep. Your metabolism lowers, and after 6 hours your heartbeat will get down to its basal rate. The whole body begins to lose tone, circulation becomes sluggish, and muscles become lax and flaccid. For every 3 days you spend in bed, you lose about 5 percent of your strength. Therefore the longer you stay in bed beyond a 9-hour maximum the weaker you will become.

If you have trouble falling asleep, don't worry. Lying in bed in a relaxed condition is almost as restful as sleeping. So rather than lying in bed beyond 8 hours because you haven't been able to sleep all that time, go ahead and get up. But promise yourself to relax the next time you have trouble falling asleep.

Myth: Work up a sweat before a contest. Wrong, wrong, wrong! Going from absolute rest to all-out exercise activity may be dangerous for a weak or unconditioned heart by causing a failure in circulation. But if you are simply going to gradually increase your activity to play a nonstrenuous game, then it is actually useless to work up a sweat, especially if your event calls for endurance.

Extended warm-ups that cause you to work up a sweat are contraindicated for two reasons: first, they use up your nutritional stores, and, second, they create unnecessary body heat, which saps energy that you could use for your activity.

Myth: Sweating gets you in shape. Many people have the mistaken idea that working out in a rubber sweat suit is a good method of conditioning because it induces sweating. In truth what you are actually doing is conditioning yourself for acclimatization to heat, which is fine if you are going to be working out or playing at the equator. But in a more moderate climate when your body works up to such a heated state, you are not likely to work hard enough to get into good condition.

The best rule to follow about working out is to avoid dripping sweat whenever possible, because it takes metabolic energy to lose heat. The activity of your sweat glands provides this energy; millions of them are located just under your skin. This energy (to secrete sweat) is taken from the total amount of energy available to the body to keep it functioning.

Your muscles also require a part of this energy in order to produce movement. If too great a share of the energy is used to secrete sweat, there won't be enough left for muscle work and other bodily functions. When your sweat glands use energy, the amount of work you are able to do lessens. When your sweat glands are exhausted and stop secreting, you are in danger of suffering a heat stroke.

There is another means of losing energy in addition to sweat secretion when you overheat—through your cardiovascular system. When you become warm and your skin gets hot, the peripheral vessels leading to the skin open. Then a large part of your blood supply is diverted to the surface of your body in an attempt to cool it down. This takes away blood needed by the muscles. In turn the heart tries to make up for the loss by pumping harder. If the load becomes too great and if it is maintained too long, you could collapse. By this point it should be clear that inducing sweat is hazardous—and does not contribute to fitness. Remember, there is no danger in being comfortably cool while you are playing or working hard. But there is danger in being uncomfortably warm. Just keep in mind that you only have a limited amount of energy available, and if you use it to dispel body heat, you won't have enough energy left to accomplish what you really want to do.

Myth: Put on a sweater after exercise. How many times have you heard this one? It is ridiculous because there is no point in prolonging heat by encasing it in unnecessary clothing. As for the belief that you may catch cold, it is possible that some parts of your body might get stiff, but you do not catch a cold by changing temperature.

After exercise that has caused you to sweat a little, you will be helping your body to recover faster if you do not put on that coat or

The "masculine" image
of female athletes is
changing today.

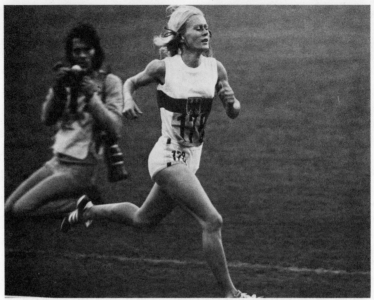

Thomas Hopker/Woodfin Camp

sweater too soon. When you have cooled down some to a more comfortable temperature and have stopped sweating, then you can put on your sweater to avoid getting chilled. You will find that if you don't stay overheated longer than necessary, you will be much more comfortable.

Myth: Women who train lose femininity. The truth is the opposite: women become more feminine. Their bodies become more *lithe* and much stronger. They develop an athlete's sense of relaxation; over a supply of power waiting to be put into action is a calm air of *languor.* If women are unfeminine after training, perhaps it is because they were unfeminine to begin with.

Women athletes who exercise a great deal will develop firm muscles, but because they have a thicker layer of subcutaneous (just below the surface) fat, they will not form bulges the way men do. Their bodies will retain their feminine contours. In addition, muscular development of the chest area will enhance the breast line, and women's main trouble spots, the hips and thighs, are slimmed and trimmed by exercise.

Myth: Big muscles make you stronger. Years ago everyone believed that, but today we know that you can increase your strength without increasing muscle bulk, and you can increase muscle size without increasing muscle strength.

Most athletes who do not need massive bodies to put against heavy loads realize and accept the fact that they should keep their muscles small. Unfortunately, this information has not reached the general public. Many still believe in the body-beautiful image that the fitness "palaces" keep promoting.

1. *How many of the myths of fitness do you still believe in? Discuss what things you do in following these beliefs.*
2. *Get together with some friends and discuss these fitness myths. Do many of your friends believe in them? Can you set them straight?*
3. *Do further research and see if you can't expose some of your own fitness myths.*

Discussion

One of the most important things intelligent men and women are always seeking is truth. This section is certainly an eye-opener. How many of the fitness myths were you guilty of following? And how many times have you heard someone repeat one of those clichés?

Throughout this chapter we've been asking you to spread the knowledge you have just acquired. How should you go about this? The most practical way is to state the facts and sources when someone makes an erroneous comment or asks a question. People will be interested in listening to someone who knows what he is talking about. So never let an opportunity go by to ask some leading questions and provide some meaningful answers.

**CONTRAINDICA-
TIONS OF
EXERCISE**

Exercise is not a panacea or magical remedy for all people. Likewise, physical fitness is not meant to be the answer to all your problems. Exercise cannot guarantee you long life nor can it promise you immunity to all diseases. In fact there are some conditions where exercise can actually be harmful to you.

**Warning Signals
and Medical
Review**

Throughout this chapter there have been several allusions to obtaining your physician's go-ahead before embarking on something new. The importance of your doctor's guardianship of your medical well-being cannot be overstressed. Therefore your doctor must be kept informed of any radical changes in your life. In addition, your physician should be informed immediately if you experience any of the following symptoms or conditions: sustained headaches, pains in the chest, blurred vision, dizziness, fainting spells, difficulties in breathing, gastrointestinal upsets, or flulike symptoms. All of these signs are warning signals that could precede dangerous situations if not treated promptly. The above conditions are usually acute ones. You will also want to see your doctor and follow his advice *to the letter* if any of these conditions apply to you: family history of heart disease, high blood pressure, extreme and constant stress or tension in daily life, heavy smoking, high cholesterol, obesity, and total lack of exercise.

Your physician deals with these problems on a daily basis and should be up to date on the latest research in these areas. It is only common sense to get an expert's advice on something as important as your health rather than accept the words of friends or relatives.

To ensure that your fitness program runs smoothly for you, there are a few precautions that you should be aware of.

Never hold your breath and strain. The glottis is a valve in your throat that must always remain open during exercise. It can be closed voluntarily, shutting off the exhalation process. When you close your glottis and then continue trying to exhale, your rib cage and diaphragm contract, causing the pressure to increase inside the chest cavity. As the pressure within the chest increases, it eventually surpasses the pressure in the veins returning blood to the heart. When that happens, the blood flow to the heart is clamped off. Shortly thereafter the heart pumps itself empty, resulting in a drop in pressure. The first organ to sense this pressure drop is the brain. The result is fainting or blackout.

Keep your water level high. We discussed this precaution when examining the myth of never drinking while exercising. Just a reminder: liquid is essential to keep the body functioning properly, and it is never needed more than when exercising.

Take a sufficient warm-up. If you start from a resting condition and suddenly switch to all-out exertion, your heart will be forced to work too hard before your coronary circulation system has a chance to adjust and respond with a sufficient blood supply. This condition, called *myocardial ischemia,* is simply an insufficient oxygen supply to the heart. Myocardial ischemia may not be hazardous to a healthy person but may cause an infarction (heart attack) for someone who isn't fit.

A warm-up should be a gradual increase of activity from a light pulse rate of 100 to a moderate one of about 120. About a minute of good warm-up is just about as beneficial as taking 6 to 12 minutes. Don't rush into your exercise following your warm-up. There is no hurry, so go at your own speed.

For sports and games the best form of warm-up is to practice slowly what you are going to do more actively later on. Once more, moderation is the key, so don't overdo it.

Is it better to walk around or sit down after exercising? Your body is restless and needs to move after exercising. The force of gravity is constantly pushing the body fluids into your lower extremities. When that happens in a quiet state after vigorous exercising, the blood drains from the brain, possibly even causing people to faint. During exercise the vessels dilate to increase circulation to working muscles. As long as you are moving, blood is kept flowing back to the heart by the pumping action of the skeletal muscles. Stopping suddenly and standing still requires the blood to be pumped by the heart muscle alone. It's a good idea to continue moving, but moderately after exercising.

Easy does it. This is perhaps the most important precaution of them all. It is not necessary to overdo. If you become stiff the following day after too hard a workout the previous day, you won't be helping yourself a bit. Getting stiff is only a sign of the working tissues accumulating lactic acid or other metabolites. It is certainly not an indication that you are getting strong. There's no need to become stiff from exercising. In fact you will be far better off if you ease into increased activity.

TAKING ACTION

1. *Make an appointment to see your doctor if you have any of the symptoms that would contraindicate exercise.*
2. *Discuss the possible benefits of warming up.*
3. *Ask several people you know who exercise regularly if they do any warm-up exercises. If so, what do they do?*

Discussion

If you are going to prescribe exercises for yourself or suggest them to anyone else, you have to know which ones are beneficial and which ones are contraindicated. In addition, you should know the warning signals to look for before, during, and after exercising. The symptoms we discussed in this section probably do not apply to you at your young, active age. But it is important to realize and think about when these conditions *might* apply to you.

Throughout this section and the chapter we have stressed the importance of constantly checking with your doctor if you plan on making any major activity changes in your life. Do you really take these suggestions seriously and are you serious when you suggest them to someone else? These suggestions, like the warning symptoms mentioned previously, may be something you assume apply only to older folks and not to you because you're young. Don't fall into the trap of false security. Just because you're young does not necessarily mean that your good health and fitness is a lasting, unalterable state. Don't gamble with something as precious as your health. Don't take chances, and don't let those around you take them either.

SPECIFIC TRAINING FOR SPECIFIC EVENTS

When you train for a specific sport event, you are following a complete fitness program in itself. Sport training goes beyond the programs to achieve minimum maintenance levels or reserves of fitness. It requires a thorough analysis of the activity. If excellence is your objective, then it's a year-round program.

If you have already decided which sport is your favorite, fine, then you can get started. But if you really want a sport you can enjoy and train for, how do you go about choosing a sport? Childhood experiences of play, sports, and games in school provided the basics of sport skills, and a small minority of you identified your serious sport opportunities from them. The majority of you only decided what you didn't want to do. Once you are out of school, decisions of participation in sports are based on the following factors: skill potential, physical dangers, individuality, and sociability.

To determine your skill potential you must realistically appraise your present sport and physical skills and then compare them with the level at which you ultimately intend to compete. If the participation opportunities available to you are suited to your ability or potential, then advancement in your sport is assured.

In checking out the physical dangers of your sport, you will have to depend on personal judgment, physical capacity, and possibly certain types of supportive or protective equipment. Some people desire to face dangerous situations as a means of balancing out their lives and giving added value to a "now" philosophy of life. If you are one who seeks a more exciting life, sports can provide that excitement to the fullest.

Sports can also be used as an expression of individuality. Many people use sports as an escape from everyday reality; others participate as a means of getting recognition. Sports offer almost endless opportunities to express yourself. Because you can be judged purely on your performance at a given time, your past experience or level of performance is forgotten as a new level of achievement is immediately recognized for its own value.

People usually need the recognition of their peers to perform at their best. This recognition makes the activity that much more meaningful. Nearly all sports involve two or more people, which makes sports an immediate social situation.

Mountain climbing—a
different view of the
world.

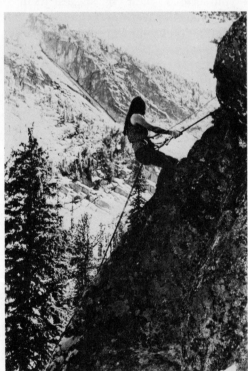

Wide World Photos

The best single way to train for your sport is to practice the sport itself. But even if you practice your sport twice a day, you won't reach anywhere near your peak level of capacity. To reach your peak you must train for each aspect of your sport. And in order to do that you must define the dimensions of your sport. The dimensions of any sport are time, distance, force, posture, skill, and concentration. From this definition will come the structure of your training program.

Time. You must establish the duration and frequency of your event. How long will it last? How often will you play in a day or in a week? Is your event continuous, or are there bursts of starts and stops? Play can vary between very active, moderately active, and slightly active even in the same sport, depending upon how you play.

Distance. Once again, your workout should resemble your event itself in order to train for your maximum. If your event takes place on a court or field, then practice should occur within these boundaries.

Force. Does your event require a great deal of force? If so, will you need total body strength to produce it or strength of some localized musculature?

Skill. In order to follow this one, break the movements of your activity down into their smallest components. Practice them separately, but remember to keep the tempo of practice as close to the actual game speed as possible. As soon as you can, put the pieces back together.

Posture. Training exercises should all be performed in the same postures that are used during the event. If this is not done, the muscle and skill development for the specific movements used during your game will not be as great as it could be.

Concentration. This important consideration involves both attitude and motivation. The essential point is to become thoroughly aware of your total environment. This includes the court, field, or room, your opponent(s), the referee, the crowd, and most of all yourself. This last one is the most important. Remember that remaining in control of your surroundings is the key to concentration.

Many of the principles of conditioning for maximum performance have already been discussed in this chapter—adaptation-deadaptation, overload, and specificity. One final guiding principle to training that should be mentioned is this: whatever your sport, to better your performance exercises should be executed in the same posture and with the same rhythm and intensity inherent in the event. You should determine all of the important phases of motion, the joint angles, and the ranges of their motion during the event.

Here are a few examples of some special conditioning exercises for many of our most popular sports:

Bowling. Arm swinging, using a bowling ball. One set of 20 to 60 executions. Forward lunging, simulating delivery. One set of 20 to 60.

Swimming. Ankle stretching. Sit on the ankles. Bend and rotate the trunk while sitting on the ankles. Four sets of 10 to 20. Lie, face up, then down, on a bench, with your arms and legs extended. Hold two cans of soup and do swimming motions with the arms and legs. Two sets of 20 to 60.

Tennis. Practice your strokes with your tennis racket. Reach for serves and smashes. Dart into position for difficult forehands and backhands. Punch out a few net shots. Keep this going at game speed for a couple of minutes. Squeeze two tennis balls, one in each hand, as hard as you can for a slow count of ten. Relax. Repeat three times.

Golf. Simulate the golf swing while holding a can of soup in your left hand. One set of 20 to 60. Put a club against your back, in a horizontal position. Hold it there with your arms, and twist your trunk. Two sets of 20 to 60.

Softball. Swing a bat. One set of 20 to 60. Circle your arm while holding a ball. One set of 20 to 60.

Skiing. Side-jump over a low barrier, with your feet together as though they were tied. One set of 20 to 60. Standing, put your back against a wall as if you were sitting in a chair. Hold the position for 30 seconds. Increase gradually to 60 seconds. Then try it on one leg.

As a final reminder, it is best to take *one* objective at a time. Work on it until you are in shape, then take on another one. You will be able to handle this easily. Take your time, take it easy, have fun, and your efforts will be successful.

TAKING ACTION

1. *Choose a sport you think you will enjoy and try it out for a period of about a month.*
2. *Develop additional conditioning exercises for your program to fit your particular sport.*
3. *Read and do some further research on your chosen sport.*

Discussion In this section we discussed training for specific sports events. Of course, we have only just scratched the surface. If you are really serious about this, you will want to do some further reading about your sport. Perhaps you are already on an organized team. Talk to your coach or other experts whose opinion about your sport you respect. Have discussions with your team players on ways to improve your training and performance. Learn as much as you can about every aspect of your sport, apply what you learn to your game, and enjoy the results!

CONCLUSION You, as a human being, move, think, and experience feelings. Exercise involves all these functions, and your conscious decision about sports participation and exercise must involve both accurate knowledge and your feelings and desires.

This chapter has given you only a small portion of what exercise and fitness are all about. It will be your responsibility to seek out new knowledge in this field as it is discovered. This is an ever-growing and ever-changing field, with new discoveries occurring constantly. How many times have you heard that old cliché that you must "keep up with the times"? That phrase is never so important as when it is being applied to your health and fitness.

As people get older, their lifestyles change, and fitness patterns and beliefs must be altered accordingly. Increasing automation and mechanization of our society, combined with increased leisure time, seem to be contributing to our lack of and need for regular exercise. But physical fitness is attainable without killing yourself in the process. Because physical fitness is such an individual matter, periodic self-evaluation of easily measured parameters (pulse-rated exercise, step tests, exercise EKGs, and so on) might help you think positively about the need to exercise.

Regular exercise can exert some positive influences on your general health and possibly increase your longevity. Older people who think of themselves as young and who also appear young in the eyes of others are often those who have remained active in their older years by choice.

Specific kinds of regular exercise can prepare you for your chosen kinds of physically demanding activities and also keep you ready for those unexpected emergencies.

FOR FURTHER READING

Johnson, Perry B., Updyke, Wynn R., Schaifer, Maryellen, and Stolber, Donald C., 1975. *Sport, Exercise and You.* New York: Holt, Rinehart and Winston.

A text exploring the reasons, motivations, and methods for developing and maintaining physical fitness.

Morehouse, Laurence E., 1971. *Physiology of Exercise.* St. Louis: C. V. Mosby.

A frequently revised text written for students of physical education.

———, 1974. Exercise and Physical Conditioning. *The Encyclopaedia Britannica.* Chicago: Encyclopaedia Britannica.

An authoritative work on considerations of physical fitness, conditioning, the modern need for exercise, and the physiological responses to exercise.

Morehouse, Laurence E., and Gross, Leonard, 1975. *Total Fitness in Thirty Minutes a Week.* New York: Simon and Schuster.

A book written especially for the general public, discussing several aspects of physical fitness and what it takes to achieve and maintain it.

Wessel, Janet, and MacIntyre, Christine, 1970. *Body Contouring and Conditioning through Movement.* Boston: Allyn and Bacon.

A self-instruction text for developing physical fitness.

part two

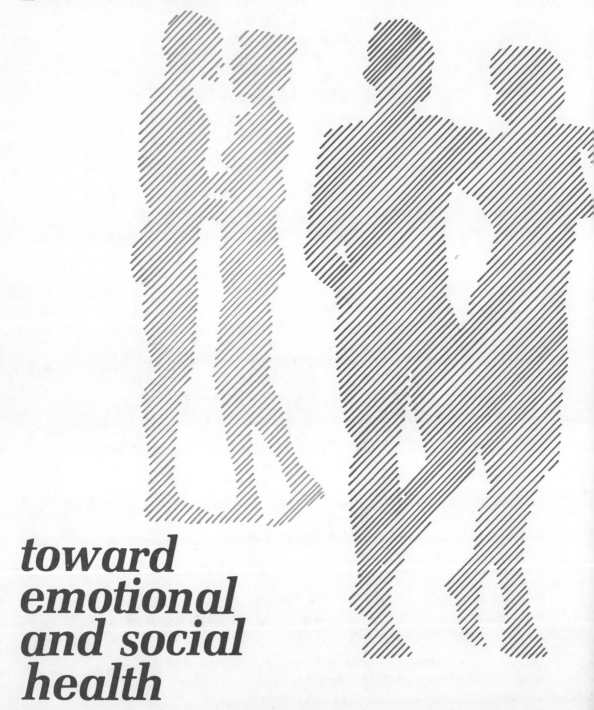

toward
emotional
and social
health

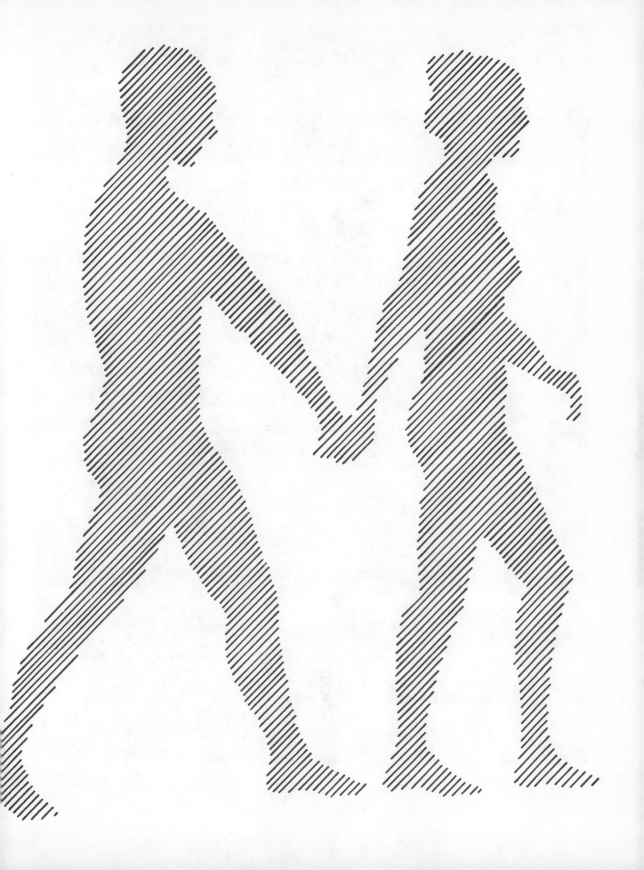

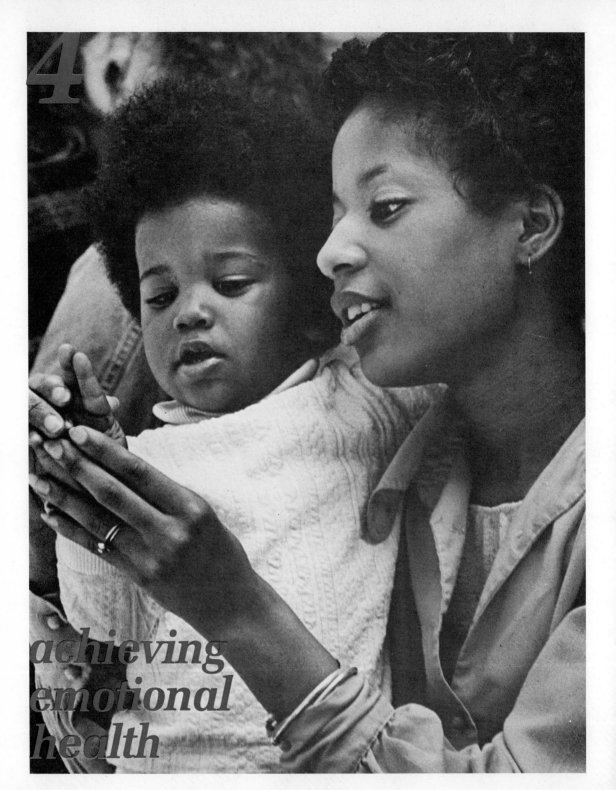

4

*achieving
emotional
health*

How can you achieve emotional health? In several important ways: first, by identifying your main goals and values in this area—for example, remaining alive and attaining a reasonable degree of happiness while living. Happy in what ways? Many, for example: just in getting along satisfactorily with and by yourself; adjusting adequately to many or most of the members of your social group; intimately relating to a few selected individuals whom you personally choose to like or love; preparing yourself for and actually working at some absorbing, enjoyable, productive career or profession; finding personally satisfying recreational pursuits; acting as a responsible citizen of your community; and acquiring a high frustration tolerance and self-discipline by stubbornly refusing to define a hassle as a horror.

We will almost inevitably associate at home, at work, and at play with a good number of moderately and seriously neurotic individuals. How can we help some of these people to overcome their emotional handicaps, understand and deal with them when they don't, and continue to remain intimate with them, if we choose to do so, even when they continue to behave in distinctly obnoxious ways? This chapter addresses itself to the important questions that follow and to the solutions of many of the problems involved. This material won't solve all your emotional problems, but if you read carefully, it well may help!

INQUIRY

1. How do we create our own emotional disturbances?
2. What kind of blocks do we consciously or unconsciously set up to interfere with our living our lives for maximum happiness and self-fulfillment?
3. What irrational ideas do we accept, create, or hold onto that tend to make ourselves—yes, *make ourselves*—needlessly disturbed?
4. In spite of our early environment and our contemporary social idiocies, can we really control and change our own emotional destiny?
5. Do we have to live with absolutistic, dogmatic *musts*?
6. How can we use high-powered cognitive, emotive, and behavioral methods of counterattacking and significantly changing our innate and acquired powerful tendencies toward foolishly disturbing ourselves?

THE GOALS OF EMOTIONAL HEALTH

Although many different systems and modes of psychotherapy exist today, including relatively passive therapies such as classical psychoanalysis and Rogerian client-centered therapy and highly active-directive methods such as behavior therapy, gestalt therapy, and rational-emotive therapy, almost all the theorists and practitioners of

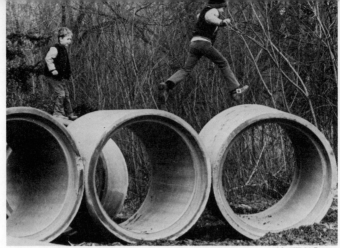

Our need to be with others is a basic part of life.

these various schools agree on the goals of mental health. Dr. Maxie C. Maultsby, Jr. (1975) has summarized these goals quite specifically, and Ellis (1962, 1973, 1974, 1975), Harper (1975), and others[1] have also considered them at some length. Let us now summarize main goals of emotional health pointed out by these and other authorities in the field.

Survival

Mental health helps you survive. As a human you almost invariably want to remain alive—and happy. But you can hardly achieve the second state without achieving the first. You can, of course, exist for 90 years and feel constantly miserable. But you probably won't choose to. If you feel anxious, worthless, and depressed enough, you may literally commit suicide. Or annihilate yourself somewhat more slowly with alcohol, drugs, or daredevil motorcycling. Or still more slowly with overeating, underexercising, or constant smoking. But if you have emotional health, you not only want to survive but feel determined to do so—and to a fairly ripe old age. Not *just* survive, but also *enjoy*.

Pleasurable and Effective Social Relations

Few of us like to exist as hermits. Normally we strongly desire to live in a social group: some kind of clan, community, or regional group composed of other people much like ourselves with whom we effectively interrelate. As humans, we tend to be gregarious. Although we enjoy solitude and privacy at times, we also want communion and sharing with other males and females. One of our main emotional goals, therefore, consists of getting along reasonably well in a social group and avoiding an undue amount of censure, ostracism, sanctions, or other severe penalties from the immediate and larger communities in which we choose to live.

---

[1]A. R. Mahrer, 1967, *The Goals of Psychotherapy.* New York: Appleton; K. T. Morris and H. M. Kanitz, 1975, *Rational-Emotive Therapy.* Boston: Houghton Mifflin; D. J. Tosi, 1974, *Youth: Toward Personal Growth, a Rational-Emotive Approach.* Columbus: Merrill.

We tend not only to group with others but also to become intimately involved with at least a few of these others—for example, members of our original families, our personally chosen mates, and our closest friends. With these few we want to effect some kind of truly collaborative, sharing, loving union. It's not that we *have* to, for we rarely will die or even feel thoroughly miserable without shared intimacy. But we usually *prefer* to, and we generally find greater joy and meaning this way than we do in most other aspects of life. If we achieve emotional health, we normally find ourselves at least moderately capable of achieving intimacy with selected others; at several notable points in our lives we somehow manage to achieve this intimacy.

Intimacy

Most of us have to earn money for the greater part of our lives. Recognizing this fact, we seek out some kind of interesting, ongoing, and decently remunerative kind of work, especially a career, profession, craft, or art. We do not necessarily feel unhappy when we are economically dependent on others, vocationally handicapped, or retired, but we usually feel happier when we have some kind of creative and productive employment. As emotionally healthy individuals, we strive for this kind of goal. Moreover, we frequently strive for some mode of avocational absorption—such as writing, painting, cabinet building, playing the stock market, music, traveling, movie-making—that we enjoy doing. Sometimes this avocation is more important to us than our regular gainful pursuits even though it may be nonremunerative or even expensive. The achieving of such a vital and sometimes almost consuming interest makes the difference to many individuals between a life of apathy and boredom and a vibrant, emotionally healthy existence (Ellis and Harper, 1975).

Vocational and Avocational Absorption

As just noted, those of us who have an engrossing interest in some field of endeavor usually feel happier than those who do not. Millions of

Recreational Activity

Creative cooking—a popular hobby today.

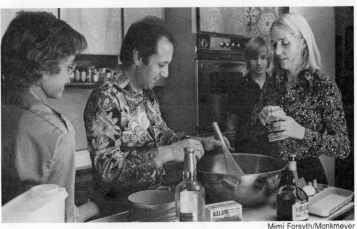

Mimi Forsyth/Monkmeyer

113

individuals, however, never become steadily absorbed in anything. Such people can still achieve contentment if they have at least one or more recreational pursuits that they can actively (or even as relatively passive spectators) participate in, such as sports, dancing, reading, sewing, cooking, socializing, cards, chess, or even TV viewing. No matter how "shallow," "superficial," or "boring" others may find a particular activity, as long as the individual who engages in it genuinely feels entertained by or preoccupied with it, such an interest can significantly contribute to this person's pleasure and emotional health.

Self-acceptance

Almost all authorities on emotional health agree that its main ingredient consists of self-acceptance. But many confuse this with self-esteem or self-confidence. Self-acceptance, when defined the way we define it in rational-emotive therapy, means that you accept yourself *unconditionally*—just because you exist—and not because you accomplish anything, perform outstandingly, or win the love or approval of others. Self-esteem normally means that you accept yourself (or rate yourself highly) *because* you accomplish, do well, gain others' approval, or have some good trait. Thus you esteem yourself or have confidence in yourself because of some achievement you have made. This kind of self-rating really makes you insecure rather than secure. Because no matter how well you do today, how about tomorrow? And no matter how much others adore you, how can you have a guarantee that they will always do so?

Self-acceptance (as opposed to self-esteem) means that you choose not to rate yourself at all. You often rate your traits, acts, deeds, and performances—such as your success in school, in sports, at work, or in love relationships. However, you do this not to show that you exist as a "better person" or "superior human" but rather to help yourself live and enjoy yourself more. If you do poorly in school or at work and

Feeling good.

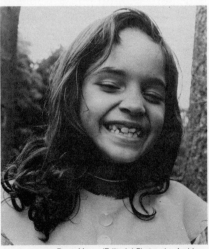

Doug Magee/Editorial Photocolor Archives

acknowledge your low-level performance as "bad" or "unfortunate," you present yourself with the practical challenge: "How can I now *change* my performance to make it better and more fortunate?" But you should not falsely conclude, "Because of this faulty behavior, I intrinsically rate as a rotten person, doomed to act rottenly for the rest of my days!" The wholeness of your person doesn't legitimately rate as anything—it has too many complexities and vicissitudes for anyone (including you) to give it a global, all-inclusive rating. What we call "you" or "yourself" consists of an *ongoing process*: a person that exists in the past, present, and future. And how can any process that has a continuing and future existence, that ceaselessly changes from day to day and year to year, ever have a monolithic, once-and-for-all rating or report card?

Self-acceptance (as we shall show later in more detail) does not consist merely of full affirmation of your legitimate existence and valid happiness no matter what flaws or handicaps you may have—a philosophy of "I exist and *therefore* I have the right to keep myself alive and to strive to enjoy myself in various ways which do not defeat myself or my social group." It also involves absence of several feelings of emotional disturbance that tend to plague most people much of the time, particularly anxiety, despair, depression, guilt, shame, insecurity, and "self-downing," that is, self-deprecation. Not *complete* absence, of course! For people rarely remain totally sane in their attitudes about themselves. But when they really accept themselves, *whether or not* they perform well and *whether or not* certain people approve of them, they relatively rarely tend to feel anxious, depressed, or insecure, since these disturbed feelings almost invariably go with some measure of self-deprecation.

High Frustration Tolerance

When people feel emotionally disturbed, they usually condemn or damn—and not merely dislike or feel displeased with the acts of—themselves and others. But they also needlessly upset themselves by unrealistically condemning the universe: demanding that it *has to* (not merely *had better*) treat them more kindly and fairly and that it *must not* (not *preferably better not*) frustrate and hassle them. They thereby create in themselves low frustration tolerance, short-range hedonism (pleasure seeking),[2] unrealistic demands, and childish whining. High frustration tolerance and long-range hedonism, on the other hand, consists of the attitude "I damned well would like things to go easier and more fairly for me, but if they don't, they don't. Now, what can I possibly do to make them go a little better?" And "I really find it hard that I have to study a good deal and take so much out from my recreational activities to do my term papers. But I don't have to view it as *too* hard or command that my teachers *must* make it easier. It would

---

[2]"Short-range" hedonism, in contrast, is thinking only of today's enjoyment and making no (or inadequate) preparation for tomorrow's.

be great if things turned out that way. But they don't *have to*!"

People with high frustration tolerance do not put up with *anything*, frequently turn activist and persevere to change what they can change. But they accept, and gracefully lump, what they cannot. And, as St. Francis of Assisi noted several centuries ago, have the wisdom to know the difference between the two!

Accepting Reality

As an emotionally healthy individual, you normally accept reality objectively, do not significantly distort or evade it, and live within its restrictions so that you do not get yourself into serious trouble. However, although you may dislike what exists, you do not pretend that it doesn't when it does. You don't continually live in fantasy (such as pretending you have ample money when you actually have little); you don't deny your mistakes and misdeeds (by alleging that you didn't perform them or that others forced you to make them); you don't act irresponsibly to other humans (by inventing special "moral" laws that enable you alone to act badly and require others to act well); and you don't claim magical or supernatural powers that elevate you above the rest of the human race. Perhaps you can survive and live very happily when you delude yourself that you run the universe and that the rest of us rate as second-best citizens compared to Great Omnipotent You, but we doubt it.

Self-actualization

You will have a limited lifetime—not to mention a limited number of hours every day in that lifetime. If you could feel sure that you'd live forever, you might well meander along, eventually get around to all the things you would like to do, and take an infinite amount of time to change your ways, develop your personality, and increase your happiness. But since we have yet to discover the fountain of youth, this possibility seems quite remote.

Self-actualization largely means that you deliberately push yourself to enjoy yourself more. You discover new experiences and pleasurable pathways; you experiment with a good number of potential joys, only to find that some of them aren't for you and some others aren't worth the effort; you wind up by somehow doing more of what *you* like to do and less of what you don't in the relatively brief span of years that you can reasonably expect to have. Not that you *must* achieve your full human potential. Any *desperate* drive in that direction will probably sabotage itself. But you might as well try. Conventional ways often seem very safe—and boring. Doing what *others* think you should may prove utterly fine—for them. Sticking mainly or only with what you first learned to do and enjoy may prove really satisfying, but low-level. Why not, for maximum happiness and mental health, ask yourself: "What *else* can I relish? What *other* satisfactions exist? Do I keep doing what I *really* want to do?" Question. Experiment. Take some risks, and see what happens.

Emotionally healthy people have a strong desire to survive and feel relatively happy. They have the subgoals of striving to remain happy— by themselves, in social situations, in intimate relationships, and vocationally and recreationally. They tend to accept themselves fully and unconditionally (though not necessarily many of their behaviors), feel tolerant toward other humans (though not always toward their deeds), and realistically accept, though often dislike, the harsh realities of the world around them and the indubitable hassles that they often face to get some of the things they most want. Although primarily interested in their own survival and well-being, they usually act tolerantly, responsibly, and sometimes lovingly toward other humans. In, and along with, their own self-interest they tend to maintain a good deal of what Alfred Adler (1974) calls "social interest." For "human" means, at least in large part, "social," and enlightened self-interest includes a significant measure of individual *and* societal concern.

TAKING ACTION

1. *Of the goals discussed, which ones do I consciously see as goals that I have selected for myself and intend to give some thought and effort to carrying out?*
2. *In what specific ways do I keep trying to actualize these goals?*
3. *Exactly how do I tend to block carrying them out?*
4. *What could I do to make my goals for emotional health clearer and help myself persist at trying to achieve them?*
5. *Compare your answers with those of others in the class.*

Assuming that emotional health consists largely of the ingredients listed in the previous section, how can you achieve it? By removing the cognitive, emotional, and behavioral blocks that interfere with its achievement and by working hard at using your potential for self-actualization that you frequently do not bother to use.

Do significant blocks to emotional maturity exist among a great many people in our society? Practically all schools of personality and psychotherapy agree that they do. Psychoanalysts, for example, hold that lack of understanding or insight into your behavior, especially repression of your early childhood experiences and feelings, causes your disturbance. Transactional analysts largely agree. Gestalt therapists hold that failure to have full awareness of your present, here-and-now feelings make you disturbed. Adlerians and rational-emotive therapists see you as choosing unrealistic or irrational goals, purposes, beliefs, and philosophies, thereby barring the achievement of saner goals. Reichian and neo-Reichian theorists claim that you disturb yourself by blocking your physical and sexual urges. Rogerian and other relationship-oriented therapists think that you refuse to accept yourself unconditionally because you make your self-acceptance contingent upon the responsiveness of others and then do not get sufficient responsiveness from these others.

In all these views, and many more could be named, you somehow (consciously or unconsciously, deliberately or unwittingly) stop yourself from achieving healthy, joy-giving thoughts, feelings, and behaviors, and in the process you bring about all kinds of self-defeating behaviors. And although devotees of various schools of therapy frequently seem to state that you get disturbed—or disturb yourself—primarily by intellectual, affective, *or* behavioral means, they strongly imply that all three (not just one) of these modalities contribute to your disturbance. Thus psychoanalysis strongly emphasizes your early emotional experiences with your family members as causative factors in your anxiety or depression. But it also insists that your early beliefs and prejudices (such as your belief that you have to get your parents' supreme attention and approval) make you neurotic and that your learned or habituated behaviors (such as your continually withdrawing from members of the other sex who remind you of your "evil," incestuous urges toward your opposite-sex parent) keep you acting neurotically.

One of the few therapeutic schools that consciously and concretely applies a tripartite emphasis on cognitive, emotive, and behavioral methods consists of *rational-emotive therapy* (RET) (Ellis, 1962, 1973, 1974, 1975; Ellis and Harper, 1975), sometimes called *rational behavior therapy* (RBT) (Maultsby, 1975). Other cognitive-behavior therapies also exist, such as those expounded by Arnold Lazurus and Donald Meichenbaum.[3] Whereas these methods had little popularity only a short while ago, they have recently gained immense favor and are now practiced by perhaps the majority of therapists in one degree or another. In this chapter let us use cognitive-behavior therapy in general and rational-emotive therapy in particular to show exactly how emotional disturbances probably arise and what one can effectively do to uproot them.

The Basic Causes of Emotional Disturbance

Although the direct cause of an emotional disturbance seems to lie in the activating experiences or events that immediately precede it (and, according to psychoanalytic theory, in the activating experiences that occur in the individual's early childhood), we have much reason to believe that other causes or influences contribute even more significantly. According to the theory of RET, we actually start from the disturbed feelings or behaviors themselves. We can quickly put them into an A-B-C framework, where C is the emotional consequence (for example, anxiety and feelings of inadequacy) and A represents the activating experiences that immediately preceded C.

---

[3]A. Lazarus, 1971, *Behavior Therapy and Beyond.* New York: McGraw-Hill; D. Meichenbaum, 1974, *Cognitive Behavior Modification.* Morristown, N.J.: General Learning.

Let us illustrate with a common example. You visit a psychotherapist, feeling anxious and inadequate (point C). He asks you, "At what times do you tend to feel most anxious and most inadequate?" You quickly respond, "Whenever I take an examination and I see, right at the beginning of the exam, that some of the questions seem very hard and I probably won't answer them well."

In other words, you feel anxious (C) immediately after you realize that the test seems difficult and you may possibly fail it (A). If he now asks you, "Does the difficult test, then, make you anxious?" you very likely will reply, "Oh, yes. The test makes me very anxious—and often very inadequate, at least when I consider it a difficult test."

"Hogwash!" he replies. "How can a difficult test possibly get into your gut and cause you to have any feeling whatsoever—including anxiety? Obviously, the test itself cannot make you anxious."

"The hell it doesn't!" you insist. "It does!"

"No," he persists, "it doesn't. Let me prove to you that it doesn't. Suppose, for example, that you took a quick look at the test and mistakenly thought it very easy when it really had many hard questions on it. Would you *then* feel anxious and inadequate?"

"Oh, no, but I see what you mean. The test doesn't really make me upset; my perceiving it as a difficult test brings on my feelings of anxiety."

"Not at all," he perversely persists. "You may see it that way, even strongly feel it so. But no!"

"How come?"

"Simple. Suppose a hundred people exactly your age, with your same kind of intelligence and educational background, all take this same test. They all see it as difficult. Would they *all* feel equally anxious?"

"I suppose they wouldn't," you say. "At least not all of them."

"Why?"

"Well, some would think they could pass it even though it seemed very hard. *They* wouldn't feel anxious."

"Right! But let's go a step further. Suppose that the whole hundred thought the test very hard and that they well might fail it. Would they *then* all feel as anxious or as inadequate as you feel?"

"Mmm. No, I guess not."

"Why not?"

"Well, they all wouldn't take failing as seriously as I do. Yes! Some of them wouldn't think it so awful to fail."

"As *you* do!"

"Right, as I do."

"You see! So A, the activating event of your perceiving how hard the test seems, does *not* cause C, the emotional consequence of your feeling upset about its difficulty. B does!"

"B? What does B stand for?"

"Your belief system—the irrational beliefs that you hold about A.

Almost every time you feel upset at C about anything that happens at A, you will know that a B exists between A and C and that this B is what makes you feel upset."

"But I don't quite understand. My belief, in the case of the difficult test, consists of (1) the belief that the test seems hard and that I may well fail it and (2) the belief that I would consider it terrible if I actually did fail it. They seem like perfectly rational beliefs to me!"

"They do? Not to me! Your first belief—or, rather, observation—seems okay: 'The test seems hard and I may fail it.' Probably correct. We'll assume that the test really has some very difficult questions on it and you therefore may fail it or at the very best get a low passing mark. Fine. This is a valid, confirmable observation, for you damned well may!"

"All right, so you grant me that sensible belief or observation. But wouldn't I also find it awful if I failed? Doesn't that belief also seem legitimate?"

"As an observation *about* your belief state, yes. You probably *would* find it awful—not to mention terrible and horrible—if you failed the test. But do you really know what *awful*, the way you use it here, means?"

"Very bad! Unpleasant! Obnoxious!"

"Oh, that would seem all right—if that's *only* what you mean by the term *awful*. But I doubt that you do. For if you merely told yourself, 'If I failed the test, that would seem bad, unpleasant, and obnoxious,' you would hardly feel anxious—and certainly not feel like a totally inadequate person for failing it. For you would then follow up with something like: 'Yes, so it would seem unpleasant. And since I find it unpleasant to fail, what can I do to succeed? And if I don't succeed this time, what can I do to succeed next time?' In other words, whenever you (or others) view something like failing a test as *merely* bad and unpleasant, you (and they) almost automatically feel *concerned* about passing it and *displeased* about failing. But concern doesn't amount to anxiety—only *overconcern* does. And displeasure at failing a test never equals a feeling of total self-downing. Only *awfulizing* and *overgeneralizing* about your failure equals that. Do you see?"

"Mmm," you reply, not a little confused, but trying to make some sense out of what he is trying to teach you. "If I understand you correctly, you are saying that if I view failing a difficult test as unpleasant, I feel appropriately concerned about it, while if I view it as awful or terrible, I feel inappropriately overconcerned or anxious. Right?"

"Yes. Exactly right, according to the principles of RET. We divide C, your emotional consequence, into two radically different kinds of emotions: first, appropriate emotions, like feelings of displeasure, dissatisfaction, annoyance, frustration, and irritation when you do something disadvantageous like fail a test at A; second, inappropriate emotions, like feelings of anxiety, despair, depression, and total inadequacy when you fail the same test."

"What makes one set of emotions appropriate and the other inappropriate?"

"A good question!" Appropriate emotions—like the rational beliefs from which they stem—help you survive and get along well in the world with yourself, others, and your general environment. Inappropriate emotions—like the irrational beliefs from which *they* proceed—help you either to die or to live and do poorly in the world. They result in failure to accept yourself, to relate to others, or adjust adequately to your environment."

"Oh, then all inappropriate emotions go along with unhappiness and appropriate ones with happiness. Right?"

"No, wrong! If something obnoxious happens to you, like failing a hard test, you'd better not feel happy! Why would *that* prove appropriate? You want to feel unhappy—meaning sorrowful, regretful, or annoyed. For such appropriate, though negative, emotions motivate you to go back to A, your activating experiences, and try to change them. If you felt happy about failing a test, why should you study for the next one? How could you get yourself to pass *any* test?"

"I see. So certain unhappy emotions, like sorrow and regret, seem appropriate. They help us to get rid of or ameliorate poor experiences, at what you call point A."

"Right. And certain *other* unhappy emotions, like depression, extreme anxiety, and self-downing, don't seem at all appropriate. For they motivate you to give up, to feel that you *never* can succeed, to consume your energies in extreme emotionalism rather than in constructively working for change. Where concern helps you do better on the next test, overconcern or panic helps you do much worse. Who needs it!"

"But can I really control or change my emotions from the inappropriate or disturbed ones, which harm me, to more appropriate ones, which help me?"

"Why not? If you change your *awfulizing* that lies behind and creates these inappropriate emotions."

"Awfulizing?"

"Yes—calling or labeling something as awful, horrible, or terrible when merely bad and unfortunate."

"But doesn't that amount to a mere semantic quibble? When something like a test that I might fail several times truly brings very bad results, can't I call that *awful*?"

"You can, but not legitimately. Stop a moment to define what you mean by the word *awful*. First, you mean that the thing you describe rates as bad—even very bad. Let's suppose it does. You fail the test several times and finally get kicked out of school. If completing school is highly advantageous to you, that result certainly seems very bad."

"Well, I feel glad you at least admit that!"

"Of course, I admit it. Badness—meaning disadvantage, discomfort, frustration—certainly exists. And enormous badness. And very enormous badness! Obviously. But when you say that something bad rates as *awful*, do you really mean that you deem it bad, even very bad?"

"Don't I?"

"Oh, you do. You do mean that—and *more*. Whenever you call a thing *awful*, you almost always mean that in addition to its badness or disadvantageousness, (1) it appears *totally* bad; (2) it really and truly amounts to *more than* bad at least 101 percent bad; and (3) because you find it so *awfully* bad, it *should* not, absolutely *must* not exist. And all these three statements, or irrational beliefs, that you have about, say, the badness of failing a test or even a series of tests amount to nonsense: they have no validity and actually consist of magical propositions."

"Magical? Come now!"

"Yes, magical."

Let us stop the conversation at this point. It is given to present the basic causes of emotional disturbance, not show you how to undo these causes and rid yourself of the disturbance. That will be discussed a little later in this chapter. What is important is showing that you have appropriate and inappropriate feelings at point C whenever something unpleasant (or, more accurately, something you *consider* or *evaluate as* unpleasant) occurs in your life at point A. The feelings you choose to have when this negative activating event occurs partly depend on prior experiences and how you reacted to them—such as similar activating events during your childhood and adolescence. But they also, especially during your early life, depend on various physiological factors such as your innate tendencies to perceive, conceive, and react to things in a highly individualistic manner.

You tend to react emotionally and behaviorally in certain vulnerable or less vulnerable ways. As Stella Chess and her collaborators and

Unhappy childhood experiences can affect us for many years afterward.

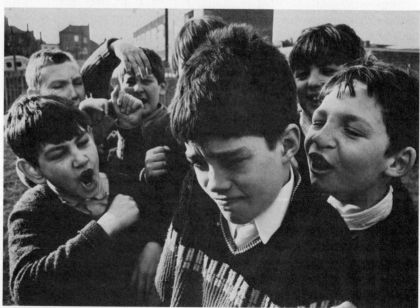

Graham Finlayson/Nancy Palmer Photo

Norman Garmezy and his associates have shown, some children "naturally" react to criticism or abuse in one manner, and other children react or overreact to it in quite a different manner.[4] As many other investigators have also shown, environmental influences and pressures on one child differ enormously from those on another child.[5] Moreover, what psychologists and sociologists often forget is that much of what we call "conditioning" actually seems to consist of *self*-conditioning. You definitely get trained or "conditioned" by, say, your mother hanging up your clothes instead of throwing them on the floor when you undress. But if you have a very strong tendency toward sloppiness you also "condition" your mother to expect less of you in this respect than she comes to expect of your brother and sister. Moreover, if at the age of 15 you fall in love with a member of the other sex who adores orderliness, you may choose to work feverishly at making yourself very tidy and after awhile may habitually and "naturally" (by what we call *second* nature) act in a more orderly way than in the past.

As many behaviorists, from John B. Watson to B. F. Skinner have shown, we get conditioned (or condition ourselves) largely as a result of reinforcement—by discovering that we find some things (such as food and sex) rewarding and other things (such as bitter substances and sex frustration) unrewarding.[6] But what many behaviorists, including Skinner, fail to note is that we, unlike rats and guinea pigs, also have a special ability to *make* "rewards" out of what others might consider serious "penalties." Thus if some professionals are severely criticized for some of the ideas about behavior that they espouse, they frequently *decide* to find this criticism "rewarding" because they consider it erroneous and choose to like the fact that they can stand up against "misguided" objections to their views. Other equally criticized theorists often *choose* to find objections to their opinions exceptionally "unrewarding" and may even surrender these opinions to get more "rewards" or "reinforcements" from their fellow professionals or from members of the public.[7] Hence reinforcement theories about why you do one thing and refrain from doing another have considerable truth, but they also work according to much more complicated rules than some of their strongest adherents admit. Besides, as Skinner himself has said in some of his later works, what he calls "contingencies of reinforcement," or the tendency of people to do something more often

---

[4]S. Chess, T. Alexander, and H. G. Birch, 1965, *Your Child Is a Person.* New York: Viking; N. Garmezy, 1970, *Psychopathology of Adolescence.* New York: McGraw-Hill.

[5]R. Benedict, 1946, *Patterns of Culture.* New York: New American Library; D. C. Glass, 1968, *Environmental Influences.* New York: Rockefeller University Press; J. Henry, 1963, *Culture against Man.* New York: Random House.

[6]J. B. Watson, 1925, *Behaviorism.* New York: Appleton; B. F. Skinner, 1973, *Beyond Freedom and Dignity.* New York: Knopf.

[7]A. Ellis, 1972, *Behavior Therapy* 3:263–274.

when environmental conditions reward them and to do it less often when they do not get reinforced for doing it, bases itself in the final analysis on our genetic endowment. This seems obvious, for if humans learn (or largely act according to reinforcement principles), they clearly have innate tendencies to do certain things. If born unteachable, they could not possibly learn anything. Consequently all their "environmental" conditioning or learning results from their inborn abilities or capacities to be externally influenced.

The ABCs of Emotional Disturbance

When any obnoxious (or *viewed as* obnoxious) experiences occur in your life at point A, and you feel or act aberratedly (meaning self-defeatingly) at point C, then A significantly *contributes to* but does not directly *cause* C. More concretely and importantly (especially for therapeutic purposes), B (your belief system *about* what happens at A) creates your disturbance. This may seem to be startling new view, especially to those who follow psychoanalytic theories. But it originated thousands of years ago, with the Greek Stoics. Epictetus, a famous Stoic philosopher, said that "people do not get disturbed by the things that happen to them, but by their view of these things." Many other philosophers and psychologists, including Marcus Aurelius, Baruch Spinoza, Ludwig Wittgenstein, Alfred Adler, Karen Horney, George Kelly, Julian Rotter, Stanley Schacter, Walter Mischel, Albert Bandura, and Aaron T. Beck, have said essentially the same thing.[8]

Rational-emotive therapy most directly and actively applies this theory to the field of emotional disturbance and psychotherapy. Its exceptionally clear premise is that whenever you feel seriously upset (for example, underemotional, inhibited, withdrawn, overemotional, highly agitated, and "crazy" at point C), don't merely look at point A which immediately preceded C to find the basic causes of your self-defeating or inappropriately emotional reactions; look for B, your belief system about A. If you find B, and clearly and concretely see what you keep telling yourself (or otherwise thinking or imagining) about A, then you will have found the "real" or most important aspect of your under- or overemoting.

Moreover, as RET theory and practice claims, the essence of B, or at least of your irrational beliefs (iB) that directly cause C, seems immedi-

[8]M. Hadas, 1962, *Essential Works of Stoicism.* New York: Bantam Books; B. de Spinoza, 1901, *Improvement of the Understanding, Ethics and Correspondence.* New York: Dunne; A. Adler, 1974, *What Life Should Mean to You.* New York: Putnam; K. Horney, 1965, *Collected Works.* New York: Norton; G. Kelly, 1955, *The Psychology of Personal Constructs.* New York: Norton; J. Rotter, 1954, *Social Learning and Clinical Psychology.* Englewood Cliffs, N.J.: Prentice-Hall; S. Schacter, 1971, *Emotion, Obesity, and Crime.* New York: Academic; W. Mischel, 1975, *Journal of Personality and Social Psychology* 31:254–261; A. Bandura, 1969, *Principles of Behavior Modification.* New York: McGraw-Hill; A. T. Beck, 1967, *Depression.* New York: Hoeber (Harper & Row); A. T. Beck, 1970, *Behavior Therapy* 1:184–200; L. Wittgenstein, 1958, *Philosophical Investigations.* New York: Macmillan.

ately evident in almost all instances if you look for a few main guidelines. Although you theoretically could have thousands of irrational beliefs to upset yourself, they all seem to fall into a very few clear-cut patterns: (1) they consist of awfulizing, catastrophizing, terribilizing, or horribilizing; (2) they almost always amount to demands, commands, insistences, and whinings; and (3) they involve some kinds of absolutistic, magical thinking that you foist upon the universe in the form of *shoulds, oughts,* or *musts.*

In other words, these studies seem to show that whenever you feel seriously disturbed, you take a highly biased or prejudiced view of some event and tend to significantly overgeneralize about it. Thus instead of concluding that one of your failings, handicaps, or even ways in which you get treated by others has distinct disadvantages some of the time, you tend to exaggeratedly conclude: "My mistake in approaching this person makes me *totally* inept. It means that I'll *never* get what I want from others. And if I never do obtain what I desire, or even get considerably less than I want, my entire life will become *terrible* and *awful*, and not merely more *inconvenienced* or *frustrated.*" These overgeneralizations do not agree with empirical reality (conditions that observably exist in the world and probably will exist in your own life). However, you nonetheless *see* them that way. In fact you have dogmatic and almost unshakable *convictions* of their truth, even though you could fairly easily find, if you *looked* for it, strong contrary evidence.

Most of your exaggerated observations, moreover, stem from either an innate and acquired tendency to escalate a desire into a need, a preference into a necessity, a relativistic statement into an absolutistic dogma, an *it-would-prove-better* into an omnipotent *must.* Thus when you feel totally inept after you approach a person and get rejected by him or her, your self-castigation actually stems from the rational belief (rB), "I would like it much better if this person accepted me, and I find it unfortunate and deplorable when he or she doesn't," *and* from the absolutistic, irrational belief (iB), "Because I would like this person to accept me, he or she *has* to do so, and because I keep failing with this individual, as I *must* not fail, I rate as a *rotten individual*, doomed *never* to get the people I like to accept me."

What we call emotional disturbance almost entirely arises from our own "*mus*turbation" about things that we would *like* to exist (or not to exist) and that we *command must* (or *must not*) exist. The three major forms of musturbation or demandingness that we continually discover in the courses of RET include:

1. "I must do well (or outstandingly or perfectly well) at tasks that I consider important and at winning the approval of people I like, and if I don't, I'll *never* get *anything* that I strongly want, and my life consequently will turn awful and horrible." This silly *must* continually leads us to make ourselves anxious, depressed, inhibited, ashamed, and self-downing.

2. "You *must* treat me reasonably (or perfectly) well, considerately, and fairly; if you don't, I won't feel able to enjoy myself, or perhaps even survive, *at all*. Again my life will turn awful and horrible." This absolutistic idea keeps making us feel angry, hostile, enraged, overrebellious, vindictive, and depressed.

3. "The world *must* arrange itself so that I fairly easily get my desires fulfilled and do not have to go through too many hassles or too long a period of waiting to get what I want. And if the world presents me with *too* many problems and frustrations, I *can't stand it.* It will *always* remain not merely hard but *too hard to bear*, and my life will prove awful and horrible." This irrational belief (iB) tends to keep making us feel self-pitying, inert, "lazy," impatient, hostile, and intolerant of any serious kinds of frustration.

Perhaps people become or *make themselves*, emotionally disturbed without employing any of these three kinds of *must*urbation. But it is doubtful. They may have other kinds of behavioral dysfunctioning such as neurological disorders like dyslexia (inability to read well) or epilepsy (convulsive seizures). And they can easily make themselves highly disturbed *about* having these disorders or any other kinds of deficiencies they possess. But when they have what we call an "emotional" or a "mental" disorder, they almost always create it themselves by profoundly and dogmatically believing in some magical should, ought, or must.

TAKING ACTION

Take a sheet of paper and write the following headings on it, leaving a few inches between each of the headings and the next one:

A (activating experiences)
rB (rational beliefs about these activating experiences)
iB (irrational beliefs about these activating experiences)
C (consequences of holding the irrational beliefs)

Now that you have these headings, start with C and write down some emotional disturbance or other symptom that you have recently experienced such as anxiety, depression, shame, inadequacy feelings, hostility, social withdrawal, a tension headache, procrastination, or self-defeating eating, drinking, or smoking. Fill in this disturbed feeling or neurotic behavior at C.

Now go on to A and fill in the activating experiences that occurred in your life just prior to your feeling or behaving poorly at C. For example: "I got rejected by a woman whom I would have liked to get friendly with," "My parents treated me very unjustly," or "I had a great deal of work to do and little time in which to do it."

Now turn to rB and fill in the main rational beliefs, usually negative ones but still quite sensible, that you had about A. For example: "How unfortunate to have this woman reject me!" "I wish my parents had treated me more justly, and I keenly dislike their treating me the way they did," "I find it quite pressuring to have all this work and little time in which to do it. Tough! I'll find it even more pressuring if I don't buckle down and do it soon. So I better do it, no matter how hard it may seem."

Now go on to iB and fill in your irrational beliefs about A. If you get these iBs down correctly, they will almost invariably include some absolutistic must and some awfulizing. Thus: "How awful for this woman to have rejected me! I can't stand getting rejected. She must somehow accept me, or else her rejection proves that I rate as a rotten person!" "My parents have to treat me justly, and I find it utterly horrible if they don't!" "How terrible that I have all this work and so little time in which to do it! Things must not turn out this way!"

If over the next few weeks you keep writing down several of the upsetting emotional consequences you feel or experience at C and then write down the activating events that precede these consequences, you will teach yourself to discover both your rational beliefs (that lead you to have appropriate feelings, such as displeasure, annoyance, and sorrow) regarding A and your irrational beliefs (that lead you to have the neurotic consequences with which you start each of these exercises). The more clearly you see your rational and irrational beliefs, the better you will feel able to differentiate them—and then go on to D (disputing them), which is explained in the next section.

OVERCOMING EMOTIONAL PROBLEMS

You can help yourself overcome your emotional problems in cognitive, emotive, and behavioristic ways. Dr. Robert A. Harper (1959, 1975), in two clearly written volumes on psychotherapy, has described most of the main systems. We will now briefly try to explain how you can help yourself in some of the major ways included in cognitive-behavior therapy or rational-emotive therapy, which are two overlapping approaches.

Rational-emotive therapy consciously and specifically includes a large number of cognitive, emotive, and behavioral techniques. It notably specializes in cognitive or philosophic methods, but it includes a large number of dramatic-emotive-evocative and behavioral-dehabituating approaches as well.

Cognitive or Philosophic Methods

RET specializes in a deep-seated philosophic approach to helping individuals with their emotional problems. It especially teaches you how to "antiawfulize" and to use the logicoempirical method of science in surrendering your absolutistic, self-defeating musts. Thus in the problem of test anxiety that we hypothesized at the beginning of this chapter it would first be necessary to show that you, and not the conditions of your taking a difficult test that you might fail, created your own anxiety and feelings of inadequacy, and that you had better take full responsibility for their creation. Assuming that this succeeded, we would proceed along the following lines:

CLIENT: I don't completely understand what you mean when you say that my beliefs that I *must* succeed in a test and that I see my whole life as *awful* in case I don't amount to a magical belief.

127

THERAPIST: But, of course, such beliefs represent magic. First of all, can you ever prove that you *must* succeed?

CLIENT: But suppose I don't succeed. That would mean that I'd fail the course, perhaps get thrown out of school, and eventually fail to achieve what I would very much want to achieve professionally.

THERAPIST: Let us assume so. But how do you find *awfulness* in all that? Admittedly, you would find it quite disadvantageous if all these things occurred. But *awful*, I still contend, really means *totally* inconvenient or disadvantageous.

CLIENT: Well?

THERAPIST: Well! You would hardly die from failing in school—or even professionally. You would not have *nothing* to work at if that proved true. And even if you had an unsatisfactory vocational life for the next 50 years, that would leave you *something*—in fact quite a lot. You could, for example, enjoy yourself nonvocationally: you could socialize beautifully, have great sex-love relations, enjoy several forms of creative or recreational activities, and actually have a lot of fun in life if you accepted yourself with your vocational handicaps.

CLIENT: Well, I guess so. Perhaps I wouldn't have to feel *totally* deprived or joyless if I failed this test and even failed vocationally for the rest of my days. But wouldn't my living on such a relatively low level still seem awful?

THERAPIST: Not unless you insisted upon *viewing* it that way. And that would amount to magic. For *awful*, as I indicated before, really means *more than* obnoxious—at least 101 percent undesirable and unpleasant. And how could anything, except by sheer magic, amount to 101 percent?

CLIENT: That sounds reasonable, but I still feel—

THERAPIST: Awful? Right! Because if you honestly look into your heart, you'll see that you truly believe that even if things in your life prove 99 percent obnoxious (which of course they could, although you have very little chance that they will, or even if they prove 70 or 80 percent obnoxious), they *shouldn't* exist. Because you find them so unfortunate, they really *must* not get arranged that way. Don't you really—honestly, now—believe that?

CLIENT: Well, yes. I guess I do.

THERAPIST: See how you command the universe to turn out the way you want it! A real Jehovah, eh? 'Because I don't want 70, 80, or 99 percent obnoxiousness to enter my life, it must not! I, the Lord, say it absolutely cannot exist in that highly unpleasant way!' Do you see the omnipotence—the magic—behind that view?

CLIENT: It does seem a little godlike, doesn't it?

THERAPIST: It certainly does!

Along these and similar lines, your therapist would continue to show you that whatever exists exists, that obnoxiousness merely amounts to obnoxiousness, and that only exceptionally nutty, unrealistic thinking would lead you (or anyone) to command the universe to work exactly the way you would like it to work. Your therapist would keep demonstrating to make you to use the logicoempirical method of science so that you could keep proving to yourself that failing a test can well prove highly inconvenient, but that it can't very well amount to more than that. Nothing in the universe can, if you really think about it! For inconvenience, frustration, and annoyance only range from 1 to 99 percent, while horror, awfulness, and terribleness *about* inconvenience range from 101 percent to infinity. They go off the scale of human reality; the fact that millions of people—indeed probably the great majority of people in the world—devoutly believe in *awfulness* and in *musts* only demonstrates how incredibly foolish and unrealistic people remain. It proves that people irrationally *believe* terribleness, or 101 percent frustration, exists, just as they frequently believe that demons, hobgoblins, and werewolves exist. But a belief in a "fact" never proves its validity; it often merely demonstrates the asininity and self-defeatingness of the believer.

So your therapist would continue to show you, in various cognitive ways, that you would almost certainly find it much *better* to pass than to fail an important exam and that therefore you *would preferably*—never *must*—pass it. You would see that whatever exists (such as a difficult test) logically has to exist, not because it fairly or beneficially exists but merely because it *does.* If your professor gives you a totally unfair test, impossible for you (or anyone else in your class) to pass, then the conditions under which he or she gave it to you—his or her viewing and doing things unfairly—make it logically necessary that the test *must* prove unfair. For how can an unfairly behaving professor actually act fairly? Of course, he can't. But you irrationally wail, "My professor must not act in the unfair manner that he or she does act! I can't stand it! How awful!"

Over and over, especially if you felt enraged about a professor giving you an unfair test, your therapist would show you that your whining about the unpleasantries and injustices of your professor's acting unfairly, and your omnipotently commanding that he or she stop treating you in that unfortunate way (1) will not change the professor's unfairness, (2) will make you feel even more frustrated than you normally do feel, (3) will give you severe emotional problems (anxiety and hostility) as well as the practical problem (passing the test) that you already have, (4) will divert your time and energy and prevent you from devoting it to looking for better solutions to this dilemma, and (5) will likely lead to all kinds of other needless difficulties. If your therapist successfully alleviates your emotional disorder about test taking and finally helps you to feel distinctly sorry and concerned, but not anxious and enraged, he or she can then help free you to approach forthcoming tests in a more efficient manner. Ideally, he can also teach you how to give up *all* kinds of demandingness and magical thinking. When at some later time in your life you confront other kinds of problems (such

as failing with your mate and feeling anxious and worthless in case he
or she may reject you), you will tend to resort to empirical and logical,
instead of omnipotent and magical, thinking. Thus you will feel
concerned rather than anxious, displeased rather than enraged.

In other words, by using the cognitive aspects of RET in relation to
your problem of failing an exam and perhaps failing at a career, the
therapist helps you to change your basic philosophy of life from one of
self-castigation, hatred of others who block you, and low frustration
tolerance for the unniceties of the universe to one of self-acceptance,
tolerance, and acceptance of grim reality when you have little or no
possibility of significantly changing it. Using this kind of a rational-
emotive approach, you will most likely not stop your present anxiety
and rage but will probably down yourself and enrage yourself considerably less in the future—even when the activating experiences of your
life seem far from fortuitous.

Can you use anti*must*urbation and antishouldism in regard to what
can be called "sexual fascism"? Definitely! Sexual fascism arises when
you do not merely wish or like people to follow the rules that you
prefer or that you think would serve society well but you also *demand*
or *command* that they do so and see them as RPs (*rotten persons*) when
they don't. Male chauvinism or sexism particularly takes this stance.
The male puts down women because they act "promiscuously,"
"unmotheringly," or "masculinely." He doesn't merely feel that it
would prove better if his mate only lusted after him, devoted herself to
him and their children, and didn't compete with him vocationally or
professionally; but he absolutistically thinks that she *must* and *should*
act in ideal "womanly" ways and sees her as a "ball breaker" or a
"whore" if she doesn't. Much of this kind of male chauvinism has
withered away in recent years, partly as a result of woman's liberation.
But a large amount still remains—a double standard resulting in
inequality between the sexes and in many kinds of prejudices and
antagonisms that ironically harm males as well as females. For if you,
as a man, denigrate women or see them as sex objects and second-class
citizens, how will you help your sex, love, or general relations with
females in general or your mate in particular?

You won't! You'd better, therefore, particularly look at your *shoulds*
and *musts* in the sex-love area, and not merely in regard to other forms
of self-downing and the hating of others. If you damn a certain person
or group, you get yourself into enough difficulty and interfere with your
relating specifically to one or more people. But if you damn an entire
sex—if you as a male despise females, or as a female, put down
males—you do even more damage to yourself and to others.

TAKING ACTION

*How can you practice point D of RET—that is, disputing your irrational
beliefs? By writing down any of the iBs that you derive from your ABC*

*analysis of one of your emotional problems—such as the ones you did for
homework after you read the last section of this chapter—and then vigorously disputing them with the kind of scientific (logicoempirical) questions
you would employ to test any other hypothesis, namely "What evidence
exists to confirm this belief? In what way can I prove or disprove it? Why does
the belief hold true? How can I support or deny it?"*

*Take for example, the irrational belief "How awful for this woman to have
rejected me! I can't stand it! She must somehow accept me, or else I rate as a
rotten person!" You would dispute this belief by asking, "What makes it awful
for her to have rejected me?" And you would answer: "Nothing makes it
awful!" I find it highly disadvantageous to have her reject me, since I would
presumably benefit from her companionship if she accepted me. But no
serious disadvantage amounts to awfulness—only to damned inconvenience!"*

*Again: "In what manner can't I stand her rejecting me?" Answer: "Of
course I can! I will hardly die of rejection. And, assuming I live, I will not
remain in intense pain forever. For the rest of my days, even if she never
accepts me, and even if no equivalent woman does, I can still enjoy hundreds
of things and probably have quite a ball. So I'll never like getting rejected by
her. But I certainly can stand it!"*

*Again: "In what way do I rate as a rotten person because she has rejected
me?" Answer: "In no way whatever! Her rejection may well prove that I have
some rotten traits—homeliness, stupidity, lack of personality, or something
else. But how do a few bad characteristics make me a totally bad person?
Obviously, they don't! And even if she happens to view me that way and sees
me as entirely worthless for having some of my poor traits, I never have to
accept her view. I merely had better accept that she has it—and rue that fact,
all right, but not take it so seriously that I defame myself entirely because she
objects to parts or all of me. A thoroughly rotten person would have no use to
anyone. And if she never approves of me, does that show that no personable
woman ever will? Hardly! Now, how the devil do I look for one who will accept
me!"*

*In this manner you can keep disputing your irrational beliefs until you
really give them up, and then discover that the disturbed consequences of
your holding them—particularly your feelings of shame and self-defamation
and your anxiety and depression—no longer exist. Try this assignment with
at least several of your irrational beliefs until you get the knack of doing it
quite well.*

**Emotive Methods
of Achieving
Emotional Health**

A therapist trying to help you with your problem about test anxiety and
rage against your professor would use various emotive, or dramatic-
evocative techniques to get you to change your basic outlook. For
thinking, emoting, and behaving intrinsically correlate with each other;
just as irrational beliefs lead to inappropriate emotions, changing your
emotions tends to help you modify your beliefs.

Your therapist would therefore first tend to accept you fully, or give
you what Carl Rogers calls "unconditional positive regard," even
though you go to him (or her) in trouble, and act foolishly in your own
life and perhaps also in your therapy sessions. He (or she) would serve
as a kind of appropriate affective model for you, showing you that he

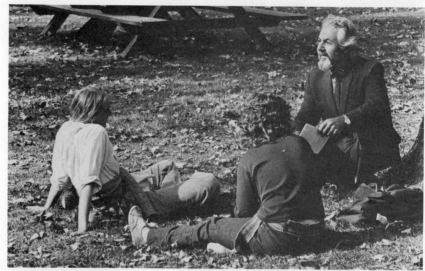

Hugh Rogers/Monkmeyer

(Top) Therapy session on campus. (Bottom left) Employee counseling. (Bottom right) One form of group therapy.

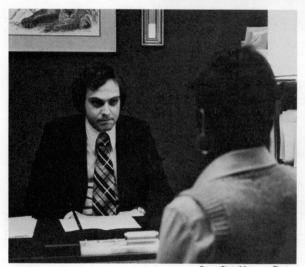

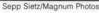

Sepp Sietz/Magnum Photos

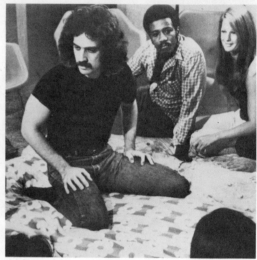

Wide World Photos

can openly face his difficulties with you (including any mistakes he might make in treating you) and that he can avoid putting himself down for his errors the way you tend to put yourself down for yours.

He would probably use rational-emotive imagery with you. In an adaptation of Dr. Maultsby's procedure, he would get you to intensely imagine yourself failing at a difficult, and perhaps unfairly constructed, test and let yourself, as you imagine this happening, feel anxious and self-downing. When you succeeded in feeling this way and fully getting in touch with your feelings, he would then have you change this feeling to one of *only* disappointment and sorrow, and not that of anxiety. When you did this, he would ask you how you did it. You would probably give him a highly cognitive answer, for example, "I convinced

myself that I would hardly see the end of the world, even if I failed in
the course, and that failing would make me an individual who had
suffered a real loss, but not in the least a totally failing person." He
would then get you to practice this kind of rational-emotive imagery—
deeply feeling inappropriate feelings, changing them to appropriate
ones, seeing how you changed them, and then continuing to repeat this
emotive-cognitive behavioral process—for at least 10 minutes a day for
the next few weeks. You would thereby learn after a while to automatically feel disappointment and sorrow but *not* anxiety and feelings of
worthlessness whenever you thought about failing or actually failed a
difficult test.

He might give you a series of shame-attacking exercises. In these
exercises, either during the therapy session or (better yet) during your
regular life, you think of yourself doing something that you ordinarily
would consider shameful, embarrassing, or silly such as yelling out the
stops in a subway or bus, wearing one black and one white stocking, or
skipping rope in a sedate neighborhood. You would then actually do
this "shameful" act, as long as you did not get arrested, fired from your
job, or otherwise seriously penalized for doing it. By doing, and
perhaps continuing to do, such a shame-attacking exercise, you would
most probably discover that shame or embarrassment exists primarily
because you not only think a certain act wrong or foolish but also
condemn yourself as a person for doing it. You would also probably
discover that you do not have to do the latter even when you do the
former.

Depending on the kinds of emotive methods that worked well with
you, he would probably use various other techniques such as dramatic
role playing, self-disclosing exercises, encounter group procedures, or
other confrontational methods that would bring you out, help you get
in touch with your dysfunctional feelings, and show you how to change
them and the irrational ideas with which they mesh.

TAKING ACTION

*Without a therapist's help you can do some of these emotive exercises
yourself. Take the RET shame-attacking exercise, for example. Think of
something that you would consider very shameful to do in public, such as
doing a jig on the street, telling a stranger that you must got out of a mental
hospital, walking with a black umbrella above your head on a sunny day, or
trying to sell last Tuesday's newspaper on Sunday. Force yourself to do this
"shameful" act—preferably several times. Then ask yourself: "How do I really
feel, now that I have done this? How did people actually react to me? Did
anyone severely penalize me in any way for my act? What did they probably
think of me? Do I have to accept the thoughts in their head and make them
my own? Of what did the 'shamefulness' of my act really consist? Must I
always have the approval of other people, even strangers? How could I keep
doing this same act and refuse to make myself feel ashamed of doing it?"
After practicing such acts several times and really thinking through these*

kinds of questions about doing them, you will feel surprised about what you learn about yourself and about the good results that you get!

Behavioral Methods

RET has always assumed that people not only think and feel in disturbed ways but that they also act or behave aberrantly, and that they get habituated to self-defeating activities which often take on a kind of autonomous role and therefore are not easily given up. Following the deconditioning and desensitizing methods originated by John B. Watson, B. F. Skinner, Joseph Wolpe, Albert Bandura, and others, it particularly emphasizes in vivo desensitization, or activity homework assignments. If you went to your therapist again with the problem of feeling terribly anxious and self-deprecating about taking difficult tests, and if you also tended to withdraw from testing situations, he would try to help you face them, persist at gradually doing them, and perhaps operantly condition yourself (or reinforce yourself) if you did persist.

He might, for example, give you a graduated series of tests to do, ranging from easy tests in courses that you did not take for any credit to more difficult tests in credit courses to exceptionally hard tests that you had even a higher stake in passing. If your professor seemed to act quite unjustly, he might not encourage you to transfer to another class and arrange to have a fairer teacher. Instead your therapist might well encourage you deliberately to stay with this unfair professor, at least for a while, until you had some practice in convincing yourself that he had a human right to act unfairly, that he didn't have to behave otherwise, and that you could fairly easily stand his injustices.

Your therapist would probably also give you cognitive homework assignments, such as the RET method of disputing irrational beliefs (DIB). Using this method, you take one of your main irrational beliefs such as the idea "I *must* pass every difficult test that I take!" and you spend at least 10 minutes a day actively disputing it with such questions as the following: (1) Can I rationally support this belief? (2) What evidence exists of the falseness of the belief? (3) Does any evidence exist of the truth of this belief? (4) What are the worst things that could *actually* happen to me if I don't get what I think I must? (5) What good things could happen, or could I make happen, if I don't get what I think I must? In thinking through these kinds of questions for a stipulated period each day, and writing or recording your answers to them, you would tend to give up or seriously modify such an irrational belief within a fairly short period of time.

Other kinds of activity homework assignments, usually of a desensitizing nature, that your therapist might give you might include (1) assertiveness training, so that you get yourself to speak up to your unfair professor early in the game rather than after you have already inordinately enraged yourself against him; (2) talking with other members of your class to see how they handle the problem of making themselves anxious and enraged about taking difficult tests; (3) the use of self-management principles (including operant conditioning) to help you discipline yourself in regard to your studying habits; and (4) skill-training procedures that might help you study better so that when you took difficult tests, you would have a better chance of passing them.

Although RET homework procedures overlap with the methods of behavior modification employed by strict behavior therapists, they differ significantly in that they are not designed only to help people change their behaviors and thereby rid themselves of their disturbed symptoms. This is certainly an admirable goal, but it can be broadened to help people undo their philosophies and irrational beliefs *by* behavioral methods. As some scientific experiments show, and as everyday observation will strongly attest, we often can change our ideas by changing our actions. In the words of John Dewey, we learn by doing. And by thinking and emoting too!

TAKING ACTION

Practice some RET homework on yourself by picking some task that you feel afraid to do, such as speaking in front of an audience, walking into a bar alone, or talking to a stranger, and assign yourself to do it, perhaps on a graduated basis. How about doing it once this week, twice the following week, and three times the week after? If necessary, reward yourself immediately after completing this task—with a good meal, listening to music, attending a sports match, or what you will—and penalize yourself—say, by burning a five-dollar bill or sending it to a cause you hate—every time within the period you set that you fail to do this project. If you balk at doing it, look at the awfulizing sentences you keep telling yourself as you balk, for example, "I would have to feel shattered if I talked to a stranger and he or she rebuffed me" and prove to yourself why this statement holds little or no validity. If you do the feared task, notice how you feel afterward; see how the doing of it disputes or contradicts your awfulizing beliefs, and show yourself how relatively easily you can perform this "terrible fearful" act in the future.

One of the great advantages of the rational-emotive approach to dealing with problems of emotional health lies in its ability to help you not

HOW TO LIVE WITH A "NEUROTIC"

---

[9]The word "neurotic" appears in quotation marks when it is used as a noun, as in "a 'neurotic' does this" or " 'neurotics' do that." It is not in quotation marks when it appears as an adjective or adverb. This is because a statement about "neurotics" implies that a class of individuals exist whom we can clearly label neurotic, whose behavior totally appears neurotic, and who will presumably act neurotically for the rest of their days. Quite an overgeneralization! To say, however, that "he has neurotic behavior" implies in a much more limited way that some of his behavior turns out neurotically some of the time. Particularly, in the field of mental health, it seems dangerous to label an individual "neurotic" or "psychotic" since such a label may type that individual for the rest of his or her life. Overgeneralizations, as Alfred Korzybski noted in *Science and Sanity* (Lancaster, Pa.: Lancaster Press, 1933), tend to lead to emotional disturbance. Therefore most of this chapter is written in E-prime, a form of language that does not use any form of the verb *to be* to minimize some of the overgeneralizations commonly employed in writings about emotional health.

only work to overcome your own light or serious disturbances but to live successfully with other "neurotics"[9] and to either help them significantly with their problems or to manage to get along nicely with them even if they remain disturbed. Here are some of the highlights of procedures outlined in the book *How to Live with a "Neurotic"* (Ellis, 1975).

The Possibility of Helping Troubled People

Don't try to help every troubled person who happens to come your way, for some have such great problems that you will not get anywhere with them and you may possibly do some harm. It would be better to refer them to a psychologist or psychiatrist. Many of your friends and relatives can be helped, but some, even though they might well benefit from psychological care, will stubbornly refuse to seek it. In most of these cases these people devoutly believe in some perfectionistic should or must, and you may have the ability to see these absolutes and to help them attack and surrender them.

Although the basic irrational ideas that people hold, to their emotional detriment, may theoretically run into the hundreds, they usually boil down to about ten. Almost all humans subscribe to this unholy decalog to some degree, but quite a few do so intensely and uncompromisingly. These we usually label "neurotics." What major ideas do they (and you) tend to hold when disturbed behavior ensues? The following are some of them.

1. The idea that you must—yes, *must*—have love or approval from all the people you find significant.
2. The idea that you must have competence or talent in at least one important area and preferably in many or all significant respects.
3. The idea that when people act obnoxiously and unfairly, you should blame and damn them and see them as bad, wicked, or rotten individuals.
4. The idea that you have to view things as awful, terrible, horrible, and catastrophic when you get seriously frustrated, treated unfairly, or rejected.
5. The idea that emotional misery comes from external pressures and that you have little ability to control or change your feelings.
6. The idea that if something seems dangerous or fearsome, you must preoccupy yourself with and make yourself very anxious about it.
7. The idea that you can more easily avoid facing many life difficulties and self-responsibilities than undertake more rewarding forms of self-discipline.
8. The idea that your past remains all-important and that because something once strongly influenced your life, it has to keep determining your feelings and behavior today.
9. The idea that people and things *should* turn out better than they do and that you must view it as awful and horrible if you do not

find good solutions to life's grim realities.

10. The idea that you can achieve maximum human happiness by inertia and inaction or by passively and uncommittedly "enjoying yourself."

If you clearly see that ideas such as these have little rationality and that devoutly believing them leads people to needlessly make themselves anxious, depressed, ashamed, self-downing, and hostile, you can frequently help your disturbed friends and associates to acknowledge their own irrationalities and the consequent self-defeating emotions and behaviors to which they lead. You can also change both the ideas and their emotional-behavioral consequences.

Assuming that you recognize, as outlined in this chapter, what constitutes emotional disturbance and how people originate and perpetuate it by their irrational thinking, you can frequently help a "neurotic" by trying some of the following methods.

Techniques of Helping Troubled People

1. Look to your own neurotic behavior and try to do something about *that*. If you act disturbed, you will have so many problems of your own and so little objectivity that you can hardly aid anyone else. So, first of all, try to understand some of your *own* foolish thinking and behaving. Accept the fact that you *have* emotional upsets of your own. Openly acknowledge them to some of your neurotically behaving friends. Show that you do not feel ashamed of these upsets, and work concertedly to overcome them by applying to yourself some of the same rational principles that you would like to use with others. Set a good model for those you try to teach to help themselves.

2. In trying to help others, recognize clearly and *accept* the fact that they have disturbances. Many of us who have rather disturbed associates simply refuse to accept the fact that these people behave unusually, and we continue to treat them as if they had perfect adjustment. If you treat them as if they can easily live up to nonneurotic behavior, you will show keen disappointment and thereby convince them that they have seriously failed, and hence you will contribute to their natural self-damning tendencies.

This means that as soon as your disturbed associates do something particularly stupid, pigheaded, or irritating, you can ask yourself, "Why did they do that?" And quickly answer: "Because of their neuroses! Because 'neurotics' frequently do that sort of thing. Not because they hate me. Not because they personally aim to do me in. Because they often behave neurotically—and *therefore* commonly do stupid or ruthless things."

3. Remember that "neurotics" rarely choose their obnoxious behavior. They partly inherit and they partly acquire a strong tendency to act neurotically. They do not *wish* to feel emotionally upset; they do not voluntarily select the path to neurosis. They mainly hate themselves. Even when they harm others, they virtually compel themselves to do

this harm by their irrational views. Why damn them, then, for having their disturbances? Why not try to help them as much as you can to overcome these troubles? If you can't help, at least tolerate *them* even if you do not wish to put up with some of their *actions* any longer.

4. To the degree that you genuinely can, try to act warmly and supportively toward "neurotics." It cannot be emphasized too often that most disturbed people down themselves mercilessly; they foolishly believe that *they* have no value when their *performances* fail or get disapproved. They can more easily accept themselves, therefore, if you unconditionally accept *them* in spite of their poor *deeds*. Emphasize their assets. Do not falsely deny their failings, but try to ignore or minimize them. Keep bringing up their good points at appropriate times. Let them know when they look especially good, when they do a fine job, when they act better than they thought they could. As you do this, don't indicate that you think them fine *people* for acting well, but that you know they *can* do well, even though they never *have* to. In other words: teach them by your words and attitudes how to stop rating *themselves* and how to only rate their *acts* and *performances*.

5. Encourage "neurotics" to do the things they foolishly fear and erroneously believe they cannot do successfully. Encourage their efforts, even though they may fail. And if they do fail, show them that the next attempt may well succeed. Try to induce them to do things at which they will probably succeed. Then point out that these successes indicate that they probably can do other things they fear. Convince your troubled friends or relatives that everyone frequently fails and that people mainly learn by trial and error. Therefore failure not only commonly occurs but has great advantages. You can also help "neurotics" see that though success may prove important, you do not see it as all-important or sacred. Show confidence in their future success, but when they fail, show that you still accept and care for them.

6. While showing "neurotics" that you wholeheartedly respect them as people, make it clear that you will not permit them to see you as an easy mark for exploitation or abuse. Adopt an attitude of *firm kindness*, and avoid pampering or babying them. With firm kindness you act nicely to people, but you set definite limits as to how far they may impose on you, and you firmly stick to those limits. You see things from other people's frames of reference but never entirely lose sight of your own vital wants and interests.

Suppose, for example, you have a neurotic woman friend who fears meeting people and insists that you stay home with her practically all of the time to protect her from her fears. Don't say, "Now look here, Bonnie, you know how stupidly you act when you refuse to meet people. And how inconsiderately you behave toward me! You never think of what *I* want to do. If you really cared for me, you'd consider me and act more sociably!"

You then would help Bonnie think herself totally inadequate, feel that you do not understand her, and think that you only consider yourself. She may well begin to feel more disturbed! Instead, try to help her see that she *can* get along with others. Gradually try to introduce her to a few new people at a time until she begins to adjust to socializing.

If, however, she stubbornly refuses to do anything about her fears, you might say, "Look, Bonnie, I really understand that you don't feel up to meeting people right now, though I know you will feel able to do it later. Meanwhile, I feel enormously cooped up and want to widen my horizons. Just because you want to remain something of a hermit doesn't mean that I have to do so too. Suppose I stay home with you most of the time but go out now and then by myself. I won't feel so cooped up, I won't start resenting you, and I can easily wait till you get over your fears and want to start seeing people with me." Working along these lines, you can stand up for your own rights and at the same time show an understanding of your partner's (or anyone else's) disturbance.

7. One central rule: *do not sharply criticize a "neurotic"!* Disturbed people largely arrive at their state by taking criticism, their own and that of others, too seriously. To tell them that for their own good they should go from point one to point two gets translated, in their mixed-up thinking, as: "Look here, you fool! You know darned well that you harm yourself by remaining at one instead of going to two. Why don't you stop acting like a dunce and do the right thing?" Your "constructive" and well-meant criticism turns to terrible self-reproach.

You can try to refrain from attacking them or even their behavior yet still hint at the *ideas* behind this behavior. If, for example, your neurotic friend fears riding on trains, don't tell him: "Oh, come on, Jim. That's silly! You know that trains have a safe record!" Certainly he "knows" how silly his phobia sounds and that riding in trains involves no great real danger. But if you emphasize these irrationalities, you label him as an idiot.

Rather, try to find the idea behind Jim's fear of riding in trains. Obviously, he believes that riding them involves some kind of danger. Thus he may have thoughts that the train will crash—and that would mean utter disaster. Or that in a crowded train he might have close physical contact with a man or woman, and he views that as unbearable. Or that if he had an attack of diarrhea in a train he might not get to a bathroom on time, and that would seem most embarrassing. If you want to help undermine Jim's phobia—especially if he will not go for professional help about it—try to discover what irrational ideas he dreams up to create this anxiety and then tackle not Jim, and not even his anxiety, but his irrational ideas.

If you discover that Jim really fears dying in a train crash, you could point out that very few crashes occur these days, that most of those that do occur result in few fatalities, that everyone has to die someday, that worrying about the possibility of a crash will hardly reduce the chances of a train's actually crashing, that preserving his life at the expense of continual worry (and avoiding trains) hardly seems worth the effort, and so on.

8. Can you induce a neurotic associate to go for psychotherapy when he or she obviously could use it but stubbornly resists going for help? Yes, but not easily! For "neurotics" often will contend that professional help costs too much. Or say they have no time for it. Or point out that they know someone who has not benefited from it. Or admit that they fear getting torn apart psychologically and not knowing how to put themselves back together again. How, then, can you help reluctant "neurotics" to accept psychotherapy? Not by nagging, but by various other methods.

First, convince them that you want to help but have less ability than a competent therapist.

Second, introduce them to people who have had therapy and have felt helped by it. Or if you know a good therapist socially, you can sometime arrange for your disturbed friends to meet this individual so that they can see what a representative of the profession looks and sounds like.

Third, introduce those you want to help to sophisticated, educated people who realize the value of psychotherapy. If "neurotics" only know uneducated, defensive individuals—many of whom themselves have run from therapy—they will keep hearing the old bromide that only "crazy" people go for treatment. Try to show them that we can hardly label most therapy clients as "crazy," but we more accurately describe them as people who have some serious problems.

Fourth, if you have had some therapy yourself, you may find it advisable to tell your neurotic friends about it and show them how you benefited from it. If one of them shows interest, you may try seeing a therapist yourself first and explain your friend's problems, especially his or her reluctance to undertake treatment. You may thus prepare the therapist to overcome your friend's doubts and help him or her to enter a full-scale therapeutic relationship.

How to Live with a Person Who Remains Neurotic

Perhaps all "neurotics" *can* get better, but many of them *will* not. Even intensive psychotherapy doesn't always produce good results, since they may resist using its teachings. Suppose you live or work with a fairly disturbed individual who simply will not accept help from you or anyone else. How can you remain with this individual without making yourself upset?

First, *fully* and *unequivocally* accept the fact that disturbed people act in a peculiar, often obnoxious manner. This may seem an unimportant point. But, no! People say, "I know that so-and-so acts neurotically. I've known it for years. Naturally I make allowances for her or his disturbance."

Untrue! These people *think* they know that so-and-so behaves neurotically; they *vaguely* know it. Actually they do not. And that makes all the difference in the world—the difference between vaguely acknowledging neurosis and *truly* knowing it.

Consider an example. A man went with a woman for two years, kept talking about her disturbed behavior, but then married her anyway because he wanted an interesting, intellectually alive companion. A few weeks after the marriage, he complained bitterly: "She doesn't do a thing. She doesn't read; she doesn't want to discuss anything interesting; she doesn't want to go visiting. She just sits all day and does nothing. How can I live with a woman like that?"

"But what do you expect," a friend asked, "from a 'neurotic'?"

"Oh, I see her neurosis, but—" And off he went into another tirade.

This man did not *fully* see his wife's disturbance. If he had, he would have expected her to act in disturbed ways: to do exactly the kind of things she did. Obviously he expected nothing of the sort and felt shocked when she acted neurotically. He said he unequivocally saw her neurosis. He thought he saw it. But no! It took quite a while for him to *really* view her as neurotic.

If you want to live peacefully with disturbed people, expect them to act in a disturbed manner. If you expect them to act sanely, rationally, and normally, what does that show about *your* rationality? For you will then keep having your hopes fruitlessly raised, then dashed. No one expects an infant to act like a grown-up, a professor like a Bowery bum. Why, then, should you expect a "neurotic" to act like a well-adjusted, mature individual?

In accepting "neurotics," don't *personalize* their behavior. Naturally, as a result of their disturbances, they will sometimes act negatively. But, as often as not, they treat you just as they routinely treat most other people and frequently just as they treat themselves. By their actions they may seem unkind or stupid. Actually, because of their neurosis they drive themselves to do unkind or stupid things.

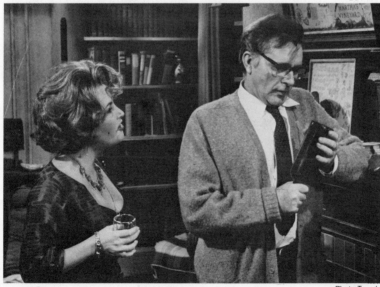

George and Martha, the neurotic husband and wife made famous in *Who's Afraid of Virginia Woolf?*

Photo Trends

Even when they deliberately go out of their way to harm someone, don't assume that they have a personal gripe against that individual. They hold something against themselves and feel driven by self-hatred to hate others. Panic-stricken people, when caught in a fire, will ruthlessly knock down others to escape. But this does not mean that they hate these others or wish them harm. Similarly, "neurotics" frequently feel indifferent or sometimes even friendly to a person while, stricken with panic, they push that person out of their way. They don't necessary *want* to act antagonistically but feel forced to do so.

If you find "neurotics" you love changeable, fine! If they will work at overcoming disturbance and at giving more love, by all means give generously to help them. But if they give up hope and refuse flatly to try to work to get better, beware. Out of self-protection, withdraw some of your attention or, if necessary, break off the entire relationship.

Usually you won't find this more drastic action necessary. Even seriously disturbed people, as a rule, have some capacity for warm relationships, and you can have limited love involvements with them. But recognize these limitations; don't delude yourself that they love very deeply. Unless you relish unrequited love, care somewhat reservedly for them. And if your relationships get too bad, wisely make a strategic retreat. Think of your own skin, for a neurotic intimate may have little regard for it!

Sometimes you cannot, emotionally or literally, get away from people with severely neurotic behavior. What can you do to live comfortably with them? Acquire a more realistic, more stoical philosophy of life. You can use your head, as well as your heart, to overcome virtually any difficulty—including those that arise in attempting to live with "neurotics."

A rational, realistic philosophy of life includes several sane assumptions. First, the world has great difficulties and injustices, but you don't have to complain or make yourself furious about them. This in no sense implies that when things don't go the way you want them or when they seem clearly unfair, you should not try to change them. Try by all means! But when you find them unchangeable, as on many occasions you will, don't become upset. Practice feeling appropriately sorry and irritated, not inappropriately whiny and enraged.

Many so-called adults demand that the world work the way they want it to work. They think it owes them a living. They insist that when things go wrong *no* justice or goodness exists. Mature adults think differently. They know we don't have the best of all possible worlds and do have much unfairness and injustice. They realize that more agreeable ways *can* come about. But they do not command that they *must*. In fact wise people avoid almost all *musts*—for *must*urbation, again, practically equals emotional disturbance.

When you have a rational attitude, you make living your main purpose: experiencing, seeing, doing, feeling, existing. You try to make the most of your 75-odd years by living them to the hilt—by discovering as many vitally interesting things as possible, by taking risks in order to gain certain pleasures, by making clear-cut goals and plans and working to achieve them.

If you want to help make the world a little better than when you came into it, great! You can choose to work for a less polluted, more peaceful, fairer world, in which you and other humans can live more happily, less neurotically. But you'd better not equate working for a better existence with depressing yourself because it does not presently exist! Our existing environment has many obnoxious qualities—and many money grubbers, tyrants, "psychopaths," and "neurotics." And quite likely will have them for some time to come.

Moreover, aside from the current unsatisfactory state of the world, humans have great imperfections. They act more ignorantly, inefficiently, and disturbed than they usually care to admit. It takes them considerable time to unlearn bad habits and acquire better ones. They forget things easily. They inappropriately make themselves both overemotional and defensively underemotional. They have a number of diseases and ailments. They frequently addict themselves to health-destroying habits. And these basic human limitations seem widespread and endless.

Take, therefore, a realistic attitude! Don't necessarily *like* the world but *accept* its reality. If you don't like things, try to change them. If you can't change them now, stop whining and keep your eye on later. Don't give up living because life has hassles. Stop commanding that goodness *has* to exist. As the philosopher Epictetus pointed out some 2000 years ago, we have practically no control over the actions of others.[10] Why, then, *must* we control them?

If you live with "neurotics," think realistically. Don't expect them to behave other than neurotically. And don't keep telling yourself, "How awful that they act that way!" So your neurotic associates behave unfairly, unjustly. Who said that they *have* to act fairly? What law of the universe states that justice *must* prevail? You certainly need not *like* their behavior. But in many cases shouldn't you gracefully *lump* it?

TAKING ACTION

What can you do, this very week, to change some of your attitudes and actions toward disturbed people? Try this RET homework assignment. Pick a fairly serious "neurotic," whom you ordinarily would avoid and complain about. For once deliberately stay *in the presence of that disturbed person. Visit or play tennis with or go on a date with him or her. Then, as you associate with that individual, keenly and clearly observe his or her obnoxious behavior. Try to see the irrational ideas (the* demands *and the* musts*)*

---

[10]M. Hadas, 1962, *The Writings of Epictetus, Essential Works of Stoicism*. New York: Bantam Books.

*that probably lie behind and cause it. Show yourself, while still in this
person's presence, that you can fairly easily accept him or her with the
obnoxious behavior, that you may never like it, but you can largely ignore or
accept it. If you want to, try to call some neurotic mannerisms to this person's
attention—in an objective, nondamning, helpful way. If this works, fine. If it
doesn't, show yourself that you can still tolerate the person no matter how
unpleasant his or her behavior remains. Then, after your visit ends, ask
yourself: "Did my neurotic associate really act that badly? Could I enjoy the
visit in spite of some of the things that occurred in the course of it? Does this
person have to act that way, or could I help him or her to change? If the
behavior truly seems unchangeable, need I still condemn him or her for
acting in a neurotically objectionable way?" Try this experiment. You may
surprise yourself with its interesting results!*

DISCUSSION   Humans significantly overlap with other animals but significantly
differ too. To a much stronger degree than any other creatures,
including the primates, we have language, we possess self-
consciousness, we know that we will have a future, we make a great
many predictions about our present and future, we possess superior
brains and thinking power, we respond less to our instincts and more to
our premeditated choices, we devise powerful cultures, and we can
even think about our thinking.

Certainly we have a potent, highly influencing biological heritage.
Most assuredly we have primitive, and important, parts of our brain
and nervous system. Admittedly we can as yet change ourselves and
our surroundings to a limited degree, and even then at notable costs to
ourselves and our environments. We never seem to actually transcend
our human limitations; we always (at least so far) remain fallible. We
frequently delude ourselves that we have attained some kind of
godhood, but invariably our actions prove this notion false.

From a mental health standpoint, the very advantages that humans
have over animals also lead to enormous handicaps. Because we have
language, symbolism, self-consciousness, unique awareness of our
errors, and the ability to see and prepare for the future, we make
ourselves not only concerned but frequently overconcerned—and thus
anxious and panicky. And because we have a wonderful ability to
abstract and generalize we often end up by overgeneralizing and
absolutizing—and thereby bring on more anxiety, as well as depression, self-downing, and extreme hostility. On an individual scale we do
ourselves in frightfully, and thus many of us wind up with neurotic,
psychopathic, psychotic, or other disturbed symptoms. On a social
scale we almost miraculously conquer the earth and the sky, but we
also fall prey to pollution, bigotry, war, political corruption, crime,
needless starvation, and almost innumerable other social ills.

What can we do? As far as we know, we can do nothing truly
supernatural or superhuman. However, many astounding, almost in-
conceivable achievements fall within the human range—including,
fortunately, enormous improvements in our emotional health.

For if the assumptions and data outlined in this chapter prove true, you can significantly understand and control your own psychological destiny. Yes, your disturbed thoughts, emotions, and behaviors most probably have some important roots in your inherited biological structure. Yes, they probably partly stem from some of the familial, educational, cultural, and other environmental factors that have assailed you since early childhood. But they also have their origin and continuance in *you*, and you consist of an ever-changing, ongoing *process*. You partly choose and decide what you will wear, eat, and do. And what you will think and feel.

On the other hand, you don't have complete free will. You can't do anything you please. Your genes, your anatomy, your community, and your physical environment all contribute to limiting and restricting you—somewhat. But you have some choice, some degree of predictability. Myles Friedman, a creative educator, holds that your basic rationality consists of this very predictability: of your ability to see the future and significantly make what you would like to see prevail.[11]

If you feel afflicted with any emotional ailment, don't merely look to the past or present. Look also to your ability to predict the future—and to some degree to make it come about. You now have the emotional consequence (point C) of some anxiety or self-downing, immediately after you have experienced some activating experience (point A). By all means get in touch with, acknowledge, and don't try to deny your negative feeling. By all means explore, discover exactly what has happened to you, at point A, just before you began to feel that way. Feel C and perceive and understand A.

But look most notably at B—your belief system. B consists of the way you healthfully or crookedly think. It includes sensible, practical beliefs about A, and stupid, absolutistic, impractical beliefs about A. Explore *both* these kinds of beliefs and separate them clearly. Do you *want* A to turn out differently, and do you feel sorry, regretful, and frustrated when they don't? Good. Wants, preferences, desires—these seem the essence of healthy human existence. They rarely lead you astray.

But do you, in addition to wanting and desiring, *need* your activating experiences to turn out well? *Must* you have them that way? Do you have to think it terrible, awful, horrible when they don't amount to exactly what you want? If so, *you* choose these needs, musts, and awfulnesses. *You* escalate your human desires to superhuman demands. You cease merely to wish that the universe will go your way and to work hard to get what you wish. You insist that you've simply *got to* have your way, work or no work. In your chronological maturity you wail as you did during your infancy. No wonder you feel miserable. No wonder you tend to get even less of what you want!

---

[11]M. Friedman, 1975, *Rational Behavior.* Columbia: University of South Carolina Press.

Look, again, to your humanness. Give up your silly grandiosity. Try, try many times for what you really want. But give up necessity. Surrender perfectionism. Forget about certainty. You do not *need* what you *want*. Remember that and you will control your emotional destiny far better than the hordes of babies on this earth who still deludedly call themselves grown-ups. A *hassle* never amounts to a *horror*. *Must*urbation means self-abuse!

FOR FURTHER READING

Adler, A., 1974. *Understanding Human Nature.* New York: Fawcett World.

A pioneering book showing how people disturb themselves by unrealistic goals, purposes, and ideals, and how they can help themselves live more happily.

Ellis, A., 1962. *Reason and Emotion in Psychotherapy.* New York: Lyle Stuart.

A basic text in rational-emotive therapy, originally written for psychotherapists but used by many readers as a self-help book.

————, 1973. *Growth through Reason.* Palo Alto, Calif.: Science and Behavior Books; Hollywood, Calif.: Wilshire Books.

Verbatim transcripts by several rational-emotive therapists of their sessions with clients, with critical comments by the author on the way they handled these sessions.

————, 1974. *Humanistic Psychotherapy: The Rational-Emotive Approach.* New York: Julian Press and McGraw-Hill Paperbacks.

An updating of rational-emotive theory and practice, showing in particular how taking a strongly cognitive approach to psychotherapy proves more humanistic than taking some of the other approaches.

————, 1975. *How to Live with a "Neurotic."* New York: Crown.

A revised and updated version of the original 1957 book on rational-emotive methods of understanding and helping disturbed individuals with whom you live or work.

Ellis, A., and Harper, R. A., 1975. *A New Guide to Rational Living.* Englewood Cliffs, N.J.: Prentice-Hall; Hollywood, Calif.: Wilshire Books.

A completely revised version of the authors' classic self-help book using rational-emotive therapy principles. Hundreds of thousands of readers have used this book to help themselves deal with their emotional problems.

Harper, R. A., 1959. *Psychoanalysis and Psychotherapy: 36 Systems.* Englewood Cliffs, N.J.: Prentice-Hall.

A lucid, easy to understand outline of some of the major systems of psychotherapy.

———, 1975. *The New Psychotherapies.* Englewood Cliffs, N.J.: Prentice-
Hall.

A clearly written supplement to *Psychoanalysis and Psychotherapy: 36
Systems*, mainly dealing with the most popular recent therapies.

Maultsby, Maxie C., Jr., 1975. *Help Yourself to Happiness.* Boston: Esplanade
Books; New York: Institute for Rational Living.

The principles and practice of rational behavior therapy and their
application to helping yourself with your own emotional difficulties.

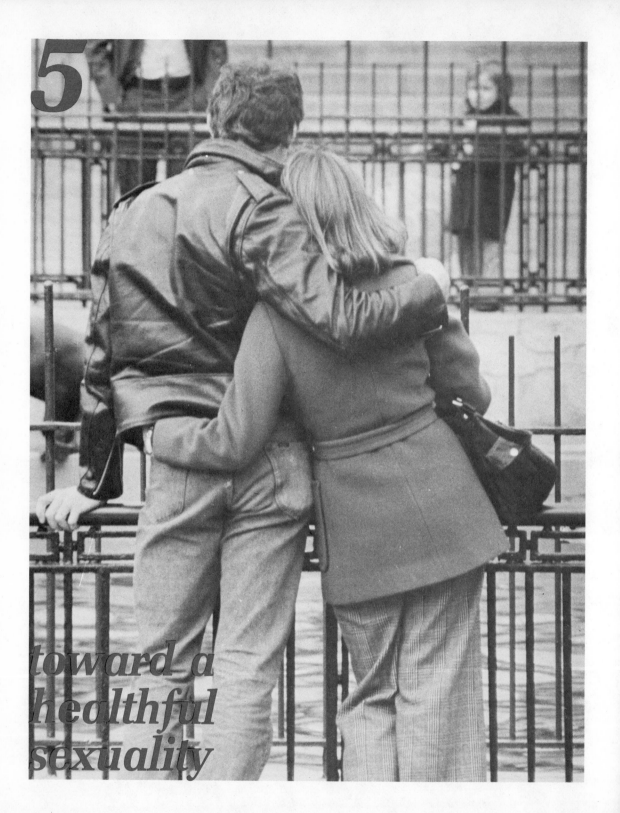

5

toward a healthful sexuality

*College and university students are now integrating sex into their
personal lives, seeking at the same time to recognize the needs
and rights of others. When it comes to making sexual choices,
they are now full-fledged decision makers. The absence of adult
supervision, the freedom with which men and women mingle in all
kinds of activities, the near perfection of contraceptive measures,
the openness of discussion, and the decline of taboos make
sexual encounters easily available if that is what is wanted.*

*The fact that many students are involved in some form of sexual
activity is accepted, and this chapter attempts to put sexual
associations, particularly heterosexual intercourse, in a context
where motives can be understood and discussed rationally. The
need for effective communication is emphasized, as is the
importance of assuming responsibility and protecting others
against needless and harmful physical and emotional outcomes.
These factors are related to sexual relationships at various levels
of emotional involvement. There is also the importance of avoiding
unwanted pregnancy and the repercussions that result.*

*The expanding dimensions of sexuality are readily apparent in
the shifting male and female roles and in the growing acceptance
of such sexual expressions as homosexuality and fantasy. How are
love and sex related and how are they differentiated? The chapter
closes with a different and unusual emphasis. The reader is
regarded as a citizen who has the obligation for creating a healthy
environment in which human sexuality can function.*

INQUIRY

1. Think of your future, your sex and love life, the kind of family you
   hope for, your continuing relations with the family in which you grew
   up. How does sex fit into that future? Do your present attitudes and
   experiences with love and sex require any modification if you are to
   achieve what you wish?
2. How would you feel about your children becoming aware of your
   sexual patterns, as they are currently and as they may be in the
   future?
3. Do you have the breadth and depth of information you need to cope
   with the sexual and love situations you are facing or are likely to
   face?
4. How do you assess your capacity to communicate effectively about
   sex? Do you find that any improvements are needed? If so, what are
   they?
5. Sexually and in your love relationships have you treated others as
   you would like to be treated? Are you committed to this pattern for
   the future?
6. What are your attitudes toward variations in sexual lifestyles? Are
   they accepting, rejecting, or mixed? Why do you have the attitudes
   that you do?

A new life begins with enrollment in college. Practically all university and college students meet new, interesting, and sometimes confusing situations. Such experiences are intriguing, but they also require some very perplexing choices. Sex and love undoubtedly occupy a very prominent place in endless conversations! The aim of this chapter is to provide helpful insights that may lead to happier college years and a more satisfying later life.

Changes Affecting Sexual Attitudes

The college environment today is quite different from that of a generation ago. Traditional views toward sexual relations, male-female roles, love, marriage, and the family are being challenged, and much controversy has resulted. New directions in behavior have emerged. As a consequence you now have to face complicated problems of decision making and choose from many options not common even 20 years ago. These changing views of behavior are the result of numerous forces. Five in particular have been influential in giving new directions to sexual attitudes, not only for college students but for the whole society.

1. *A much greater openness about sexual matters now exists.* People hesitated to express even a general interest in sexuality 20 or 30 years ago. To admit they had had sexual relationships except in marriage was certain to invite criticism. Complete honesty seemed possible only when close friends confided feelings and experiences to one another.

Whether you are male or female, it is certainly much easier today for you to say straightforwardly that you are interested in sex or that you have had sexual encounters. Barriers still exist, however, and there are still persons before whom one remains silent. Parents or persons in authority are generally included in this category.

More tolerant attitudes—and an openness that makes discussions of sexuality easy—are increasing. This greater freedom is a marked help in decision making. Wisely used, it is all to the good. Sexual activity can have various outcomes, some exciting and enjoyable, others disappointing and disturbing. All activities, sexual and nonsexual, entail risks, but these can be recognized and minimized through honesty, frankness, and sincerity. A sexually active person should insist upon an adequate knowledge of sexuality for himself, the use of effective contraceptive methods, a willingness to say to a partner just how one feels about sexual relations and what experiences are the most or least acceptable, and a readiness to call immediate attention to any evidence of venereal disease or pregnancy and to take needed preventive and protective steps. These are advantages that come from openness and frankness.

A Gallup poll of 55 campuses, reported in May 1970, indicated that 75 percent of all persons interviewed no longer believed it important that they marry a virgin. Another Gallup poll taken in May 1975 asked, "Do you think it is wrong for people to have sexual relations before marriage?" Among the freshmen, 76 percent said no. This increased to 85 percent of the seniors. While studies done to date probably do not accurately represent the overall national scene, they do point to an increase in the acceptance of nonmarital intercourse.

Studies have been conducted to determine whether intercourse prior to marriage is increasing or decreasing. The results range from probably little or no change to a definite increase. More significant, however, than sheer percentages or numbers showing participation is the importance of showing how sexual experience affects relationships. We need more information regarding motives, communication, and happy and unhappy outcomes of sexual associations. The next two changes indicate why this new direction is necessary.

2. *Control over outcomes of sexual activity is growing.* More and more, people are able to decide what will result from sexual relationships; the physical consequences can be largely decided by accurate information and by an exercise of caution in crucial situations. In your lifetime this sense of control has always existed; you have not known a time when it did not. It has come largely from a wider use of contraceptives. Even though many young people do not have access to contraceptives, they still know about them and so have the sense of being able to decide on outcomes. While there is no absolutely foolproof method of contraception, there is very little reason for unwanted pregnancies. Furthermore, if social attitudes could be changed and adequate medical measures taken, venereal diseases could be wiped out. Control here, however, particularly in casual relations, is less sure than when unwanted pregnancy is the issue.

Young people are generally more optimistic in their attitudes toward controlling the outcomes of sexual activities than more mature adults are. Parents ordinarily do not encourage this optimism, at least in their children. Parents usually warn of the serious dangers of entering a

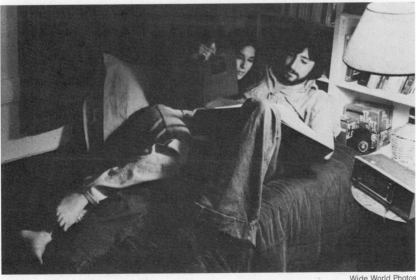

Living together has become a more accepted practice in college dormitories.

Wide World Photos

sexual relationship. There is evidence to support a pessimistic approach, for there are always cases to be cited of venereal infection and of unwanted and unhappy pregnancies. But even as their elders warn them, young people are aware that these consequences do not necessarily follow.

Contraceptives are becoming increasingly available. With a little inquiry, with a bit of exploration, both contraceptive information and devices are generally available, even to teenagers. They may be purchased over the counter, although some can be obtained only through a doctor's prescription. There are Planned Parenthood clinics which tend to be especially helpful. In many colleges and universities the health service offers gynecological and contraceptive services, or advice on how to obtain them. Moreover, there is an increasingly large amount of information on all aspects of sexuality, particularly through peer conversation, books, and classes.[1]

3. *Unmarried couples on college campuses are now living together for extended periods.* One now finds on practically all college and university campuses couples who share apartments, spend weekends together, or otherwise arrange their schedules so they are closely associated for prolonged periods. This practice is apparently growing, and students may well find they will have to decide whether or not to participate in such an arrangement.

4. *The relation of males and females in their sexual and love relationships is changing.* Typical arrangements in your parents' youth discriminated severely against women. In the first place, the man took the lead in male-female relationships. The boy asked the girl for a date, he made the arrangements, and after the date was over he decided whether there would be another. Sexually he was permitted, even expected, "to be on the make." The girl had to be enticing enough to encourage him to return, yet diplomatic enough to fend him off without hurt feelings before "things went too far." Furthermore, the male was not really faulted if they did "go too far"; he was simply "sowing his wild oats." The female, however, lost her virginity, and this might well raise serious questions about her moral standards.

The girl was also supposed to have "falling in love" as a paramount interest. The romantic concept of love was quite in vogue, and for a woman, marriage and becoming a housewife was really the major objective. This role patterning was part and parcel of the double

---

[1] A special reference should be made to numerous books and pamphlets now published for students and often prepared by them. They are very explicit about anatomy, birth control, abortion, sterilization, venereal diseases, pregnancy signs and tests, and gynecological problems. Since there are so many such publications and since they are relatively inexpensive, we have bypassed any extended treatment of these and similar physiological topics in this chapter. To obtain an extended listing of these handbooks, order *A Guide to Sexuality Handbooks.* This pamphlet has been prepared by Youth and Student Affairs, Planned Parenthood Federation of America, 810 Seventh Avenue, New York, N.Y. 10019. These handbooks are sold only in multiples of four; the price is $1.00 per set of four.

standard: one rule for males, another for females.

The feminist movement, however, has brought about great changes. Women are no longer the retiring, diffident creatures of yore; they expect different conditions in the family, in education, and in the business and professional world. Men now recognize that they too have been living stereotyped roles. Consequently a similar kind of questioning about role patterns is now developing with men, and male-female relations are being reexamined on campuses throughout the nation.

5. *The definition of sexuality has been broadened; it now includes concerns not formerly associated with sexuality.* Certain matters not of particular importance even a few years ago have now assumed great significance. Among them are changing attitudes toward maleness and femaleness and what is appropriate in sex roles, the question of unmarried couples living together, casual sexual relationships versus those of longer duration, abortion, and a more accepting attitude toward homosexuality. There are still others. Formerly sexual discussions centered mainly on reproduction, genital growth and development, and certain sexual acts, particularly masturbation and premarital intercourse. The presentation of physiological facts was the central concern. If options or choices were possible, they were not discussed; young people were told what was the approved way. No effort was really made to weigh alternatives. Today more and more young people make their own decisions. This chapter is intended to help you with the decision-making process.

6. *Sexual pleasure, including that produced by masturbating, is increasingly viewed as a legitimate part of life, even a kind of human right.* This development has occurred in the face of the dour Victorian attitude—a view that disapproved sexual pleasure generally, especially for women, and justified marital sex only for procreative purposes. Moreover, masturbation was firmly believed to be devastatingly harmful, causing diseases, insanity, death, and even damnation. Few people now believe such nonsense, and masturbation is therefore far less often a cause of anxiety or guilt feelings than formerly. In fact many specialists now recommend it for both sexes at any age as a totally harmless source of pleasure, different from but not inferior to sex with another. Sex therapists often recommend masturbation to certain clients not only as a pleasurable release from sexual tension but also as a step toward learning to enjoy sex with another.

TAKING ACTION

1. *In class or small group discussions ask fellow students to explain what their parents or other adults told them about intercourse outside marriage, the dangers of venereal disease, pregnancy, and homosexuality. How does that compare with what you were told? Then let each student say what he expects to tell his own children. Will it be different from what his parents told him, and in what way?*

2. *Check your health service to see what kind of assistance in sexual matters
   is available to students.*
3. *Ask a group of class members to engage in an informal conversation on
   changes now affecting the lives of both males and females. First let the
   men talk on male roles and women on female roles. Indicate what seems
   desirable and undesirable. Without announcing it beforehand, reverse
   roles. Males will assume they are females, females that they are males, and
   all will discuss their feelings toward possible roles. Analyze how the class
   feels about what was said before and after the reversal.*

AN EXPLORATION OF HETEROSEXUAL RELATIONS

New books, articles, films, and research studies on human sexuality are coming to public attention daily. Therefore any exploration of sexual concepts confined to a single chapter must be limited. Here we will concentrate on selected mental health aspects of sexuality common to the late teens and early adulthood.

The Intercourse Continuum

Interest in intercourse is common in the late adolescent to early adulthood years for several reasons. This is the age when hormonal secretions make both male and female bodies extremely sensitive to physical stimulation. The erogenous zones—especially the abdomen, the pelvic area, and certainly the genital organs themselves—are highly responsive, particularly to those stimuli that have become associated with sexual activity.

"Do you think it is all right for young people to have intercourse?" No helpful answer can be given to this highly general question, which becomes even more difficult when a "yes" or "no" answer is wanted. The question itself focuses on intercourse as an act; it ignores important social and psychological meanings. It assumes that intercourse has the same techniques and qualities, the same expectations, and the same consequences whenever and however it occurs. Presumably both male and female react to it in the same way. It seems as though intercourse is viewed as a circumstance in which male and female join sex organs simply because each has a body that will accommodate the genitals of the other.

Our language is similarly limited. It would be clearer if we had several words describing the qualities and emotional significance of the sex act. The single word "intercourse" cannot and does not make these differentiations. Even though two persons may be antagonistic to each other, they may still bring their genitals together. In this case, rather than "intercourse" a better word would be "copulation," a joining of parts. Intercourse could then convey the idea of partners giving and receiving, the concept of interchange being involved. A person might have many experiences in copulation but never have had intercourse.

Simplistic ways of looking at intercourse are very defeating. They provide no means for describing the subtleties and intricacies that actually go along with intercourse. Even though the sex organs are joined in intercourse, a wide range of feelings from hostility to a deep and well-established love may be experienced.

We are accepting intercourse as an all-inclusive word. However, we will discuss it from the point of view of showing how intercourse can convey different meanings at different times. This will be done by using an intercourse continuum (see Figure 5-1). In this way we can look at

EXTENT OF EMOTIONAL INVOLVEMENT IN INTERCOURSE

Level 1	Level 2	Level 3	Level 4
Hostility–rejection	*No affection*	*Some affection exists*	*Much or deep affection*
All relationships renounced	A casual, episodic relationship	A relationship with chances of persisting	A strong relationship exists

Figure 5-1

The intercourse continuum. (An adaptation from the continuum used in Lester A. Kirkendall, 1961, *Premarital Intercourse and Interpersonal Relationships.* New York: Gramercy Publishing.)

sexual associations from several standpoints. The continuum is divided into four parts, or levels. Each one indicates a different degree of emotional involvement or noninvolvement existing when intercourse occurs. The involvements range from situations in which the partners clearly reject one another emotionally (Level 1), to casual relationships in which no affection exists (Level 2), to associations in which they care somewhat for each other (Level 3), to associations in which they care very deeply (Level 4).

Then three personal characteristics that individuals use as they relate to others will be correlated with the levels of emotional involvement. The purpose will be to see how these characteristics change and how they influence behavior from level to level.

The characteristics used in this examination are:

1. *Motivations.* As we study motives, we become aware of the various reasons that cause people to enter or to reject a sexual relationship.
2. *Communication.* Communication, both verbal and nonverbal, is extremely important, for it gives people the chance to understand each other, and if they wish, they can change their relationship. Communication itself will not solve problems, but it is an essential first step toward any solution.
3. *Protective measures.* These are the efforts each partner makes to protect the other from unpleasant or harmful consequences, which include possible pregnancy, prevention of venereal disease, discovery, guilt, and other emotional reactions of a negative nature.

The question being explored is this: "When one examines these personal characteristics closely, will intercourse, or a rejection of it, be

regarded differently as emotional involvement changes? If so, how?"
We are convinced that it will be, and through making this analysis it
can be understood more clearly.

Attention will be given to Level 1 only when by doing so a definite
point can be made. Major attention will be given to Levels 2, 3, and 4 of
the continuum. Unquestionably these are the levels of greatest interest
to our readers.

This discussion relates to circumstances surrounding the male-
female relationship, that is, heterosexual intercourse. Much of what is
said will apply to same-sex relations as well. Space limitations,
however, prevent the same analysis of homosexual relations.

TAKING ACTION

*Before reading further, list ideas indicating how you think each of the three
characteristics will be affected as intercourse occurs at various levels of
emotional involvement.*

Motivation One needs to understand motives if one is to judge
accurately the meaning of intercourse to the partners. The kind of
communication that occurs, the concern for protective measures, the
appraisals made of intercourse, the length of time the relationship
continues, and other matters as well are determined by existing
motivations. Furthermore, as motives change, these other factors will
change also.

Sexual motivations are not always easily determined. Any aspect of
behavior is complex, and sexual behavior is probably more complex
than most. In matters of sex people are taught to remain silent and to act
as though they were quite devoid of feelings. Yet sexuality is a part of
one's personality; it cannot be discarded like a coat. The consequence
is that almost all of us keep most of our sexual feelings hidden and
private. In public we tend to live as though we are nonsexual beings.
But private and public lives cannot be so neatly separated, so many
sexual motivations are repressed and denied. As a consequence they go
into the subconscious, the deeper recesses of the mind, and may well
produce behavior that is quite unexplainable either to the individual
involved or to those about him. In other words, the conscious and
unconscious become intertwined in a complicated way, so the interpretations of motives become just as intricate.

The way to become aware of one's own motivations is to discuss
them openly with some objective, rational person concerned with
helping people understand their own behavior. A friend may be helpful
at this point, but a much more likely person would be one trained in
counseling. Most important of all, however, are a readiness to be
objective and a willingness to engage in discussions which will probe
motives.

Yet certain statements about sexual motivations at the various levels can be made with some assurance. At Level 1 where there is a rejection of, or possibly a feeling of hostility toward, the other person, the motives of the hostile person are self-centered and are focused on circumstances beyond the sexual association itself. Level 2, with its casual and episodic experiences, is less rejecting but clearly self-centered. In most situations persons are interested in the physical sexual experience or see it simply as a recreational experience. Moving past Level 2 and to Levels 3 and 4, individuals show a growing concern for the sexual partner as well as the welfare of others. Concern with self is more and more merged with a concern for the other.

Usually a concern for the welfare of a sexual partner is built over a period of time. Barriers are broken down gradually, persons disclose themselves psychologically to each other, and each invests in the other emotionally. As a consequence each comes more and more to conduct himself in a way that expresses a deepening interest in the other. The greater one's emotional investment in a partner the more pronounced is his concern for that person. Sometimes, however, the investment is not really where it seems to be. An illustration taken from Level 1 experiences, discussed in the research study cited in Figure 5-1, will explain one such "investment" complexity. In this study a group of 38 high school and college males who had gone to prostitutes were interviewed at length to understand their experience. In many instances what happened hardly sounded like a sexual experience in the typical sense. The men began by challenging each other, boasting, daring, and casting doubt on each other's masculinity, until no one could back out and still save face. The interviewer soon realized that this was essentially a male group experience; the prostitute was there simply as an accessory, and the men evidently regarded her as such, too. They avoided the pronouns "she" or "her," resorting to the neuter pronoun "it" instead.

For some of the fellows this was their first experience in intercourse, and they were frankly frightened. If they could have gone to a room and no prostitute had appeared but they could have come out with a rattling good story, they would have been very pleased. The story is what counted, and these men were viewed as authorities on sex by the other fellows.

Apparently the prostitutes themselves felt like an accessory. They were to provide intercourse, but that was as far as their services went. One fellow had always wanted to discuss with a prostitute her attitudes toward herself. So he asked if any kisses were ever exchanged during intercourse. Her reply was, "No, I'm a whore, not a lover."

However, it is important to remember that prostitutes are human beings; each is different, behaves differently, and perceives herself differently.

Motivations for engaging in the casual, no-affection (but nonprostitute) experience in intercourse (Level 2) has some variation according

157

to whether one is female or male. One of the common motivations, particularly for males, was to satisfy their desire for the physical pleasure of intercourse and to satisfy curiosity. The sharing of these experiences with other males was still a motive, but less so than at Level 1. At Level 2 they were now much more concerned with extended sex play. They liked partners who at times were quite seductive, actively enjoyed the experience, and placed no obligation or responsibility on them.

Until recently, however, no unmarried female in her teens or twenties would have admitted to similar motives. Possibly they were there, but to acknowledge this openly was too threatening. Consequently it had to be denied or, if accepted, had to be associated with feelings of love and a desire for a relationship. Many girls must sympathize with the following comment made by Helen, who is now in college. After high school graduation, Phil invited Helen to spend the night in his camper. He could and would use condoms, and she had just finished menstruating, so there was very little risk of pregnancy. Her reaction was:

> Here, suddenly, was a situation which I had been arguing should be as fully open to women as men—in fact women should feel free to invite men sexually as well as to be invited by them. But I suddenly found the old Victorian attitudes I had lived by for so long standing in my way. I heard myself saying, "But I've known you only this evening. It has been a nice evening, but we have no relationship going. I don't think we should." He was quite understanding and accepted my decision.

TAKING ACTION

1. *Complete Helen's case history. Provide a rational and reasoned support for the position you take. Would you be willing to announce your position publicly? What qualifications, if any, would you make for other young women?*
2. *Comment on Phil's approach and your feeling about his reactions to Helen's decision. How would you feel and act yourself if you were in a similar situation?*

Certainly not all Level 2 motivations center so clearly about the physical pleasure of the sexual relationship or around curiosity. Sometime the persons who have been associated in affectional relationships find themselves rejected. They may then turn to casual relationships, which may or may not include sex. Their motivation may be a desperate hope of finding in the casual relationship what they lost in the other. Revenge for their rejection may be a motive. Whether the other person knows it or not, the one rejected has his angry feelings relieved and the need to retaliate satisfied. Sometimes an individual will feel he has extended his love unwisely; from now on he will engage in only casual and transitory associations, and hopefully there will be no further hurt.

For some a casual relationship holds the possibility that from it a continuing affectional relationship may emerge. In other words, hopes are focused at Levels 3 and 4, though behavior is essentially at Level 2. Seemingly women more than men cling to this hope, and this in turn causes more trouble. In such circumstances a woman too often misjudges the evaluation a man is likely to make of casual sexual experience. Her belief is that sex is very important to him, and that having experienced intercourse, even at the casual level, he will then extend love. All too often the male supports this rationalization by voicing affection when there is little or none.

Motivation at Levels 3 and 4 comes to be increasingly "each-other" centered. As this occurs, one sees his or her partner in a different way. The needs and desires of the total individual are now central, and the participation in intercourse for physical pleasure of lesser importance. If the movement into an each-other centered relationship comes at the same time for both, and if personalities are reasonably well matched, the chances for the association to be satisfying and permanent are good.

The female ordinarily expresses affectional-emotional feelings sooner than the male, especially during the years between adolescence and early adulthood. This probably results from the teaching to which boys and girls have been subjected. For females the need for building a relationship and finding a mate has been stressed. The male has been taught to find his satisfaction in other ways—in aggressive striving, success in athletics, preparing for an occupation, or kindred activities. Furthermore, he is expected to be more interested in the physical aspects of sex than the female is.

The current repatterning of masculine-feminine roles is altering sexual attitudes and the meaning sex conveys. Today there is more free discussion, and both male and female can acknowledge their enjoyment of sex more easily. Free communication also enables partners to express dissatisfaction with the sexual relationship—for example, feelings of guilt, fear of discovery. If motivation is genuinely concerned with the other person, then open discussion may result in either a reordering of the intercourse relationship or a decision to forgo it entirely.

Finally, sexual contacts at Levels 3 and 4 are prized for the physical nearness they provide. Whereas sexual experience at Level 2 may provide an opportunity for penetration and an orgasm, at Level 3 and especially Level 4 touch and prolonged body contact assume great importance. Males particularly comment on their enjoyment of such contact once they have experienced it. Usually their early conditioning has been essentially at Level 2, where attaining orgasm is the prime objective. Adding the pleasure of touching and a longer time for the entire experience increases enjoyment and satisfaction for both male and female.

As each-other centered motivation develops, the sexual attitudes of both male and female change, often in opposite directions. As the female feels love and tenderness infusing the relationship, she becomes more and more ready to accept intercourse. At the same time, the male becomes less and less sure that this is what he wants. He becomes more concerned over what this would mean both to himself and his partner. Men with considerable casual sex experience often feel that intercourse will result in a loss of respect for the female.

Communication   Just as motives change from level to level, so does communication, both verbal and nonverbal. Clear, honest, and direct communication will certainly help in coping with sexual problems. This may not be easy, however, since personality characteristics greatly affect the ability to communicate. A loss of self-respect, anger, hurt and repressed feelings, or a tender ego can easily make discussion very difficult if not impossible.

First, look at Level 1. In any relationship, sexual or nonsexual, if hostility or a feeling of rejection exists there is likely to be little or no verbal communication. Under those circumstances whatever is said may simply be a demand, "Take your hands off me," "Lie down," "Take off your clothes." There may be much nonverbal communication, for example, staring, sulking, angry glances, or turning away. If the persons are in direct body contact, physical force may be used by one to obtain what he wants; the other will likely resist. If this sounds like rape it should, because this is rape (although it is not so defined when it occurs within marriage). Rapist demands are the most obvious illustration of hostile communication at the sexual level, though there are rejecting contacts with lesser degrees of hostility.

Couples who copulate as a commercial matter may not be hostile, but certainly they have no intention of carrying the relationship further than that occasion. A vast emotional gap exists between the two, and neither intends to close it. Of course communication may be honest and very direct; the kind involving buyer and seller in any business transaction. "We will go to this room." "The price for a straight screw is $50.00. Anything else will be more."

Even though money is exchanged for service, contemptuous attitudes still exist. The men regard the women as whores or sluts, and the women are aware of this. They are likely also to resent legal discriminations. The prostitute's patron is seldom as liable before the law as the prostitute herself.

Commercialized intercourse does exist at levels where the buyer and seller of sexual services are more nearly equal in terms of educational and cultural backgrounds. There are also situations in which there is a very indistinct dividing line between outright commercialization of sex and giving and receiving sexually as a part of some other exchange. The expectation may be that a gift or a dinner for which one person pays the entire bill will be followed by intercourse. This is often so taken for granted that no discussion is needed. Even in some marriages sexual favors are given or refused as a way of gaining some other end. Sex can be used for advantage taking and exploitation at any one of the four levels.

Sometimes hostility and rejection are replaced by aggression, for example, when one person completely dominates another. Then one is apt to say a "violation" has occurred that some male or female has been given a "snow job." The person getting the "snow job" may be either male or female. In the movie "The Graduate"[2] Benjamin Braddock, meets at a party an older woman, Mrs. Robinson, who is the wife of his father's business partner. Mrs. Robinson soon seduces Benjamin. However, he very soon realizes that Mrs. Robinson has no interest in him as a person. For example, he suggests ". . . do you think we might do a little talking?" Mrs. Robinson is uninterested. She needs someone to satisfy her ego and Benjamin is simply an accessory, just as were the prostitutes mentioned earlier. These circumstances finally lead to a traumatic break between Benjamin and Mrs. Robinson.

Here a male is being violated. But are not both the aggressor and the victim violated? The victim, Benjamin, is violated emotionally and physically, but the aggressor, Mrs. Robinson, has destroyed the better, more generous side of her character. In the end she is completely rejected by Benjamin, and as a consequence she feels deeply violated herself. Her reaction is to become even more vicious and disparaging of Benjamin and others around her. At the end of the movie she is more isolated and alone than at the beginning.

Communication at Level 2 is becoming easier as people become more tolerant. If people are interested in sexual relations, they are more likely to be straightforward about it. Formerly, and for some even yet, if a couple wished to participate in a casual sexual relationship, they used subterfuges and ploys to determine the intent and attitude of the other person.

This conversation was reported by a boy who was trying to "make" a girl, said to be "an easy lay." At one point in their conversation this exchange occurred:

MALE: *What does your father do?*
FEMALE: *Oh, he's a carpenter. He makes things.*
MALE: *Yeh? I make things too.*
FEMALE: *Oh, I like people who make things.*

And so with this evasive interchange the situation was resolved in favor of intercourse without it even being mentioned.

Homosexuals seeking nonaffectional relationships are caught in the need to be coy and evasive as well. "Have you a match?" "Haven't I met you somewhere before?" "What time is it?" Such comments are used to avoid feelings of rejection that might occur should a direct statement of sexual desire be made. The tabooed nature of same-sex relationships make evasion and indirectness in expressing homosexual interests seem even more necessary.

Advances are sometimes invited by nonverbal means. Dress and the way clothing is worn, particularly among women, is the best illustra-

---

[2]Charles Webb, 1971, *The Graduate.* New York: New American Library. The story in paperback.

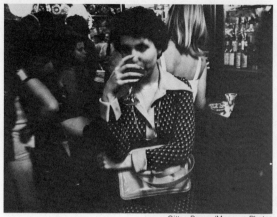

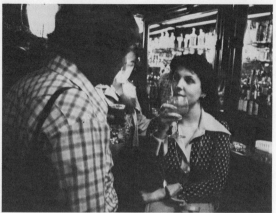

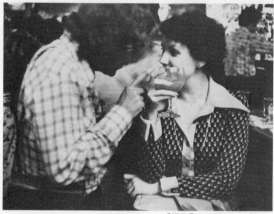

Casual encounter
in a bar.

tion, though men's clothing may convey the same message. What is most wanted is something that will cause a comment, as an avant-garde dress design or an unusual sweater. This provides a point of contact, and so a conversation can begin. Sometimes these messages are so blatant there is no mistaking them. For example, open messages on T-shirts, V symbols for vasectomy, sexy ornaments, and so on.

Straightforward, face-to-face verbal communication about sex is still not easy for many. At the casual level physical contact even to the point of intercourse is sometimes easier to accomplish than to verbalize sexual desires or feelings. When one boy was asked "Well, have you ever asked her whether she experiences an orgasm with you?" he looked up in astonishment and replied, "Why, I couldn't ask a question like that. We aren't very close friends!"

At Levels 3 and 4 there is much more concern for the overall relationship and more desire for open communication. Whether this occurs is another question. At Levels 1 and 2 two inhibiting factors stand in the way. One is the self-centered character of motivation. The

162

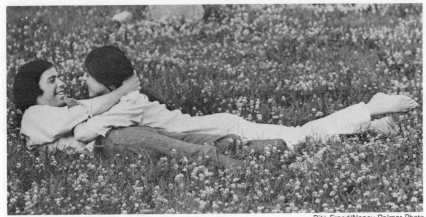

Rita Freed/Nancy Palmer Photo

lack of any special concern for the partner means little interest in communication. The other is the ever-present inability to talk freely about sex itself. In Levels 3 and 4 the first inhibiting factor has pretty largely disappeared. If it is a genuine affectional relationship, the inhibition has been replaced by a desire to support and help the other person. But this too is an inhibiting factor, particularly for males. Most have not been expected or encouraged to speak openly about their sentimental feelings, whether they involve a sexual partner, love for a child, for a buddy (for a buddy most males would never use the word "love"), or for a warm, tender response to their parents. Nor have men learned to express themselves tenderly about sex itself; four-letter words are more their forte. Furthermore, the male is supposed to know what to do sexually without having to converse about it. So men still face difficulty in communicating about sex in ways they would sometimes like, especially at Levels 3 and 4.

Females have not had it easy either. In the past they have had to stand back, often wanting to talk about sex attitudes and relationships with male partners but hesitating because traditionally men should take the lead. For women to take it might result in undesirable consequences. First, the woman would be threatening male dominance. Second, it might make her seem overaggressive and so deeply concerned with sex that her motives might be questioned. The new openness is rapidly altering this, however, and women are finding themselves more and more able to manage their sexuality in harmony with their needs and desires.

Protective Measures and Acceptance of Responsibility A survey of both motivations and aspects of communication show how these two personal characteristics change from level to level on the intercourse continuum. The same is true for protective measures and the acceptance of responsibility. As motivations become each-other centered, these changes occur.

163

Protective measures include contraceptives for the prevention of pregnancy and prophylactics to prevent venereal diseases, the utilization of knowledge which will help ward off threatening possibilities, and effective communication. These measures are emphasized for this reason. Personal and sexual fulfillment will come, not through denying or renouncing all sexual expression but through exercising personal and group responsibility. This becomes increasingly clear as knowledge and control over sexual associations are utilized by more and more persons. Situations that arise through the irresponsible use of sex can and often do cause much unhappiness and many regrets. Experienced counselors have noted that whenever people think they have been protected and responsibly dealt with, they are appreciative and pleased.

At Level 1 and in many of the associations at Level 2 protective measures are solely for self-protection. The man will use the condom or other prophylactics to prevent venereal infection. The woman is concerned with preventing pregnancy and uses a diaphragm, the pill, or an interuterine device. In any event in most Level 1 and 2 contacts each person is usually on his own. Neither cares particularly about the other, as these comments illustrate. "I (a female) have the feeling that I've caught the clap but I didn't say anything to him (a recent sex partner) about it. It's up to him to protect himself." "I (a male) figured she had been over the road before and could take care of herself. So I didn't pull out, nor did I use a condom. It was her life, not mine."

The long-existing double standard has traditionally shifted the burden of responsibility to women. Using this concept the woman is held to be accountable for upholding moral standards. Males are not expected to observe the same rules. In one rap group some discussion occurred concerning a "gang bang"—a situation in which males one after another have intercourse with a single, willing female. After the last one had finished and was adjusting his clothes, he turned to the girl and asked, "Don't you have any morals?"

Protective measures and responsible conduct in casual associations become complicated when partners have different motives and expectations. One partner may simply be hoping for an enjoyable experience; the other may want the same but also hope that a long-lasting relationship will result. The one with the stronger attachment may think that there is more affection than is the case. The more emotionally involved partner may feel exploited or "used" and think the other unfair. He or she may feel hemmed in and possessed.

Sometimes subtle (or not so subtle) hints about spending more time together or the possibility of marriage occur. Thoughts that pregnancy might make marriage necessary may be entertained. The male or female may no longer take precautions against pregnancy, the female may pretend pregnancy, or pregnancy may actually occur. The crisis that follows will doubtless alter the relationship drastically.

People tend to hope for too much from a relationship in too short a time. Even people who seem matched from the first still have much to

learn about one another. The best safeguard is honesty and straightforwardness about expectations and the satisfactions one finds in the
association.

One of the best protections for both sexes is adequate knowledge
about sex, about themselves, and about the other sex. The traditional
practice of trying to keep youth "innocent" by keeping them ignorant
leads to disaster over and over. The following is an example of how not
being "innocent" can pay off. Contrast this girl's experience with that
of others you have known.

*My parents were very open about sexual matters. With two older brothers
and a sister, there was nothing we couldn't talk about. We saw and
discussed movies, read books and commented on them, and thoroughly
analyzed situations as they involved friends and relatives in the community.
Moreover, our friends knew this, and at times they were included in the
conversation. As a consequence, though I didn't realize it at the time, I was
never pushed by anyone to enter a sexual relationship nor were my brothers
or sister so far as I know. Actually the other kids asked us many questions,
and we were sex educators for a lot of our friends.*

*At college this background helped as it had before. I never really started a
sex discussion because I felt quite adequately informed anyway, but I did
talk readily if the subject came up. If I told how our parents handled our sex
education, everyone was pleased but astonished. I think the boys I dated
played their hands very carefully. I know one girlfriend told me that one
fellow had told another, "Don't try any sleight-of-hand stuff with her. She's
wise to it all!"*

Enjoying the physical stimulation of the entire body even to the
point of orgasm without inserting the penis into the vagina is a
protection against pregnancy. It is an intensified pleasure also. In our
culture people (particularly males) are taught that unless penetration
occurs and climax follows, there has really been no sexual relationship.
Our semantics, for example, are built on that concept. "Sex" means
"intercourse"—penis in vagina. Ejaculation is spoken of as "the
climax," If there is no ejaculation, the whole experience has been
anticlimactic. "Foreplay" is body touching and contact preceding
intercourse, not a part of it. "Play" is a better word. It would include
the joyousness couples find in loving, whether or not penile penetration occurs. In fact intercourse might be anticlimactic. Our language
focuses far too heavily on the physical aspects of sexuality and too little
on the emotional.

Cultivating the sensitivity of the entire body has another advantage
for both men and women. It helps to extend sexual activity throughout
life. Men in particular will find this much to their advantage, for the
genital reactions as experienced in youth slow down with aging.
Erections are harder to attain and are less prolonged; orgasms are
reached more slowly and lack the intensity of those experienced in the
teens and twenties. But the pleasure of touch and physical closeness
between partners who enjoy each other means more and more with
each year that passes.

The Principle of Fair Play

Whenever discussions about sexual conduct occur, questions about morality will be raised. The common ones are, "Is this right?" or "Is that wrong?" It is well that they are, and we will consider them also. Often these discussions take a traditional cultural or religious approach. Generally some type of authority tells us how we should conduct ourselves. This code of behavior gains its authority from antiquity, and the implication is that it should remain unchanged.

This is not our approach to morality, but we feel the views we have presented represent a sound framework for moral decision making. Instead of thinking of an inflexible code of behavior and specific acts, certain basic principles should be kept in mind in decision making. These principles are applicable to all aspects of behavior, though our concern has been with sexual conduct. A major problem is that sexual morality has not been regarded in the same way as the rest of our behavior. This results in many contradictions, which can be eliminated when all conduct is judged by the same standards. This can occur when various principles based on an understanding of human needs and desires are used in analyzing behavior and decision making.

We will discuss one very important principle—the principle of fair play. All others are subordinate to it. It can be stated this way: No person should intentionally use any human capacity—his intellect, physical strength, creativity, sexuality—in a way that would put any living individual—or one yet to be born—at a disadvantage. With this principle as the foundation for ethics, one then stands firmly and steadfastly against the misuse and exploitation of himself and others.

Moral attitudes and behavior are to help people wherever they live to survive with dignity and satisfaction. Day by day the world is becoming more and more interdependent. People from different cultures and races are now able to meet each other and build and maintain either temporary or long-lasting friendships. Unless people find ways of building understanding, in working together and establishing mutual respect, humankind is likely not to survive. A world-encompassing morality that brings all people and all their capacities under one ethical umbrella is necessary. The principle of fair play is such an umbrella.

We do not have to think in such global terms every time we make a sexual decision; it does mean, however, that each person is a part of humanity and therefore has more to think about than himself. If we use the principle of fair play, decisions are no longer precise and clear-cut. Sexual intercourse outside of marriage or participation in casual relationships will elicit differing opinions from people who are quite important to the decision maker. Each individual will have to learn how to reconcile differences in his own mind and how to balance desirable or undesirable forces one against another.

Even in days when decisions seemed simple—"right" versus "wrong"—they were never actually so. But today it is even more complicated. In very few situations will it be possible to satisfy every person or every existing principle. But here we add another important principle—one that will provide direction: when the short term has to be balanced against the long term, the best decisions are those that help more and more people over time to reach out to one another in understanding and with confidence.

Actually a number of points that can be crystallized as principles have now been made. Four illustrations are (1) moral decisions must be based on knowledge and understanding; (2) effective communication is an important first step in decision making; (3) when partners have differences in expectations that they have not expressed, trouble may follow; (4) the extent of emotional involvement conditions human behavior in many ways.

TAKING ACTION

Develop several principles that will apply to sexual decision making. Make them not simply a word or phrase, but state them in complete sentences as in the preceding paragraph. Then apply them to issues and disputed points concerning sexual choices and conduct.

Perspectives on Unwanted Pregnancy[3]

It was only a hundred years or so ago that medical scientists ascertained that the days midway between the menstrual periods were the days when conception was most likely to occur. Until then the occurrence of pregnancy seemed to resemble a lottery. With knowledge about the optimum period for fertilization and the control that came as contraceptives were developed, couples have found it more and more possible to decide when they want conception to occur. They can then act on that desire with hope of success.

Medically it is now possible to determine when ovulation has occurred and to time intercourse so that pregnancy is likely when wanted. Along with such knowledge, we are learning more about optimal conditions of pregnancy and birth, stimulation of infants, the role of father as well as mother in child rearing, and so on. We are becoming aware of the urgent need for educating for parenthood.

This expanding awareness has another dimension—the unwanted pregnancy. With scientific and medical developments such pregnancies are largely unnecessary. The overriding concern is the future of the unwanted child. The usual discussions about an unwanted pregnancy focus upon the pregnant, unwed girl and what choices she has before her. Sometimes concern is expressed for the father, but usually the pregnancy appears to be another example of the Immaculate Conception. The father is usually ignored, bypassed, and according to his own view delightfully or forlornly forgotten.

Until the pregnancy has actually occurred, even more ignored is the

---

[3]The physiological and technical details of pregnancy are better known than are the mental-emotional health aspects. Therefore we have chosen to emphasize the latter. The former are readily available in books and pamphlets. Several are listed at the end of this chapter. See also footnote 1.

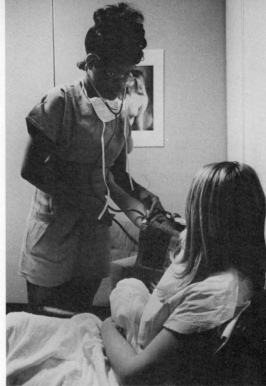

Abortion clinic.

Al Kaplan—DPI

fate of the unwanted child. It is brought into the world with no awareness of what lies ahead and certainly with no voice in the matter. In the end this may turn out well for the child, but if it does, it will take the careful planning and effort of a good many people.

An unwanted pregnancy can hardly take place without involving various family members, relatives, and friends. These people may be involved in many ways; some will be helpful, others definitely not. Some may spend time trying to assess blame for a situation that can no longer be changed; others may suggest alternatives with varying degrees of objectivity and emotion. Parents or others may find themselves caught in making financial arrangements. Persons outside the family may be approached for counseling, legal, or medical help. On the other hand, the couple, or the girl alone, may attempt to stumble through this morass unaided. Of course, the best way to deal with unwanted pregnancy is to avoid it in the first place, if not by abstinance, by nonvaginal play or contraception. However, if it does occur, the four options most commonly mentioned are the following.

1. *Abortion.* This option has been much debated in the last several years. It has been used for ages but in the past was fraught with danger for the woman. In many societies and groups abortion is illegal or, if not illegal, strongly disapproved. As a result abortions have been done surreptitiously, and often by persons who were completely unqualified. The unsanitary conditions under which such abortions often occurred added to the danger.

The circumstances were further complicated by the secrecy that surrounded the act. Since those involved feared to talk, the diagnosis of pregnancy often came much later than it should, particularly if abortion was to be the option chosen. All this added to the danger, cost, and inconvenience and likewise made other arrangements more complex.

There is now more openness about abortion, and medical techniques have been developed so that abortion in the first 12 weeks of pregnancy is a routine and legal though still controversial procedure. Physical complications seldom occur at this time. For many years the most common method was called "D and C" (dilation and curettage). A general anesthesia was usually given, after which the opening to the uterus was dilated. Then the lining of the uterus was scraped with the curette, a spoonlike instrument, until all fetal matter had been removed. The procedure ordinarily takes around 15 minutes. The woman can return home the same day and be back at work within a day or two.

Another method is *vacuum aspiration.* This too can be done on an outpatient basis. The cervix is dilated, and a metal or plastic tube attached to a small vacuum pump is inserted into the uterus. Then a vacuum is established, and the resulting suction draws the fetal material out of the womb. This can be done in 5 minutes or less.

A third method, the *saline treatment*, is used when pregnancy has progressed beyond the trimester stage. The physician inserts a needle through the abdominal wall and into the uterus. The amniotic fluid in which the fetus floats is drawn off and is replaced by a salt solution. The fetus is destroyed, labor is induced, and the fetus is expelled. This is a more complex procedure than the other two and emphasizes the importance of early diagnosis if abortion is contemplated.

The selection of abortion as an option has other complexities as well. Currently a bitter controversy has arisen around its legal and ethical implications. There are those who argue that a woman should have the right to control her own body and to decide whether she wishes to bear the fetus she has conceived. Then there are those who see the fetus as an already living child and argue that destroying the child is killing a person. Handling feelings of guilt, coping with the sense of being legally forced into an intolerable situation, dealing with family dissension—all these and still others may be part and parcel of choosing abortion. Still, many risk abortion even though effective means of contraception are available.

2. *Keeping the child.* More and more unmarried mothers apparently are deciding to keep their babies. It may be argued that the child was actually wanted, or it may indicate simply that the mother's view changed as the pregnancy progressed. The motivations for keeping the child may vary greatly just as will the outcomes. The many girls in early adolescence who are keeping their infants is a disturbing circumstance. The reasons voiced by a girl in such a situation for keeping the child, her financial inability to support it, her lack of emotional

support—these almost always suggest hard days ahead for all. Many of the "child mothers"[4] see the future through rose-colored glasses, however. To them, keeping their offspring is the "right" thing to do. Many of them have been reared in poverty and have lived lonely, isolated lives. Keeping the child therefore serves two purposes. First, they feel it gives them something to live for. Second, it seems to serve as a form of "love insurance" for the mothers.

Today there are over a million women in the United States who, as unmarried mothers, head one-parent families, and half of them are teenagers. Admittedly the picture painted here is a bleak and unhappy one, especially for the babies, who are often mistreated because of the mother's ignorance of child care and development. Undoubtedly some women, especially those in later adolescence who have a better education and/or supportive parents, can be more successful as mothers. Still, for the sake of those immediately involved and for society itself a more responsible attitude toward sexual activity is needed.

3. *Entering marriage.* If the child was unwanted, then entering marriage means simply another "unwanted" situation. This has long been a solution, with the rationale being that marriage would erase the stigma of illegitimacy and provide the child "a name." In some states birth certificates are now issued with no indication of illegitimacy if such was the case. Community opinion has also mellowed a great deal. For this reason the urgency to marry to avoid the "illegitimate" label has eased.

If marriage does occur, it should be a desired union. The couple should also have the maturity and a degree of readiness that offers it a reasonable chance of succeeding. What all too often happens in a forced marriage is that the couple remains together for several years, has more children, and finally abandons the marriage anyway. Under such circumstances every year only adds to the disastrous consequences of an event that was a mistake from the beginning.

4. *Adoption.* This solution has been more used in the past than currently, since so many mothers are now keeping their children. Although an emotional wrench is often involved in giving up a child, the solution may be the best one in the long run for many unwanted children. Certainly there are more requests for children to adopt than there are children available. This is a reflection of the greater readiness among those interested in adopting children to disregard racial and ethnic barriers. These lines are now being crossed with increasing frequency.

TAKING ACTION

1. Prepare a much fuller report than is given here on one or more of the four options.

---

[4]Lisa Connolly, 1975, *Human Behavior* 4:17–23.

2. Visit child care agencies or homes for unwed mothers to find more about the problems these agencies face. Are there any agencies or counselors working with unwed fathers?
3. Prepare a questionnaire or survey to be used with teenage males. How many are fathers or might be fathers? What would be their attitude toward the girls they made pregnant? A caution: Before you begin this survey talk it over with your instructor to determine whether sponsorship is needed—and if so, its nature.
4. Conduct a role-playing situation. (a) You are an unwanted fetus. You are aware of the arguments going on concerning your future. Voice your opinions about what should be done. (b) You are an unwanted fetus. You have just been listening to the various views and rationalizations of men who father unwanted children, such as "It's the woman's responsibility to prevent pregnancy," and so on. Set up a dialogue around these reasons. (c) You are a male who has fathered an unwanted child. No one has paid any attention to you in the whole matter. Express your feelings and get a dialogue started. (d) You are an unwed mother. Discuss your feelings with a social worker or your parents about keeping your child.

Barriers to the Use of Contraceptives   We have noted that the number of unwanted pregnancies is high and is increasing from year to year, with a disproportionately high number of the women involved in their late teens and early twenties. At the same time we have insisted that very few undesired conceptions need occur if people would make effective use of available information and contraceptive devices. What then is the reason for the widespread failure to use the knowledge we have?

One problem is that practically everyone has learned to avoid sex as a topic of conversation. Most people feel that references to sexuality, particularly around such worldly matters as the use of contraceptives, is in poor taste, especially in the home. Consequently youth, even those who are sexually active, have no feeling of approval for the use of contraceptives and little information about their use. Without effective contraceptives it is only a short step to unwanted pregnancy.

Many young people avoid purchasing contraceptives even though they know they need protection. "I didn't want it said all over town that I was having intercourse." This diffidence also prevents partners from speaking directly to each other about what they do or fail to do to prevent conception. "I had expected to pull out before I 'came,' but I didn't make it. I didn't mention it to her, though." "I missed my period something like six weeks ago, but I kept hoping I would menstruate. But I just can't keep quiet any longer. I'm going crazy!" When something is amiss, it should be acknowledged at once; the chances are much better then that potential problems can be coped with. If pregnancy is a possibility, measures taken early will be less drastic and have a better chance of success than those taken later.

Inadequate or erroneous knowledge results in people protecting themselves ineffectively. "I had heard that a good hot shower would kill the sperm and make it impossible to knock a girl up. It didn't work." "I thought there were only three days between menstrual periods when the egg could be fertilized. There must be more days than that."

Not only may an individual fail to understand his or her own anatomy, he or she may be even more ignorant concerning the anatomy of the other sex. Moreover, many young people are poorly informed about the effectiveness of methods of contraception. Many a girl has had intercourse with a boy who wore a condom, yet she has never seen one. Nor does she know why or to what degree condoms are effective. A boy may feel everyone is protected if, when he asks a girl if she is taking the pill, she replies yes. He may not know whether she started the day before, whether she has been taking them consistently, or whether they were prescribed to fit her needs.

Some young couples are now going together to doctors or clinics where birth control methods are discussed and prescribed. With both being a party to the planning, they know how each is involved in effective birth control. This sharing should be encouraged, for responsible planning includes both male and female; it is not the responsibility of one person alone.

All contraceptives depend on proper use for their effectiveness. Sometimes one or both of the partners are so eager for intercourse that they "cannot" wait for better circumstances or even to use the time they have effectively. Putting a condom on hastily, inserting a diaphragm haphazardly, or forgetting to take the pill can easily mean failure. Some females are hesitant to touch their own genitals and so avoid the use of any contraceptive measures requiring this.

Casual intercourse often takes place under unfavorable circumstances. This is one of its problems. Intercourse should occur only when adequate time is available, when there is no fear of discovery, and space and circumstances permit the proper use of contraceptives.

Everyone uses rationalizations to excuse what he does. In automobile driving an attitude toward accidents is clung to with great persistence: "It won't happen to me!" This same rationalization holds concerning unwanted pregnancy, and it is one that certainly blocks any effective use of contraceptives.

Still other myths interfere with the effective use of contraceptives, for example, the desire for pleasure and spontaneity. Obviously sexual intercourse can be very enjoyable, but it is also a forbidden fruit. As a result people are in conflict and so seek ways of enjoying the fruit while pretending they found it just by chance. This results in the argument that "we were so carried away by passion we had no chance to plan. We were just swept off our feet." Spontaneity and pleasure in having an enjoyable experience is certainly not violated by planning. If one wishes to play in the fresh-fallen snow or cavort in the falling rain, there is no argument that dressing to protect oneself from the cold and wetness spoils spontaneity.

Sometimes conflicting attitudes distort motives and block effective contraceptive procedures. A male may insist he doesn't want to produce a pregnancy yet continually wonder about his own ability to reproduce. In the end he proves his capacity by causing a pregnancy. Rather than seeking to prevent pregnancy, he feels a sense of achievement when it occurs. This attitude is a significant one in cultural groups emphasizing the "macho" image for males.

A female may insist that she wants no pregnancy. However, she may simultaneously feel that if a pregnancy should occur, then the marriage she desires will follow. Whatever its disadvantages, being involved in a pregnancy may also be taken as an evidence of maturity. In the eyes of society, once a young person (male or female) is involved in a pregnancy, he or she is no longer a child. These people are now regarded as adults, perhaps prematurely and without a full realization of what is now demanded of them, but nonetheless they are adults. Some females may feel very guilty over participating in intercourse outside of marriage. As a consequence they punish themselves and dispel their guilt feelings by becoming pregnant. In this way they atone for misconduct and are punished for what they have done.

TAKING ACTION

In cooperation with your classmates draw up a checklist of motives used as reasons for failing to use contraceptives. Give it to individuals or groups and present your findings to the class.

FURTHER SEXUAL CONSIDERATIONS

Sexual concerns have moved far from the concentration that formerly focused attention on physiology and heterosexual intercourse; many new and varied concerns are now being given considerable thought. We can consider only a limited number in this section. You should, however, be aware of this ever broadening and expanding range.

Changing Concepts of Masculinity and Femininity

What is required in being a man? What does it take to be a woman? Until a few years ago this knowledge could be rather neatly packaged and distributed quickly to all who wanted to know. There were a few people, of course, who didn't fall neatly into a particular package, but they were considered oddballs and not acceptable models for others to follow. Of course, in other cultures role patterns were different, and well-informed persons knew that. But these were strange arrangements found in other societies and not really suited to an advanced civilization like ours.

The views in the preceding paragraph expressed the attitudes of many people only a few years ago. Even now many feel that role concepts and patterns have become "unglued," and undesirable consequences have resulted, with probably even more serious ones to follow.

A clearer understanding of what is happening now may come by tying in a bit of historical knowledge. Down through the ages women have been discriminated against in many ways; in relation to men they have been placed in a subordinate role. Thus "woman" means the "wife of man" and the implication seems to be that there is no such thing as a woman separate from wifehood.[5] Man has been physically stronger than the female. This, plus the fact that women during their reproductive years were often pregnant and occupied in caring for children, simply meant that men have been in a position to work out social arrangements that fit masculine wishes and needs. Even though they were subordinated, women contributed to society in many ways, through locating and preparing food, making clothing, cultivating herbs and grains, and working with basketry and weaving. They sometimes assisted men in hunting; they even aided them at times in warfare. But the woman's unique and indispensable role was to bear the man children.

In the sexual field, throughout recorded history women have been more discriminated against than men. We noted that in prostitution the legal penalties have typically been assessed against the woman. She has been the one prosecuted, not the man. Under the double standard the female has been severely faulted for the same sexual behavior for which the male achieved recognition from other males. Generally, not nearly such strong demands for virginity have been placed on males. In rape cases the woman has had to prove her sexual virtue, and if she had violated conventionality in any way, the man could go free. This approach is only now changing. Traditionally the penalties for adultery have been much more severe for the woman than for the man. Also a menstruating woman has been considered "unclean." Even in the New Testament this uncleanliness existed for seven days after menstruation, and anything she touched, sat on, or lay on became unclean. She was therefore essentially an outcast during this period. If any man had intercourse with her, he was unclean for seven days also.

The conditions cited come from the distant past, but there are illustrations much nearer in time. In 1881 men were told in an etiquette book:

> When addressing ladies, pay them the compliment of seeming to consider them capable of an equal understanding with gentlemen . . . they will appreciate the delicate compliment. . . .[6]

Even now, women are taught to be passive and subordinate to males. This begins when they are children. For example, studies of stories in readers prepared for children in the lower grades have found boys pictured as innovative, imaginative, and active even in childhood. Girls, on the other hand, usually stood back, watched, and admired the males. They often asked for male assistance in even the simplest tasks.

---

[5]Vern S. Bullough, 1973, *The Subordinate Sex*. New York: Penguin Books, p. 3. This history of attitudes toward women provides worthwhile supplementary reading for both men and women.

[6]Cited by Judson T. and Mary G. Landis, 1973, *Building a Successful Marriage*, 6th ed. Englewood Cliffs, N.J.: Prentice-Hall, p. 13.

The highest praise any girl could receive was to be told that she behaved as competently as a boy.

In the past century many things have changed, yet women even now find the cards stacked against them in many ways. It is only in recent years that educational opportunities have become more available. The right to be freely admitted to a college or university of one's choice came slowly to females. Scholarships and grants have gone more readily to men. At one time the question arose as to what educational degree should be conferred upon women. The awarding of a bachelor's or master's degree did not seem proper, so for a time such degrees as "Laureate of Science," "Maid of Philosophy," or "Mistress of Polite Literature" were conferred.

A serious problem for women still exists in the business world. For many years and in some states a married woman could not own property in her own name. Even now laws on this matter vary from state to state. The extension of credit or charge accounts to a married woman had to be approved by her husband. This is still the case under certain circumstances. Many other instances of legal discrimination against women can be found in the business world.

Vocationally men have had many more career openings available to them; the woman's role has been that of being a housekeeper, wife, and mother. Throughout the early years of this century there were few places for women in the work force. The range of occupations acceptable for women was limited. For example, they could be teachers (men were the administrators), clerks in stores (men were the managers), librarians, and nurses. Even when the jobs were essentially the same, women were paid lower salaries than men. Women either did not receive promotions, or if they did, their promotions were fewer and given after longer periods of time.

Within the home the major portion of child care was the mother's responsibility. Biologically, of course, only the female can breast-feed the child; beyond that, however, loving, playing, indulging in little jokes, listening to childish secrets, kissing a hurt finger, and tucking the child in bed were all essentially the mother's responsibility. The man could love the child, but as a man should. He might say, "Be a big boy. Big boys don't cry," or "You're going to be a little rascal." He was decisive: "Father's word is final." Discipline was the father's province: "Wait until your father gets home." This description was not true for every family, but neither is it a caricature.

According to custom the female should be appropriately ignorant concerning sex. Her concern was in establishing a relationship; one of her main objectives was "to hook a man." Since women were supposed to be innocent and before marriage sexually uninitiated themselves, they often expressed the desire to marry a sexually experienced man. Males were expected to be interested in the genital aspects of sex and, through prior experience, would know what to do. In this way female naiveté would be both appreciated and overcome at the same time. The double standard accepted this as a legitimate distinction between male and female behavior. For the men, however, it gave them freedom to experiment sexually without being severely criticized.

A few decades ago all this was more easily accepted by women since their expectations were at that level. For example, their education had not led them toward professional lives or business careers. Women are now moving toward a new social position. Although many of these inequalities still exist, women are now protesting them—asserting, even demanding, their rights. Erasing these inequalities is an important plank in the women's movement. Once this is achieved it will surely be to the advantage of both sexes. Not in large numbers as yet, but women are functioning successfully in virtually all professional, technical political, service (for example, police), and construction occupations. There are even women jockies, wrestlers, football players—and as of 1975, a professional league baseball umpire!

This has not been a women's movement alone, however, It has affected men as well. At times and in certain ways men feel restricted and discriminated against too. There is no formally organized men's movement, though here and there small local liberation groups are found. Males generally see their problems from a different angle than do women. Their dissatisfaction most often centers upon being walled in emotionally in other ways. They are concerned with the rigorous demands that they be aggressive, competitive, achieving, and unflappable in any emergency. They hesitate to express tenderness and sentimental feelings.

Many men regret these stereotypes. While the desirable male stance is to "be tough" and "play it cool," these men are asking something more: "If a man wishes to cry, why can't he?" "If two men love one another and wish to kiss each other, why not?" Some men want a very different role in child rearing. They feel that the typical pattern pretty largely excludes them, except as they become "strong men" or disciplinarians. Would not children, and society itself, profit by having men

Women's lib demonstration.

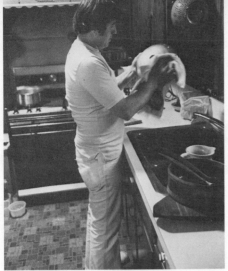

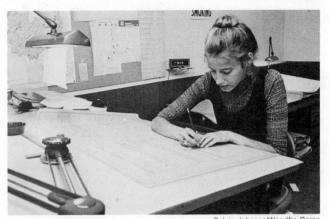

Richard Kalvar/Magnum Photos   Sylvia Johnson/Woodfin Camp

who could express their tenderness more openly? These are questions that some men are asking; these are ideas on which a few are acting.

Occupationally men have moved into activities formerly reserved to women. Male kindergarten teachers, nurses, telephone operators, dressmakers, typists, and stenographers have been featured in news stories. In some instances husband-wife roles have been reversed. The wife has moved into some professional or business occupation, while the husband has assumed the role of househusband.

An excellent illustration of the complexity of some new developments is the readjustments that became necessary as young women entered the sports world. For a girl to go down to the corner lot and play ball with the boys was not too much of a wrench. Something more was involved though when she wanted to play in Little League. When she wanted to participate in high school and college football, basketball, track and baseball, a great deal more was at stake, particularly if males and females were to be treated alike. As college sports like football and basketball became "big time" events, the income from admissions assumed great importance. The money was used to provide male teams with first-class equipment and athletes and their coaches with chartered planes for trips, medical care, and other needs. Thus while women held cake sales to get the equipment they needed, the men were able to dip into the cash register and use the money paid as admissions to equip themselves. Was it right, was it equitable for women, when their sports did not pay their own way, to ask for an equal division of the money? Was it right, when they have not been provided sports activities and have been accorded only the role of cheerleaders, for women to be denied these funds for their sports? This became a significant issue.

What arrangements are needed before something becomes a woman's sport? Do both sexes play on the same team, or do we have men's basketball and women's basketball teams? Will intramural sports do for one sex while the other engages in an intercollegiate schedule?

Here, of course, erasing discrimination is far past the "change in attitude" concept. Can we hope that the various revisions in role patterns will produce men and women who are proud and pleased to be male or female but are not mere puppets to existing role models? Can we agree that we need intelligent and outreaching women, men who can feel deeply and express their emotions, individuals who are first of all genuine, loving human beings and secondarily male or female? ["Androgynous" (Greek, male and female) individuals are people who behave as they deem appropriate to the situation rather than as stereotyped "male" or "female" behavior dictates.]

TAKING ACTION

1. *Conduct a survey among students to ascertain attitudes toward the arrangements they would like to see exist in sports as they relate to feminine participation. Extend this survey to high school students or to older people (your parents, for example). What problems do coaches emphasize?*
2. *Do you see any problems arising as women are taught, as men have been, to get into the highest-paying, top-rung occupation?*
3. *What problems will arise as men express tender and sentimental feelings openly? Can men hug and kiss each other publicly or walk down the street holding hands? Conduct a survey to find what attitudes exist toward this kind of masculine behavior.*

Same-Sex Attraction and Experience

For the general public homosexuality is usually defined as an attraction towards members of one's own sex, with a heavy emphasis laid on genital relations. While we will accept this definition, we plan to push beyond it, laying a heavier emphasis on emotional ties and a deeply caring relationship. The emotional aspect should be recognized as essential in any prolonged homosexual association. Certainly there are numerous casual genital contacts; this we all know. Then too some people are deeply attracted to other same-sex individuals with whom they have never had genital relations. Genital involvement may not have seemed feasible for one reason or another, even though one or both might have desired it. These people are expressing a homosexual attraction, however.

Generally people are friendly to one another simply because they are human beings, not because of genital anatomy. This is especially true of children. As they grow older, they receive increasing pleasure from the sex organs, and genital contacts that permit touching and physical closeness become more and more meaningful. Depending on past experiences these can come from same-sex or other-sex persons.

There is a continuum for homosexuality that duplicates the intercourse continuum used earlier. Persons who have little familiarity with how individuals with homosexual preferences relate often feel that the big majority of, if not all, homosexual associations are either casual or at the exploitative, advantage-taking level. On the contrary, many are tender, loving relationships in which deep, sincere, emotional feelings are expressed. An understanding of homosexual relations is seriously hampered since most people think in terms of common social myths and misconceptions. They try to fit homosexual expression to their prior concepts and as a result arrive at traditional views.

A bit of historical background may help in understanding homosexuality. In ancient Greece a sexual relationship between males was common. Sometimes the partners were the same age. A more idealistic form occurred when an older male selected a boy nearing adolescence and, with the consent of his family, became his sponsor or mentor. This was thought to be the acme of love, ranking ahead of heterosexual love. An older man could have an emotional and sexual relationship with the boy, but at the same time be associated with a woman who bore his children. As the younger man himself matured, his mentor would often help him find a wife, while the younger man in turn became the mentor for still another boy. In Greece this was not thought of in homosexual or heterosexual terms as is the case in our culture. It does dispel the myth, however, that a person must be either homosexual or heterosexual—one or the other.

Interesting illustrations are found today in cross-cultural comparisons, particularly those involving males. A traveler in the Philippines or in an Arab country may well have seen two adult males holding hands as they walked, or when they parted engaging in a warm embrace and kissing each other fondly, lip to lip. This now and then happens in our culture, but a very different interpretation is placed on it here. With all the myths we subscribe to we are apt to regard this as evidence of homosexuality.

The distaste and dread of homosexuality as it exists in American society is demonstrated by a common attitude. Whether male or female, most heterosexual people think it a compliment when they are regarded as sexually attractive by a person of the other sex. If someone of their own sex suggests they are sexually attractive, however, it may be taken as an insult. This is particularly true for males. Why does this occur? This is a matter of social conditioning. Some men learn to accept a homosexual overture as a compliment but simply decline it if not interested—just as women may gracefully decline male overtures.

Far more concern and interest has focused on the homosexual activities of men than of women. Research data, case histories, and general investigation of conditions concerning male homosexual activity are easily found. Much of this reflects the severe disapproval of homosexuality among men. Female homosexuals, or Lesbians, find much more tolerance, even acceptance, than do men. Two women can live together with nobody giving their lifestyle more than a passing thought. Two men doing the same would be regarded with suspicion and probably criticized. Therefore more information is available about male than about female homosexuality. The numbers differ also. About 3 percent of the male population and about 1 percent of the female population are exclusively homosexual.

Data from the Kinsey research indicate that, for some, homosexual activities begin prior to puberty. Many individuals in their late teens and early twenties are still worried over experiences in same-sex genital play occurring in late childhood or early adolescence. They wonder if this indicates homosexual tendencies. The mere fact that it occurred, however, tells nothing. At that particular stage in development many individuals have had same-sex experiences, which the great majority later dropped.

Disregarding prepubertal activity, the Kinsey studies indicated that by age 45 about 37 percent of all men had had at least one homosexual encounter leading to orgasm. For women the corresponding figure was 13 percent.

In his first report Kinsey found that 18 percent of the males in his study had "at least as much of the homosexual as the heterosexual in their history for at least three years between the ages of 16 and 55," while 13 percent had "more the homosexual than the heterosexual" in their histories.[7]

Women too combine heterosexual and homosexual experience but not to the same extent as men. In the second report[8] two comparisons of females and males between the ages of 20 to 35 show the same difference: 4 to 11 percent of the women had as "much or more homosexual experience than heterosexual experience"; for men the percentages were 9 to 32. Those having "mostly homosexual experience" included 3 to 8 percent of the women but 7 to 26 percent of the men. This is to be expected, however, since women have not been permitted to be as sexually active; repression bore down upon them more heavily.

Irrational Beliefs about Homosexuality   A rational, objective understanding of homosexuality cannot come until certain myths are dispelled. Here are five common ones.

1. *Homosexuals and heterosexuals are very different from one another, and this difference can be clearly distinguished by the fact that one has a same-sex partner.* Most people have assumed that one same-sex genital experience serves to classify an individual homosexual. The readiness with which this statement is accepted shows the intense feeling and deep rejection felt for homosexuals. If an individual who had had a number of homosexual experiences now had one heterosexual experience, no one would then insist that that person should now be regarded as a heterosexual.

Data from the Kinsey study were just cited to indicate that both homosexual and heterosexual experiences are a part of the sexual

---

[7]Alfred C. Kinsey et al., 1948, *Sexual Behavior in the Human Male.* Philadelphia: Saunders, p. 650.

[8]Alfred C. Kinsey et al., 1953, *Sexual Behavior in the Human Female.* Philadelphia: Saunders, p. 488.

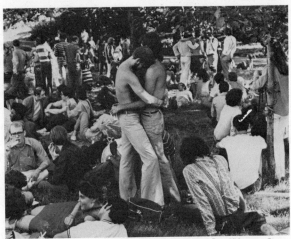

Leonard Freed/Magnum Photos

patterns for many people. With the greater willingness to express sexual preferences and behavior openly, more and more persons also seem ready to say they have had sexual experience with partners of both sexes. Some authorities are now suggesting that all persons have the capacity to respond as ambisexuals (a more accurate term than bisexual) and that in the future there will be more and more of this breaking across gender lines. No firm data are available to establish or disprove these claims; only the future will provide the answer.

2. *One consciously chooses to be a homosexual.* This myth can be answered with the question "Does one consciously choose to be a heterosexual?" Thinking of sexual preferences in this manner, it becomes clear that they are learned, or at least largely learned. One may decide not to engage in the activity associated with his sexual preference, whether it be homosexual or heterosexual, but still the preference is there.

This becomes clearer as we study how these two patterns of conduct are learned. Our society is arranged to encourage heterosexual behavior and to discourage homosexual behavior. Generally speaking, parents, teachers, the mass media, and peers provide cues and arrange situations in which relating to a member of the other sex seems the right or natural thing to do. This begins at an early age when a child is praised for being "a nice girl" or "a big boy." Furthermore, they are urged, sometimes forced, into activities or ways of thinking which are proper for "nice girls" and "big boys." Typically these patterns fit into long-existing sex roles, and they lead toward heterosexuality as the approved sexual pattern. The child is not offered the homosexual role as a possibility, and any movement in that direction is discouraged.

But if this is the case, how does anyone develop a homosexual preference? One answer is, by being unsuccessful one way or another with one's efforts to become a heterosexual! At one time this failure was laid very largely to an inability of the child to experience and adapt to the traditional sex roles. Succinctly the pattern was stated this way. The male homosexual came from a family in which his father was aloof and disassociated himself from the boy or when he was absent. The mother was dominating and demanding. These disturbed relations combined, perhaps with other factors, gave rise to homosexual desires in the male. For the female the conditions were just reversed. This viewpoint has been accepted by many and is still accepted by some. Certainly this pattern is true for some homosexuals, but nobody knows to what extent they are cause and effect.

That concept has been expanded, and various other causative factors are suggested as occurring with some persons. Two comments, one from a female and the other from a male, are illustrative.

I (female) grew up in a home where I had two older sisters, both of whom became premaritally pregnant and so married unhappily. What I heard from them left me determined never to become closely associated with any male. I found a close girl friend whose attitudes and interests paralleled mine in many ways. We loved each other, spent hours together, slept together, and ultimately we became sexual partners. It was a simple and logical movement into Lesbianism.

As a boy I had a father who had many aspirations for me and tried to make the things he liked come true for me. Because of his striking appearance and his athletic ability he apparently had his way with women. He wanted the same for me. I wasn't up to it either in athletic ability or my interests in women. Sexually I matured quite early. By the time I was 15 I had had sex with several boyfriends. Later I had intercourse with girls too but never found that as enjoyable as with males. I liked athletics but not the competition, the roughness, or the continual emphasis on practice. I couldn't live up to my father's expectations, and while we remained reasonably friendly, I decided I must live my own life. By the time I was a high school senior I knew I belonged in the gay world.

3. *Homosexuality represents an illness.* This view comes from at least two sources. The first arose from the idea that homosexuality was the result of hormonal imbalance and it would disappear if the proper hormonal balance was restored. Efforts to treat homosexual patients with hormones had little success, and when a change in sexual interest did occur, there were questions. How long would the change last? What caused it? Was it the consequence of the hormones or of a strong wish to change? Today very little attention is given to the hormonal imbalance theory.

Another belief is that homosexuality is "unnatural" and a mental illness. Since men and women are biologically designed to mate for purposes of procreation, any other use of the genitals was regarded as a perversion or a deviation. As more and more is learned about both homosexuals and heterosexuals and their capacities and effectiveness as persons, this view is falling by the wayside too. We have the story of one psychiatrist telling another that "All the homosexuals I see are sick." The other psychiatrist replied, "And so are all the heterosexuals I see." As evidence of the growing acceptance of the latter view there was the 1973 decision of the members of the American Psychiatric Association to drop homosexual behavior from among its list of mental disorders.

4. *Certain personal characteristics distinguish homosexuals from heterosexuals.* The standard list for males includes a swishy walk, limp wrists, effeminate gestures and mannerisms, and interest in certain occupational fields. The list could be expanded, but the answer would still be the same: some males within the gay group do fit this stereotype, but many more do not. (And some exclusively heterosexual males do!) Some judged by traditional views are very masculine.

Neither do Lesbians fit any particular role pattern. Lesbians are often thought to be very masculine and the terms, "butch" and "dyke," are used to describe them. "Femme" (or 'fem') is used to describe those who play the passive and subordinate role in a Lesbian relationship.

All these are stereotyped ideas and fit only a small proportion of either male or female homosexuals. The evidence continues to mount: homosexuals are people, and beyond their sexual patterns they have the same feelings, emotional needs, desires, and capacities as do heterosexuals. Everybody will benefit as this concept gains acceptance.

5. *Homosexuals are a threat to society in several ways.* An idea persists that homosexuals, male or female, are seductive and in their relations with same-sexed youth will take sexual advantage of them. The prevalence of this view works against placing any known homosexual in a teaching or coaching position or in any other where he might be in close contact with children or youth. No research data comparing seduction activities of heterosexual and homosexual individuals are available, but if they were, we may be sure that there would be advantage-takers in both groups. This issue will have to be decided on an individual basis, however, just as would decisions about honesty or truthfulness. That a particular individual expresses a certain sexual preference does not say what to expect in his relations with others.

The government services, especially the military and other branches dealing with security matters, have long regarded homosexuals as security risks. The point commonly made is that they are subject to blackmail and to avoid blackmail they might reveal any secrets about which they had knowledge. This is theoretically true, of course, in that the homosexual may be vulnerable to threat. The circumstances are not of his making, but so long as the social stigma exists and his job or community standing are in danger, blackmail is possible. The way to remedy this is to change the social situation so that sexual preference can be openly expressed and honestly lived.

More and more it is becoming clear that many of the homosexuals' problems are either created by or made worse by social attitudes. Finding employment, retaining it if homosexuality is known or thought to be the case, finding suitable living quarters, meeting other people with a homosexual preference and openly associating with them—these and other circumstances have greatly complicated the problem of homosexual living. Things have changed for the better in the last few years, but there still are many more changes needed.

TAKING ACTION

1. *Interview persons who have traveled in other cultures to ascertain what expressions of affection they have seen there. Report this to the class.*
2. *Look into the gay situation in your community. Are there counseling facilities to help homosexuals find a place in the community? Could they be hired as teachers? Are there places where they can meet? Would they be accepted in a church? Is the prevailing attitude one of accepting homosexuals as they are, or is the desire to change them?*
3. *Ask college males and females if they have experienced a homosexual approach. How did they feel about it and how did they handle it? (Did you have any personal feelings about this as a suggested activity?)*

**Fantasies or
Daydreams**

People very seldom, if ever, mention their sexual fantasies. They are a form of mental sexual activity that almost everyone experiences. However, they are filed away in the darker recesses of the mind—away from the awareness of all, even those closest to us. The fantasizer often feels guilty and tries to repress these imaginative excursions. Repression more than anything else one can do, however, ensures their return. Dealing with fantasies effectively comes from understanding them and the function they perform.

Fantasies, or daydreams, occur about almost everything in life: one's stunning success in his business, profession, or politics, one's capacity as a host or hostess, one's withering sarcasm toward some objectionable person, one's tenderness with a disturbed child, or the profound wisdom of one's comments. And so fantasies occur about sex as well.

Sexual fantasies may result from a variety of stimuli. Some may occur simply as a result of having a fertile imagination and others from those sexual thoughts that drift in and out of mind. They may be provoked by things heard, seen or smelled. This is, of course, an individual matter, for some persons are susceptible to certain stimuli, some to others. Fantasies are very likely to occur as a person engages in masturbation or intercourse.

One researcher[9] found that masturbatory fantasies differed to some extent between males and females. Whether these variations reflect differences in the way boys and girls are taught no one knows. Boys, however, had more fantasies in which they were forcing someone to submit to sexual activity or were themselves sometimes being forced to submit. Sometimes sadistic or masochistic exchanges occurred. Boys fantasized intercourse with more than one female, group sexual experi-

---

[9]Robert C. Sorenson, 1973, *Adolescent Sexuality in Contemporary America.* New York: World Publishing.

ences, and oral and anal intercourse. Girls generally reported fantasies of sexual relations with someone they liked or of being forced into sex. They sometimes thought of inflicting forms of light violence. Some persons, more females than males, can fantasy themselves to orgasm.

Sexual fantasies serve the same functions that our other daydreams serve. First, they are short vacations from reality, safe excursions into territory we are unlikely to traverse. They serve as substitutes for action. Thus they allow some degree of satisfaction for desires that may never be satisfied otherwise. In this sense they relieve sexual frustrations, although they may be frightening at the same time. For example, to image that you are overpowering another for sexual reasons may make you feel this could actually take place. Yet you can fantasize these overpowering situations in other things, as in sports or hand-to-hand struggles, without feeling you will be pushed into doing them. This is another illustration of the fear built up around sex.

In the second place, fantasies also grow out of deprivation. In wartime concentration camps where hunger was always present, there was much fantasizing of food. When a person one loves is absent, one imagines what it would be like to see him, to hear his voice, to touch him. Perhaps if there were more openness about sexuality, sexual fantasizing would diminish.

Fantasies may also center about possible or actual forthcoming events. Thus a young woman who anticipates intercourse immediately ahead may imagine possible circumstances, and dream of conversations that may, or that she would like to, take place. She may rehearse various events several times, thus lessening anxiety and preparing herself to meet diverse situations. (One thing she should remember: the male is likely to be indulging in such fantasies himself. Should they exchange fantasies?)

Kaplan,[10] a sex therapist, notes how fantasies can serve a purpose at one point yet may become a liability at another. Even when it seems a liability, it can still be an asset or at least acceptable to the fantasizer if he can fit it into his total pattern of living. She described the case of a young man, Mr. D, who imagined himself a heroic superman as he masturbated. As an adolescent he intensified his fantasy by wearing a superman costume. When he married, his fantasy during intercourse made him impotent, but he could not drive it from his mind or confide in his wife. With professional help he got the courage to tell his wife about it. She not only took it in stride but was presently turned on by it. As his anxiety declined, the fantasy reoccurred only occasionally.

An exploration for the source of this fantasy took Mr. D back to his own childhood. Then strict childhood prohibitions against expressions of sexuality gave rise to anxiety and guilt. It is likely that these guilt

---

[10]Helen Singer Kaplan, 1974, *The New Sex Therapy*. New York: Brunner Mazel, pp. 217–219.

feelings associated with fantasy were not dispelled but were repressed. They were still there, ready to be attached in some manner to later expressions of sexuality—in this case Mr. D's experience in inter-course.

Fantasies, then, are normal. The need is to accept them as another phase of life that serves a useful purpose.

Love and Sex
We have challenged the traditional view of sex with the hope of expanding traditional concepts and giving them deeper roots. Now we wish to do the same for love.

As a word, "love" is used in many and confusing ways. It has been overused, misused, and misunderstood. It is used in referring to things as well as to people. We say, "I love football," "I love my new clothes," "I love peppermints," and "I love her." However, as is pointed out (Kirkendall and Osborne, 1968):

> Surely not all these "loves" are the same. If we could be more precise in our choice of words, more honest and aware in recognizing our feelings for what they really are, instead of saying "I love" we might more often say "I enjoy," "I desire," or "I get gratification from." Love has become a beautiful, lazy, cover-up word for all kinds and degrees of feelings, selfish and unselfish. "I love you" can mean "I want to dominate," "I want to possess you," "I feel dependent on you," as well as "I care deeply for you." "Making love" often refers merely to petting or physical sex expression, and a "love affair" may involve no love at all.

This is all a part of the romantic view of love, a tumultous upheaval of emotion that apparently comes from the wild, blue yonder. Consider the following (Kirkendall and Osborne, 1968):

> For years it has been portrayed in song and story as "mysterious," "everlast-ing," or "true"; one "falls" into or is "hit" by it. Love occurs "once in a lifetime"; and "your heart knows" when the "one and only" comes along. When love "strikes," everything must be sacrificed to follow wherever it leads. We are told that love will automatically solve problems, and if it is "true love," then "lasting happiness" will follow.

Love has been much exploited by commercial interests. Advertise-ments of all kinds assure you that this perfume will make you irresistible. If you gargle with Listerine, you will become lovable. This deodorant or body wash will make a male "smell like a man" and attract women.

There is a reason for this emphasis on love, however. The stimula-tion, excitement, and responsiveness we give and receive in being near to others is necessary for satisfying growth and development, and, of course, these same experiences provide the foundation from which love grows. So we can understand the enthusiasm for and concern with love. It ministers to one of the deepest needs of humans—the sense of acceptance and belonging. Looked at it this way, love is no longer so "mysterious," nor does it "hit" you. We no more "fall" in love than we "fall" in hate or grief.

Love with meaning is based on qualities of character, such as straightforwardness, sincerity, dependability, consideration, and concern. Friendship can be understood in these terms also. In fact we define love as a deep and abiding friendship, one that has grown so satisfying and fills so many needs that those who are parties to it wish never to give it up. It is a friendship that has become ever more meaningful and ever more intimate.

There is no one particular approach typical of all who come to love others; neither is there a single way for developing friendships. Nor is there one way and only one way for appreciating a beautiful sunset; some will view it calmly and temperately, others rapturously and exuberantly. Yet all enjoy it. Likewise some will form their friendships or love relationships slowly, taking their time and testing each experience and every step. Some may have been hurt in previous experiences and are defensive. They have much difficulty in extending themselves, and if they do they may pull back very quickly if the situation seems threatening. Others admire some particular personality quality or find certain experiences exciting and move into close relationships easily and very quickly.

The "fast movers" are frequently said to be infatuated ("to be made foolish"), and the implication is often that their judgments are questionable. Such relationships are usually expected to be of short duration, and infatuated persons are sometimes said to be in love with love and to ignore reality. Such judgments should not be made offhand, however. There are too many qualifying circumstances.

Whether or not a relationship growing out of infatuation has endurance may depend upon several things. One is the willingness of people to reveal themselves and the extent to which they do. Some people are quite ready to express their thoughts and feelings. Too, there are differences in the accuracy with which people judge personality characteristics in others. Surrounding circumstances are important. Crises, accidents, unexpected events may bring out the best and/or the worst in an individual. For example, Maurice and Emily became very fond of each other as they danced and played in many ways. Then Maurice visited her at her home in another town and had the opportunity to watch her at work (Kirkendall and Osborne, 1968):

> Watching her work with children and seeing how she dealt with parents was a revelation; for me an entirely new personality developed. Her patience, her ingenuity in meeting situations, her straightforwardness with the parents gave me a different view of her. I now realize that actually I had been infatuated, but now I left knowing I loved Emily, and that my values were in a better perspective.

Diagrammatically, Figure 5-2 explains Maurice and Emily's experience. The steep rise in the infatuation curves represents the pleasure

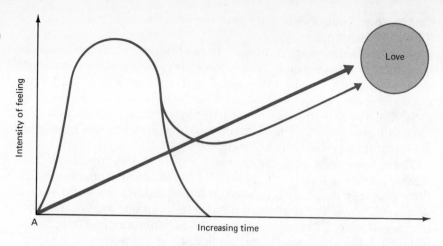

Figure 5-2
The difference between
love and infatuation.

Intensity of feeling

A

Increasing time

Love

they found in social and recreational activities and from physical attraction. The activities they were enjoying to begin with did not have the same significance in building a long-term relationship as those qualities Maurice observed during his summer visit. Had this visit not occurred, the infatuation might have collapsed in the end.

In contrast, everyone has seen relationships in which the infatuation curve fizzles after a time. At first there is "falling in love," physical attraction probably soon leading to intercourse, but then there is an unwinding and a slow moving apart. "No hard feelings, but each of us found other interests and other persons."

Thus far the relation of sex and love has been discussed as an aspect of the physical attraction found in infatuation. There is more to it, however. As noted before, stimulation, responsiveness, and sympathetic interchange are essential for satisfactory maturation. This is possible only as people are in close proximity, can touch, and be near to one another. This involves the highly important fifth sense—skin-to-skin contact, the response that comes through physical nearness. Sexual contact through the sensitive erogenous zones of the body provides the maximum in body responsiveness. So it is no surprise when persons like one another that they feel a physical attraction. This may or may not end in a sexual relationship.

Physical attraction includes other things than simply genital activity, of course. There is the grandparent who hugs the grandchild, friends who put their arms around each others' shoulders, or kisses extended to a loved one. These expressions can and sometimes do move into genital contacts. Customs and family backgrounds have established various boundaries and barriers that limit these outreaching expressions in certain ways. As examples there are differences in age, race, the sex of potential participants, the extent of previous intimacies, or the way and extent to which people are related, as in the case of parent and child, especially, perhaps, father and son. Many barriers are loosening.

Active enthusiastic physical contact is greatly enjoyed in a sexual relationship. Even in casual relationships, Level 2, comments were enthusiastically approving when there was vigor, cooperation, and full-body participation. Actually, at this level physical activity must provide the major portion of the enjoyment. The two illustrations are from Level 2 experiences.

(From a female.) This was a very casual relationship, but very enjoyable. We were both very active, could say freely what we enjoyed, and both had exciting orgasms.

(From a male with a prostitute.) She just lay there. There was no feeling about it at all. I could hardly tell I had had a climax.

While those in love appreciate the physical dimension also, the emotional dimension tends to add greatly to their pleasure. Evaluations of a sexual relationship often refer to the sense of closeness and to the depth of feeling which occurs when the emotional and the physical aspects are combined. When the emotional element is so included, intercourse becomes a part of an even deeper experience. It may occur less, but when it does it may mean more; for example (see Kirkendall and Osborne, 1968).

Happily married couples maintain various physical expressions of affection, usually including intercourse, throughout marriage and into old age. This is a fact that young people often have trouble believing, since physical expression, especially sexual, is so commonly associated with youth. What happens is that as couples live, learn, and grow together, they find many ways of expressing their affection. Their understanding deepens, they plan projects of mutual concern, and they enjoy the same friends. Affection is expressed in a variety of ways, although the physical side becomes relatively less important than it was when the relationship was young.

Broadly speaking, then, love involves relating to the world together. The most satisfying closeness in life often comes from such experiences as working for a common cause, enjoying a poem or a sunset with someone for whom you have a deep affection, and simply knowing that the loved one is near. Antoine de Saint-Exupery in Wind, Sand and Stars *wrote, "Life has taught us that love does not consist so much in gazing at each other but in looking outward together in the same direction."*

Discussion: You as a Citizen and Healthful Sexuality

College and university students reading a chapter on human sexuality directed to them will hardly expect to be addressed as citizens. Yet you are; you are a voter at 18, and as an educated person you are influential in the formation of public opinion. Your influence will increase. Here you can make a needed contribution, for we need better ways of dealing with human sexuality. We need attitudes based on adequate knowledge to cast off taboos that interfere with discussion, interfere with happy human relationships, and prevent sound programs.

News stories dealing with sex appear in print almost every day. They often suggest desirable changes. Yet they are read simply as news, even as curiosities. If one reads them as a citizen, however, one's feelings toward them might very well be changed. Here are some illustrations.

1. The Equal Rights Amendment, the proposed twenty-seventh amendment to the United States Constitution, states that "Equality of rights under the law shall not be denied or abridged by the United States or by any State on account of sex." Though intended to provide women with equal rights, it will also apply to the rights of men as well. Suppose that your state was considering ratification. Would you favor or oppose it? To whom should you express your opinion?

2. In 1974 the city of Cocoa Beach, Florida, passed a city ordinance making it unlawful for women to wear topless bathing suits on the beach. If you had been on the council, what would your position have been? Suppose that the ordinance dealt with men, not women—would that have changed your vote?

3. In Snow Hill, Maryland, in 1975 the advisor for the high school newspaper was removed from her position as advisor. She had failed to stop an issue of the paper that dealt with birth control, contraceptives, and abortion. It advocated sex education beginning in the sixth grade to help prevent teenage pregnancies. Six high school student staff members interviewed doctors, a psychiatrist, social service and public health officials, teenage mothers, and two 16-year-old unwed fathers. The reaction of people in the community was 90 percent negative. Suppose that you were to talk to a group of protesting parents. What would you have said? If you were a member of the school board, what would your position be? Do you have adequate evidence to support your position? Enough nerve?

4. In several high schools the administrators have faced demands that a teacher who is suspected of, or has admitted to, homosexuality be dismissed. No evidence was presented to indicate that the teacher had approached or exploited anyone. Would you approve or oppose these demands? What avenues would be available for voicing your opinion?

5. In Stanfield, Oregon, a farming town and community, the city council passed an ordinance in 1975 assessing a fine against the owner of animals mating where people could see them. (A few years ago, a national campaign was launched to require covering the genitals of all animals in public.) This referred to dogs, cattle, and horses. Suppose you were on the city council, would you have voted aye or nay? Why?

6. In 1975 two WACs in the Army openly stated that they were Lesbians and in love with each other. The announcement was made by Pentagon officials that they would be discharged. The women then said they would take their case to the courts and fight the decision to discharge them. Do you support the position these women have taken? How can you make your voice heard?

7. In several cities the shelves of school and public libraries have been searched for books that have obscene words or sexually explicit discussions. The demand is then made that these books be destroyed. Do you support these demands? If so, to what extent?

The recital could go on and on. The real concern is that informed citizens help in making sexuality a human capacity that can be dealt with like any other.

Thinking of yourself as a citizen, prepare a citizen's platform with several planks that you would like to help achieve during your lifetime. Collect these from other class members to note the scope of their concerns.

FOR FURTHER READING

Hettlinger, Richard F., 1974. *Sex Isn't That Simple.* New York: Seabury.

Interesting to read, with excellent illustrations. Discusses recreational sex, commitment, homosexuality, sexual liberation, and the future of marriage.

Johnson, Warren R., and Belzer, Edwin G., Jr., 1973. *Human Sexual Behavior and Sex Education*, 3rd ed. Philadelphia: Lea and Febiger.

A small book but with extraordinary coverage of historical, moral, legal, linguistic, and cultural aspects of the subject.

Katchadourian, Herant, and Lunde, Donald T., 1975. *Fundamentals of Human Sexuality.* 2d ed. New York: Holt, Rinehart and Winston.

A textbook for human sexuality classes. Covers anatomy and behavior and explores the erotic as expressed in society.

Kirkendall, Lester A., and Heltsley, Mary, 1972. *Understanding Sexuality.*
——, 1973. *Understanding Dating Relationships.*
Kirkendall, Lester A., and Osborne, Ruth F., 1968. *Understanding Love.*
Kirkendall, Lester A., and Tumbleson, William C., 1973. *Understanding the Other Sex.*

These four pamphlets are published by Science Research Associates, 259 East Erie Street, Chicago, Ill. 60611. All are simply written, with case situations used for illustrations. Each deals with a special concern.

Kogan, Benjamin A., 1973. *Human Sexual Expression.* New York: Harcourt Brace Jovanovich.

A textbook on human sexuality, covering usual anatomical and behavioral topics. One chapter on marriage. A delightful style.

McCary, James Leslie, 1973. *Human Sexuality.* New York: Van Nostrand.

Discusses the education of youth about premarital sex, sexual attitudes, and some social issues. The heavy emphasis is on the human sexual system and the sex act.

Morrison, Eleanor S., and Borosage, Vera, 1973. *Human Sexuality: Contemporary Perspectives.* Palo Alto, Calif.: National Press Books.

A reader with selections on new directions in male-female roles, heterosexuality, homosexuality, some public issues, common misconceptions. Emphasis on relationships.

6

pairing and bearing:
for and against

This chapter reviews current trends in family formation, continuance, and dissolution—marriage, parenthood, and divorce—in relation to health and mental health. The impact of improved family planning, abortion, liberalized attitudes toward nonmarital sex, and equality between the sexes are discussed.

Relationship issues in marriage are presented, emphasizing the advantages of delay in contracting a lifetime obligation. Parenthood, similarly, has been accepted for too long as a necessary condition of normal adulthood. Reasons are given for questioning earlier assumptions about timing of the first child, spacing of births, family size, and adoption.

Although changes in the family are anticipated, it is not an obsolete institution. On the contrary, it will probably hold its place as the primary institution of society, but on an improved basis: it will be formed later, by older and wiser young people; it will be smaller, with wider birth intervals; individuals will cope better with each other and the outside community; and society will help families more while hindering them less. A larger proportion of our population will be able to elect nonmarriage and nonparenthood without stigma, and those (still the majority) who choose a conventional family lifestyle will be more likely to do so with truly informed consent.

INQUIRY

1. Doesn't the high divorce rate prove that the concept of lifelong marriage to one person is unrealistic?
2. "My parents would die if they thought I would never have children! How can I make them understand that I have a different set of goals in life?"
3. By allowing young people to live together without benefit of marriage, don't we undermine the basis of family life and the morals of society?
4. Would you rather be widowed or die before your spouse? Why?
5. What should a marriage contract include?
6. Does divorce always mean that a mistake has been made?

Hasn't modern medicine put the family out of business as a health care source? Doesn't new knowledge in many fields of science and health make most parents unreliable teachers and examples for their children? The answers to these questions are partially "yes" but fundamentally "no." The family is still an important source of health education, example setting, and health care itself.

Think for a moment where your patterns of nutrition were established—where your first accidents occurred and how you learned to be careful of life and limb. Where did habits of cleanliness, dental

**FAMILY AND
HEALTH**

care, exercise, and choice of shoes get started? Where did we get our attitudes toward smoking, drinking, and drug use? And last, but by no means least, where did our patterns of forming relationships emerge from? For most of us these patterns were established at home. The family may not be the total health care delivery system—far from it—but your parents laid the foundations, and many of you in turn will do so for the generation that follows.

Is Marriage Hazardous to Health?

Married people are generally healthier than other categories: single, divorced, or widowed. This fact, however, can be interpreted in more than one way and, as with other statistical generalizations, needs to be considered with caution. For example, people who are basically healthy are those who elect to go to the altar. Those with major physical illnesses and mental problems would be less likely to end up married, and thus they would represent a high-risk population for physical and mental illness in the single population. This is more true for men than women, as we shall see.

In the past few years more young Americans are remaining single longer. Since more healthy people have delayed marriage, the average health of the single population as a whole must have improved. It will take considerable time, however, for this recent trend to be reflected in the overall picture. The reason for this is that the married population consists of all persons now married who entered that status through all past years, some over half a century ago. Thus changes that have occurred rapidly in the past few years, affecting mainly young people, will not be reflected in statistical summaries of the whole population for some time to come.

An important phenomenon relating to health status in marriage also has its amusing side. This is the "marriage gradient," which describes the situation in which women marry men who are older, taller, and smarter than themselves. This has been the case in American society for some time: one could call it traditional. Only about one-seventh of the wives in 1960 were older than their husbands, for example. We don't need any research on height in marriage, but we do know that the educational status of husbands generally is higher than that of their wives.

Why do we have a marriage gradient? It derives from another tradition in which men were, and were expected to be, dominant in the home—the protector, the manager, and the boss. In the not so distant past women had few rights in the economic, social, or psychological spheres. It was definitely a partnership of unequals. Nowadays matters have shifted toward a partnership of equals, but the old tenets take time to change, and it is still rather unusual to find a couple, married or otherwise cohabiting, in which the woman is taller, better educated, or older than her partner.

One of the important consequences of the marriage gradient is that in the never-married minority of women and men in this country quite

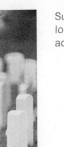

Surviving a spouse is a lonely and difficult adjustment.

Wide World Photos

different characteristics are found. Among spinsters, you expect and do find taller and better educated women than the average for their time. Conversely, among the lifelong bachelors, one finds more who are short, but more important, more who are undereducated and less affluent. To sum up, never-married women are often outstanding among their sex in social and personal achievement, while never-married men are more often on the bottom rungs. This fact is reflected in mental hospital admission rates, which show single men with a much higher rate of serious mental illness than their married counterparts.

The marriage gradient, while amusing in some respects, has contributed to an immense problem among the elderly. Because men are generally older than their wives and because males' life expectancy is less than that of women, wives generally outlive their husbands by five or six years. In the United States we have about 9 million widows but only 2 million widowers. Most wives who are younger than their husbands can expect to live their last years as widows, without the relationship that has been most important to them through their lives. Most men escape the pain and suffering of bereavement, letting it fall to their women.

If you think that it is worse to die first than to be widowed, ask some people in their middle and older years what they wish for themselves and why. Marriage itself is not hazardous to health, but certain patterns of marriage—such as this age gradient—clearly contribute to a variety of health, mental health, and social problems.

Another serious imbalance in relations between the sexes is that traditionally as men grow older, they are freely able and expected to pay attention to all women younger than themselves, whereas women are expected to pay romantic attention only to those men older than themselves. Thus as we age, males have an ever-increasing scope of romantic interests, whereas women have a constantly shrinking scope. Of course, people don't have to abide by popular and prevalent, but unjust, notions of what is proper. But such expectations, even if "unofficial" or unspoken, amount to social pressure, largely to benefit

195

and protect men. First, it protects their prominent leadership status for men to marry downward in age and status. Second, men who are older have a wide range of eligible women to protect them against loneliness and the threat of obsolescence or rejection. Nevertheless, women must suffer these pressures precisely because men do not have to. Finally, men escape the ultimate injustice of bereavement by dying first.

Caroline Bird points out that the marriage gradient "has always been around. What is new is that there are now so many exciting alternatives to marriage . . . that the brightest women no longer have as much incentive to play dumb."[1] Her implication is, of course, that in order to get married many women who were brighter than their partners pretended they were not. It is also quite well known that women with leadership ability had to act submissive even though they often wielded considerable influence in a discreet and covert manner.

TAKING ACTION

Make a survey of at least four people in each of three generations, two of each sex in each generation. Ask them whether they consider it possible for a good marriage to result if (1) the woman is taller than the man, (2) the woman is better educated than the man, (3) the woman is older than the man. For a larger survey set down a number of statements in "true/false" or "agree/disagree" format so that the respondent can simply make a check mark. Analyze the responses by age, sex, and marital status.

Stress, Health, and Illness

In recent years as more understanding has developed about the relationship between emotions and bodily function, a whole new field of psychosomatic medicine has been defined. A number of illnesses are now known to be related to stress, such as gastric and duodenal ulcers, asthma, high blood pressure, and migraine headache. Other conditions are more surprising: tuberculosis, thyroid disease, and diabetes may be influenced by various life stresses. It is often assumed that a variety of mental disorders are also associated with stress, but research in this area is far from conclusive. It is known, however, that many people use medical services of various kinds during stress periods, desperately seeking physical remedies for complaints that stem from problems at home, at work, or in personal relationships. These patients have a variety of vague or specific complaints, for which no physical basis can be found. It is the doctor's job and inclination to exhaust all physical tests in such cases before referring the patient for psychological help. Indeed, that is often the patient's wish as well, and some will not accept a'referral to a mental health professional except as an extreme last resort. Others accept such a recommendation with appreciation and relief. The upshot of the matter is that a great deal of time, effort,

[1]H. H. Hart, ed., 1972, *Marriage: For and Against.* New York: Hart, p. 172.

and money are spent on situations that are essentially stress conditions, most often family-related but unrecognized as such until the physical tests are completed.

In the past decade or so a number of researchers have studied life events and stress in relation to health and illness. They have attempted to find out what kinds of health problems are associated with various events, normal and abnormal, that occur to people either in the normal course of events or as the result of bad luck. Some of the items from one of these tests are listed in Table 6-1. It can be seen that most of the items regarded as stress events are related to family life.

You should not assume that to avoid stresses one should avoid marriage and parenthood (although for some this is good advice). Family life entails stress; so does living outside a family. The stress events of separation, bereavement, arguments, dependency, loss of status, and loss of income are relatively well known and quite familiar to everyone, even those who have not experienced them directly. As a result, people have ways of estimating how serious stress would be, and the agreement of many different classes of observers is very great.

As an exercise, ask people to rank various events in terms of stress

SOCIAL READJUSTMENT RATING SCALE					Table 6-1
Rank	Life Event	Mean Value	Rank	Life Event	Mean Value
1	Death of spouse	100	24	Trouble with in-laws	29
2	Divorce	73	25	Outstanding personal achievement	28
3	Marital separation	65	26	Wife [or husband] begins or stops	26
4	Jail term	63		work	
5	Death of close family member	63	27	Begin or end school	26
6	Personal injury or illness	53	28	Change in living conditions	25
7	Marriage	50	29	Revision of personal habits	24
8	Fired at work	47	30	Trouble with boss	23
9	Marital reconciliation	45	31	Change in work hours or	20
10	Retirement	45		conditions	
11	Change in health of family member	44	32	Change in residence	20
12	Pregnancy	40	33	Change in schools	20
13	Sex difficulties	39	34	Change in recreation	19
14	Gain of new family member	39	35	Change in church activities	19
15	Business readjustment	39	36	Change in social activities	18
16	Change in financial state	38	37	Mortgage or loan less than $10,000	17
17	Death of close friend	37	38	Change in sleeping habits	16
18	Change to different line of work	36	39	Change in number of family	15
19	Change in number of arguments with spouse	35		get-togethers	
			40	Change in eating habits	15
20	Mortgage over $10,000	31	41	Vacation	13
21	Foreclosure of mortgage or loan	30	42	Christmas	12
22	Change in responsibilities at work	29	43	Minor violations of the law	11
23	Son or daughter leaving home	29			

Source: T. H. Holmes, and R. H. Rahe, 1967, *Journal of Psychosomatic Research* 11:216.

and compare that with the values obtained by the original researchers. (This scale was begun with marriage as the midpoint, and many different groups of judges, including college students, agreed remarkably on the relative stress values of various other life events.) Check off those events that have occurred in your life over the past 12 months. A mild life crisis is indicated by a score of more than 150, a major life crisis by a score of more than 300. Onset of illness is much more likely to occur in the presence of increasing life crisis. The Holmes scale is a useful tool in health education with special emphasis on family life and mental health. In some hospital and clinic studies it has become a health education instrument, and patients coming for checkups have found it helpful in gauging the level of stress under which they are living throughout the year. If their score goes up, they can then take steps to reduce the level of stress in their lives in hopes of lessening the chance of exceeding their own stress tolerance, physical or mental.

Prevention, Treatment, and Rehabilitation

Public health defines the preceding terms as primary, secondary, and tertiary prevention. The first is avoiding illness altogether and promoting health. The second is finding cases of disease or incipient illness early on and rendering prompt treatment to cure the ailment before it becomes very serious. The third is the restoration of health to the seriously ill where possible, and the limitation of disability among those in whom the illness has already taken a serious toll.

In all three categories the family is of great importance. Earlier we pointed out that habits of nutrition, safety, cleanliness, and so on are generally established in the home. All of these are related to primary prevention. During the course of life all of us become sick at one time or another, and our first treatment experiences generally occur at home, not in clinics or hospitals. We are nursed back to health from the usual diseases in the bosom of the family. In times past and in other cultures today the extended family—that is, the more distant relatives—were or are actually involved. In some cultures extended family members move into the hospital compound to cook for the patient and allow him or her to enjoy both the company and the customary routines that family members provide. Childbirth at home is a relatively new innovation in our own culture, although it is actually a return to an earlier mode. It emphasizes the normality of a health event. Rooming in at hospitals is also relatively new and not universal, but it enables family members to stay with children to decrease stress of separation, which may only add to the trauma of illness or accident.

In the early years of life by far the most common cause of death and disability is accident. In our society from the first year of age onward to age 35, this is the chief cause of death, the most common being the automobile accident. Young children must be taught not to run in the street and to avoid other hazards of modern life; thus the family plays a role in primary prevention of accidents and the establishment of lifelong habits of reasonable caution in a society in which new dangers are always being introduced—dangers that offset in many ways the advances in sanitation and health care that allow us to live longer. Between ages 1 and 5, accidents kill more children than the six leading diseases combined!

Rehabilitation, or restoring the partly disabled or ill person back to productive functioning, is also affected by family status. Persons do better if they have close and caring relatives to return to. Unfortunately, our society lacks adequate intermediate care facilities. Persons without homes or family support are often caught between prolonged, expensive hospital stays and being relegated to a "human warehouse," such as a poorly staffed convalescent home.

TAKING ACTION

1. *Interview, individually or in front of the group, class members or acquaintances who have experienced any hospitalization or death in the family within the past year. Inquire about the course of treatment, the involvement of family members, and the expectations and wishes of the individual going through the crisis.*
2. *Visit a clinic, hospital, and/or nursing home, and interview staff and patients (who volunteer) about family relationships, strains, and the support that develop during the course of illness and recovery.*

The oldest and most universal of human institutions, the family, is now widely being questioned as a sound and sensible arrangement for the future. More has been written about family life than any individual can read in a lifetime, and no attempt in this chapter is made to be comprehensive. Some themes of current interest will be summarized to give an overview. It must be remembered when discussing statistics on social phenomena that there is a time lag between the events and the publication of data. As a result, rapidly developing trends of great significance may not be evident for some years after they have occurred, and even then interpretation may be complicated. This is definitely the case in U.S. vital statistics and those concerning marriage.

IS THE FAMILY A HEALTHY INSTITUTION?

The *nuclear family* is the major family form in our society and is defined as parents and their children usually living together in a household. The *extended family* includes other relatives—that is, grandparents, uncles, aunts, and cousins. The extended family appears to have lost its influence in American society of the twentieth century. High mobility, urbanization, and economic independence have made it possible for individuals to determine their own futures regardless of the location of extended family members. However, it is also true that with easier transportation and communication family members several hundred or even several thousand miles apart in our country today may be in contact as frequently as extended family members used to be in villages only a few dozen miles apart.

Much has been said to deplore the fragmentation of extended

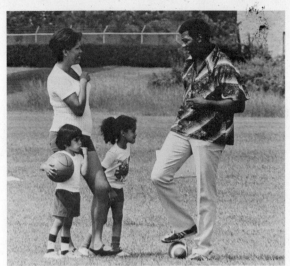

A nuclear family.

Mimi Forsyth/Monkmeyer

families because they represent an important support system. However, the primacy of the nuclear family and independence of individuals from extended family ties can be regarded as an increase in the freedom of personal choice for association and forming of relationships. With the decline of the extended family we also have a decline in clannishness and perhaps an increase in mutual tolerance across ethnic, religious, and social boundaries.

TAKING ACTION

1. *Discuss the allocation of your own current family contacts as compared with those of your parents and grandparents. What percentage of time do you spend with relatives as compared with those in earlier generations? Include telephone time and correspondence. What level of enjoyment do you experience with family and nonfamily associations? What family traditions have disappeared, and which ones still exist or have been newly created (such as the summer camping trip or Sunday bowling)?*
2. *Gather some data on and discuss the merits of extended versus nuclear families.*

Even the nuclear family seems, to many people, to be disintegrating in view of high divorce rates that have occurred in recent years. This phenomenal divorce rate must be regarded in the context of several facts. (1) Marriage in the United States is an almost universal expectation, or has been up until the last few years, with 95 percent or more of eligibles exchanging vows. (2) The most common characteristic of divorced individuals is that they remarry, and usually within a year or two. Dissolution of a marriage obviously does not mean disillusionment with matrimony. (3) The rising consciousness of equality between the sexes, the increase of women in the work force, and new divorce legislation have contributed to the high divorce rate.

Since divorces occur within the total of marriages contracted in previous years, we are witnessing in any one year the demise of

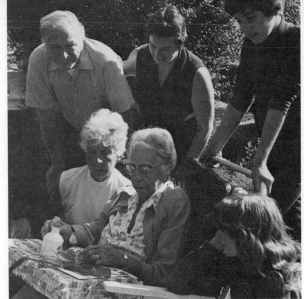

Elinor S. Beckwith

marriages contracted in all previous years. Among teenage marriages, divorce rates are much higher than in older couples going to the altar. In the 1960s and before, a large proportion (40 percent) of teen marriages resulted from premarital pregnancy, usually accidental. The high divorce rate for these young, "forced" marriages affects more than the two parents: most have children too. Since age at marriage is now going up, we can expect that the decisions being made in the very recent years are sounder and will be followed by longer-lasting marriages.

A related phenomenon is delay in parenthood, made possible by such factors as contraceptive technology, better sex education, and the availability of safe medical abortion. Abortion in particular is a crucial health issue affecting marriage and parenthood because the chief users of abortion have been first-time-pregnant (primigravid), single young women who were deliberately delaying parenthood after a birth control failure. As time goes on, abortion should decline in importance while primary prevention of unwanted pregnancy becomes the usual practice. But it is only in the past few years that most first births in the United States were planned for their timing. Until recently many couples were pregnant at the time of marriage, and many others married because of the need to legitimize a birth or to avoid the sin of fornication. Nowadays cohabitation is not so frowned upon—less so, perhaps, than marrying to legitimize sex. When unions are formed, it is for something other than sexual gratification. This phenomenon is in itself a radical departure from the previous basis on which marriages were commonly formed.

Although many people think that premarital sex undermines the foundation of marriage, it can be argued instead that it strengthens the foundation since the decision is made on more rational grounds than could have been the case in the past. Neither argument, however, is more than a generalization, nor can either be applied across the board or in any individual case without considerable knowledge, empathy, and reflection. To urge couples to try sex before marriage is as hazardous as urging them not to. Some couples will be unable to give sex a fair test outside of marriage, and trying it would create an unnecessary failure. Others may find premarital sex good but lose their enjoyment after marriage because for them the excitement of something forbidden was a necessary part of erotic stimulation. (Counseling or psychotherapy is indicated in such cases.) Suffice it to say that directives for or against sex must be replaced by a more tentative approach.

Interpreting Recent Trends

People who are critical of the family in modern society hasten to conclude from recent trends that this doughty and familiar institution may be on its way out. The same trends, however, can be interpreted to mean that there is a retrenchment of the family as the primary, but not uniform or universal, social institution; that is, not everyone should be expected to participate in it in the same way. Thus in the late 1960s and early 1970s the age at first marriage went up, and the number of marriages went down—as did the birth rate. At the same time the divorce rate went up, but so did the remarriage rate. And more couples were living together openly without sanction of legal marriage.

Thus new families were formed at a slower rate, old marriages were broken up at a faster rate, and fewer children were added to families. But a predictable characteristic of people who are divorced is that they will remarry; most do so within a year or two of their divorce. One wit referred to this as "the triumph of hope over experience." In fact it is a testimonial for marriage as a worthwhile institution while showing that some—indeed many—marriages do not work. In a society where more than 90 percent marry, one marriage in three will end in divorce at current rates. It is no wonder that many fail, at least for lifelong marriage. If social pressures in the past had not forced so many people into marriage, especially young marriage, the divorce rate of today would undoubtedly be lower. We can therefore predict that with fewer marriages contracted at an early age and more people being free to remain single, those who marry are more likely to remain so and happily than in the past. Chesterton once said: "Don't blame the ills of the world on Christianity, because it has never really been tried." The same can be said of the nuclear family in America, because until now family formation has been a matter of habit or yielding to social or sexual pressure rather than a mature choice of free and equal adults.

It is indeed remarkable and fortunate that with the advent of good birth control methods (including safe medical abortion for cases in which contraception fails) the birthrates and fertility expectation of young Americans are congruent with zero population growth—that is, a leveling off of population growth so that one generation replaces the next rather than increases the numbers. Thus it appears that the decline in procreative sex (as contrasted with conjugal sex) tends toward stabilization of population—a much overdue societal necessity.

Factors that have contributed to the delay in marriage, which in the long run should have a favorable effect in lowering the divorce rate, are the following: more women enrolled in college, more women gainfully employed, and for a period in the late 1960s more women of marriage-able age than men, as the result of the post–World War II "baby boom." Also, from about 1965 to 1972 the annual absence of a half-million men, mostly single and of marriageable age, in Vietnam had a retarding influence on marriage rates. The movement for women's liberation and the public discussion of alternatives to marriage and parenthood also contributed to these trends.

With all the discussion of increased divorce rates it is helpful to realize that the portion divorced in the population in 1970 was 3.6 percent for men and 5.5 percent for women in the age group 35 to 44. These are people divorced and not remarried, and they are a small percentage of their age group. About five-sixths of divorced men remarry, as do three-fourths of divorced women. Factors contributing to increased divorce, besides a higher personal standard for happiness in marriage, include the increase in jobs and therefore economic independence for women, an increased tolerance of divorce in society (even national political figures can be divorced), and the passage of no-fault divorce laws. Under such a law a couple may end a marriage by mutual agreement without penalty as long as they can settle reasonably the division of property and arrange for the care of children. Such laws are being passed in a number of states, although it should be kept in mind that in states where no-fault divorce is only one of several options one spouse may charge fault against the other but agree to a no-fault divorce in negotiations for a better settlement. Thus the adversary concept may still persist even where no-fault is one of the alternatives. Women who are divorced from their first husbands were married on the average two years earlier than same-age women who are still married to the first husbands. A "rational" remedy would be to set an age minimum at which marriage would occur—for example, age 21, which is the age of "majority" stipulated for certain legal contracts. This would increase maturity at marriage and decrease the major factor associated with later divorce.

Should there be such laws? Would it undermine the structure of family life or improve it? Would it increase nonmarital cohabitation, and if so, with what consequences for individuals and society?

TAKING ACTION

Discuss whether a divorce agreement should be written up by couples entering marriage as a test of rationality. What should it include?

When divorce trends in relation to family forms are discussed, the status of children must be considered. In 1970 about 70 percent of **Children of Divorce** children under the age of 18 were living with their two natural parents, and those parents had been married only once. In other words, being the child of divorced or separated or widowed parents is not so unusual in our population since about 30 percent are so affected. The death of a parent is now rather a rare cause of a child growing up in a one-parent family, whereas divorce, separation, and the never-married state are increasingly associated with this atypical family form. Since 30 percent of children do not live with both their biological parents, they are not as isolated or uncommon as was the case even a short time ago. This is to the advantage of youngsters, since being the child of a divorced couple is hardly a stigma today, even though it is still a difficult hurdle in life to overcome. Various kinds of physical and social handicaps may affect us during our life cycle; at least we can hope that social stigma will not be added to what is already a difficult circumstance.

Because the birthrate has been declining, the average number of children involved in divorce has been decreasing (down to 1.22 in 1971). But because of the vast increase in divorces, the overall number of children involved in divorce is going up, at least as recently as 1971, when it was 946,000. This number represents far more children than can be treated by all the child psychiatrists and psychologists in one year, just as the number of couples divorcing—over 1 million—is far more than can be even briefly evaluated by all the mental health professionals in the country. Most of the families undergoing divorce therefore do not have the benefit of professional counseling or support during this life crisis; this is a matter of concern in regard to health and in particular to preventive psychiatry. In many states, for example, it is required that a lawyer participate in the divorce action, but hardly ever is it required that a health professional or counselor concerned with human relations be involved.

TAKING ACTION

List reasons for and against compulsory evaluation and/or counseling of couples undergoing divorce. Consider the civil rights issue of invasion of privacy along with the possible health and mental health benefits to adults and children. Discuss ways in which the matter could be made discretionary with a judge or with some other third party, such as a trained arbitrator or mediator. Who should pay for such a service? And how should it be organized so as to avoid complications where religious considerations exist? If conciliation is clearly impossible, how can there be economic justice and how can child custody solutions be found? Is there a need perhaps for a subspecialty in the helping professions called divorce counseling? At what age should children have some say in regard to their own custody? Who is best equipped to resolve custody disputes?

**Living
Arrangements**

204

A little known but certainly important change reflecting on the family is the trend in household size since the turn of the century. At that time the average household consisted of five persons; from 1920 to 1950, four persons; since 1960, three per household; and slightly below three in 1970. One in every six households consists of one person living entirely alone. More elderly people live apart from their adult children, and more young people live away from home and "off campus."

In 1970 there were 143,000 unmarried couples (of opposite sex) sharing living quarters. Many of these were widowed persons cohabiting unmarried in order to retain pension or survivor benefits, which would be lost in remarriage. Others were young adults in a trial marriage situation. In all there was a remarkable eightfold increase in reported cohabitation during the 1960s. It is more permissible now to have and to acknowledge this living arrangement: more are doing it, and more people are willing to tell the census interviewer about it. The eightfold increase suggests a radical change in social permissiveness; however, 143,000 couples is a relatively small proportion of the approximately 50 million U.S. households.

MARRIAGE AND NONMARRIAGE

Marriage is a very complicated affair. Much has been written about mate selection, problems of money and sex, child rearing, in-laws, vacations, and how to properly squeeze a toothpaste tube. All of these problems and joys of marriage provide grist for the mill, not only for counselors, business and loan offices, and travel agents but also for novelists, advertisers, and architects.

It is safe to say that the cloud over the institution of marriage in our society is due in large part to the haphazard way in which marriages have been put together, not to an inherent weakness of the marital relationship. It is also a by-product of the fact that practically everyone marries—or has done so until recently in our society.

The Contract

Can we expect teenagers, or very recent ex-teenagers, to make a contract with each other that is supposed to last a lifetime? If at age 20 you decide to marry someone after a year of dating, you are in effect making a contract that is supposed to last 50 years, if you live out your expected span of 70 years. That year of dating might represent 25 to 50 percent of your lifetime dating experience, since not many people start intensive dating before age 16 or 17. It is no wonder that the divorce rate for marriages contracted in the teen years is double the divorce rate for those formed later.

When 95 percent of the population marries, it is no surprise that 15 percent of couples have broken that contract within 10 years. It is perhaps more surprising that 85 percent are not broken. In recent years there has been a delay (an increase in average age at first marriage), with an attendant increase in the proportion not married at subsequent ages and ultimately an increase in the proportion who will never marry. This represents an expansion of personal alternatives: if you marry at an early age, you lose the nonmarriage alternative (the same applies to

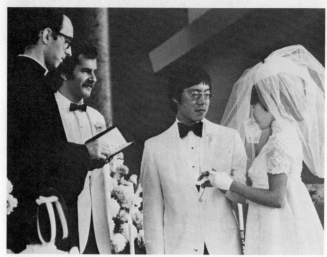

Phiz Mezey—DPI

parenthood and many other choices). If you remain single longer, you
keep options open either for marriage or nonmarriage. This may seem
obvious; but over the years marriage was socially impressed upon
people as the only way to go through the adult years (the same for
parenthood). Only in the current decade can it be said that nonmarriage
and nonparenthood are serious and unstigmatized alternatives that can
actually be implemented without, for example, being considered
abnormal or being a hypocrite.

Obviously, making nonparenthood and nonmarriage viable alternatives required both technological and social progress: effective birth
control for the former and acceptance of alternative lifestyles for the
latter. If we accept the fact that many people who wish not to marry at a
given time have normal sex drives, what options do they have? Until
recently abstinence was the only socially approved choice (not even
masturbation). Nonmarital cohabitation is the current description of
what in the past would have been called "living in sin" or "fornication." Having acceptable alternatives for healthy sexual expression, for
intimacy, to be able to form an important and perhaps lasting heterosexual bond without matrimony does not necessarily detract from the
institution of marriage. On the contrary, the denial of such alternatives
forces into marriage people who should have time and experience to
make a mature, informed choice rather than be forced to conform in
order to enjoy any intimacy at all.

In days gone by, although few would admit it, people were motivated to marry in order to have legitimate sex. With cohabitation more
accepted, marriage no longer has that as a major motive. All the more
remarkable, then, that people who cohabit often go on to marry. This
gives the lie to the caustic aphorism "Why buy a cow if you can get free
milk?"

As an illustration of trends in family formation (a formal term for marriage, with or without children) ascertain the approximate ages of your grandparents and your parents at the time they married. Choose, if possible, the date on which they were married for this exercise. Look up a major newspaper and a local newspaper or magazine of that date in a library, and read it thoroughly with attention not only to news stories but to advertising, obituaries, features, and editorials. Thus you may better be able to reflect upon lifestyles at the time in which your family of origin was being established. Look in particular at newspaper items relating to health, heterosexual relations, and family life. Write out a plausible marriage contract that might have reflected the actual views of partners being married at those two dates separated by a generation.

The Pleasure Bond

Given that sex, even ideal sex, is not the driving force in getting married today, we nevertheless must look at sex as an important factor in keeping the intimate relationship together.

In spite of all our knowledge, the ways of body and mind are still mysterious. We do not know why sexual fidelity is important to people, whether married or not. We are not sure why fidelity or the ways in which it is maintained, or trifled with, differ often between men and women and between people with different educational, social, and cultural backgrounds. Yet in everyday experience, in the world's great literature, and in the counselor's knowledge of marriage breakdown, sexual exclusivity is a major issue. Let us explore a theory that cannot cover every case even if it is generally correct but will allow the reader to approach the issue with some objectivity.

In early human relations attachment behavior is a major feature to be observed. Infants know who the primary care-giver is, and although some children are more tolerant of substitutes than others, depending on the quality and number of such surrogates, a strange person introduced at about a year of age may cause the child to react with great anxiety. Separation problems and stranger anxiety are the manifestations of a normal but sometimes heightened (and then pathological) response in early childhood.

Attachment and separation issues in the first year or two of life may be related to the need for continuity and stability of attachment later on. Nevertheless, there are many traits of infancy that we modify or change if they prove to be dysfunctional later in life. If fidelity to a particular relationship in adult life means we must live in misery, then that fidelity is dysfunctional. In such a case the ability to make that deliberate separation in a bad relationship is a sign of maturity. On the other hand, the ability to maintain a valued attachment and to make some compromises, even sacrifices, to maintain a basically good relationship is also a sign of maturity, particularly where that attachment allows for a greater productivity (as on a farm), greater economic efficiency, and greater effectiveness in important tasks such as child rearing. It is reasonable that there be a form of relationship that adults

207

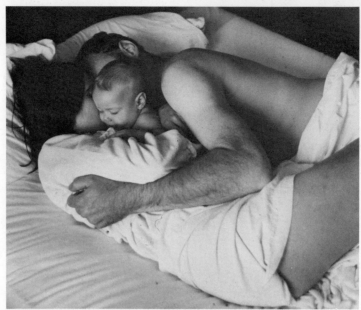

Joanne Leonard/Woodfin Camp

regard as a matter of personal commitment—one that is expected to last and provides not only for efficiency and effectiveness but also for such intangibles as companionship and emotional security.

We saw earlier that irrational customs have led us to the sorry state of having surplus widows in our population (9 million as compared to 2 million widowers). This is perhaps the greatest failure of the institution of marriage! Such statistical failure can be remedied by rationalizing the ages at which people marry. The point of such an approach is that most people who marry for life have companionship as one major value in marriage. If a marriage is good enough for three, four, or five decades, then reduction of the period of separation from the spouse at the end of life should be welcomed. This may require unusual rationality in the beginning of the married life cycle, but it is no harder to induce that rationality than it is to continue an irrational custom that increases the widowhood disparity and distress.

Theoretically, companionship in late life is an important factor in the marriage commitment. We all will, if we live long enough, grow less attractive in conventional terms, become ill, and in some ways lose certain capacities. At the same time we gain knowledge, experience, depth, and perhaps a different kind of attractiveness. The fidelity bond implies that members of a couple will not depart from their relationship merely because another relationship becomes possible with someone who is temporarily or permanently more attractive than the spouse. When people marry, they are saying in effect that they are no longer shopping for a better relationship. They are essentially closing out certain options.

What are the benefits to be gained by closing out other options forever? One is that shopping becomes tiresome, especially for a mature person who has made up his or her mind. Another is that we do not like to know that someone we cherish is continuously shopping to improve upon us! There is mutuality in the commitment, which means that we are not constantly vulnerable to being replaced or to finding a replacement. This emotional security is valued by us not because it allows us to become complacent—that is a pitfall to be avoided—but because it allows us to be more vulnerable in other important ways. If we are constantly on trial, we can never let down our guard. If we know that basically the spouse is committed to remain with the other spouse, then the sense of commitment allows us to let down the guard and participate as more open, vulnerable human beings than we can in any other relationship.

It appears that sexual vulnerability and sexual competition are incompatible with each other. Good sex is perhaps the most mutual expression of two different, but complementary, biological and psychological needs. The expression of these needs cannot take place effectively where anxiety or hostility is strong. This is not to say that competition itself is bad or that it is bad to want to have sex appeal and to be a good lover. But these strivings can have their place in the life cycle without being dominant and egotistic. To make an analogy, sprinting is a fine form of competition, but sprinting carried through one's life as a form of personal transportation is an encumbrance rather than a pleasure. One cannot sprint and at the same time enjoy the countryside, much less converse with a companion.

The pitfall of marital commitment is taking the spouse for granted. This, however, was more likely to occur in situations in the past where divorce was stigmatized or forbidden than in a present-day situation where divorce is allowed as a reasonable last resort for a failed relationship. Although we deplore excess competition, with its anxiety and hostility, we also deplore laziness or carelessness in the maintenance of a relationship. We should be kept on our toes to the degree that caring for a partner means taking responsibility for our own behavior and extending ourselves toward making the other person happy. The essence of companionship, whether friendship or marital commitment, depends on the capacity to interact mutually in ways that maintain a firm but delicate balance between concentration and relaxation. Commitment means that growth and change are expected and encouraged, and mistakes can be tolerated if made in a context of good faith.

In a lifetime of companionship, or even after a few years, there will be times when the partners are less equal than when they first made their commitment. During illness one becomes dependent on the other, much more so than when both enjoy good health. The ability of the two partners to adapt to changing roles reflects their sense of commitment. This commitment and the principle of fidelity mean that you will not

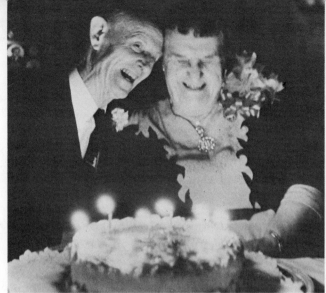

Celebrating married life together after 50 years.

Elliott Erwitt/Magnum Photos

desert your partner at a time of stress or need, and you can be confident that you will not be deserted at such a time.

The ability to maintain sexual fidelity, to regulate sexual life in a mutually satisfactory way, is a special symbol or paradigm for regulating the relationship as a whole. Neither spouse demands immediate, continuous, or guaranteed sexual satisfaction from the partner; respect for the other requires that emotional and physical readiness be taken into account. The absence of such readiness does not mean that the one with greater need can simply go and find another partner, nor does it simply mean accepting less sex. Instead it means that they work the matter out with self-respect and mutual respect within the relationship on the presumption that they are going to find a comfortable solution. The adaptation of a couple sexually is a delicate balance of passion and trust that grows and changes through the years. It should not be taken for granted or become fraught with anger or tension. Good sexual intimacy, of course, helps, and is helped by, mutual accommodation in other spheres of life.

Jealousy has been singled out by some as an undesirable and unhealthy emotion. Probably, however, it is inevitable in love relationships because it signals one's vulnerability to loss of the partner or loss of self-esteem. If you are incapable of jealousy, you are also incapable of making that moderate effort that is required to keep a relationship at its best. The absence of jealousy suggests either that someone is taken for granted or that someone is using intellectual arguments to deny feelings of vulnerability. Of course, pathological jealousy is a different matter. An argument for the normality of jealousy does not mean that marriage partners possess each other or control all other relationships the partner has. Fidelity may be expected, and it can be earned, but it cannot be ordered, any more than old King Lear could command his daughters' love.

Far more has been written on the subject of fidelity, jealousy, and vulnerability than can even be alluded to here. Any very broad generalization may run afoul of individual differences in matters this personal. Some people can handle situations that would be overwhelming to others. Sometimes, however, the process of "handling" a situation—for example, having two lovers at once—may be a sign that feelings have been numbed already or are in the process of so being.

Some people define fidelity as a situation in which spouses never have to lie to one another. Others object to this, because "keeping one's own counsel" can be a way of protecting the feelings of another and thus is more loyal and loving than always telling the unvarnished truth.

TAKING ACTION

Can you think of a situation in which the telling, rather than the feeling or the action, is hurtful? Define fidelity in marriage and friendship. Interview three people in three different decades of age on fidelity, commitment, and jealousy. Discuss meanings these words may have.

Alternative Lifestyles

In the book *Beyond Monogamy* (Smith and Smith, 1974) a range of lifestyles is considered, including extramarital sex, group marriages, communes, and swinging. Although some of these new forms of intimacy and sharing have created quite a stir and received widespread publicity, they are not as common as their renown suggests, and they should not be regarded as a threat to established forms even though they may be alarming to defenders of the establishment. These new lifestyles are mostly experiments, but some will persist and grow. There is no reason to deny these forms a right to exist, and the sensationalism surrounding them will decrease with time.

Henri Cartier-Bresson/Magnum Photos

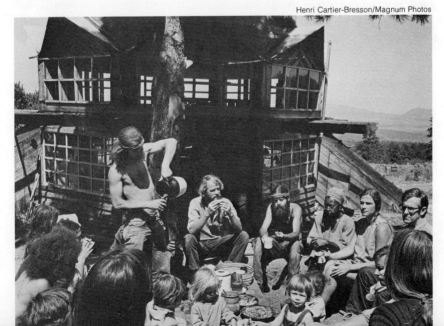

Communal living.

211

Of course, it is no more reasonable to suggest that these forms are ideal for everyone than it is to suggest that conventional marriage is ideal and right for everyone. Both these directives are overgeneralized. If there is one thing that can be learned from recent controversy about the future of marriage, it is that no one who is adult enough to enter into such a contract need be told exactly how to do it. These contracts are not routine matters, and young people in particular should not be brought up thinking that they are simple. If people will delay marriage until a certain degree of maturity is attained, then whatever style they adopt is more likely to be well chosen.

The ability of individuals to try or to adopt different lifestyles depends not only on their backgrounds and experience but also on the particular personal and social circumstances in which these choices are made. For example, infidelity or extramarital sex was long accepted, at least for men, who in many societies have been tacitly liberated from the marital bond, if only with a prostitute. However, the wife was expected to remain faithful, often under severe penalties of law, custom, or biology (that is, a pregnancy caused by someone other than her husband). It was expected under those conditions that the straying male was not deeply emotionally involved with his outside partners. However, it was assumed that for a woman to have sex outside marriage she would have to be deeply involved. Thus male infidelity was presumably less a threat to his wife than female extramarital sex was to her husband. Supposedly, women did not have cause to be jealous if their men merely engaged in pelvic release, while men would have every reason to be jealous of their women who presumably were involved heart and soul with an illicit lover.

Now with a women's liberation movement articulating careful criticism of the stereotypes and advocating a freer stance for women with regard to sex, we hear arguments that women as well as men should be able to enjoy sex for its own sake without deep emotional commitment. One side effect of this change is a shift for both sexes so that men more often find themselves "turned on" with emotional commitment in sex as women characteristically were in the past. Women in their effort to emulate a male "Don Juan" sometimes take on the less desirable features of "masculinity." For their part, males may find women's readiness for uninvolved sex a turn-off or a threat rather than something to be wished for; again, men will vary in their responses just as women do. It will be a while before these matters settle down in our society, if they ever do. We can be grateful for the increased freedom of choice that we enjoy, but we must also remain somewhat awed by the responsibility of choosing well when so many alternatives are available.

TAKING ACTION

Perhaps the most challenging new lifestyle is homosexual marriage. Discuss the following aspects. Are there good reasons why it should not be endorsed by state and church? Apart from bearing children, are relationship issues any different from those in most marriages, such as commitment and companionship? Should homosexuals be allowed to adopt children? Be foster parents? (Incidentally, most homosexuals can be biological parents, and many are.)

Some of the changes that affect sexual freedom are also reflected in other areas. Researchers on the family talk about such matters as companionship, sex roles, and power structure in marriage in relation to such matters as child rearing, marital happiness, and even health. Lois Pratt[2] found that more attention was paid by couples to both preventive medicine and medical care in marriages where there was flexibility of sex roles rather than rigid conformity, where there was equal sharing in decision making, and where there was more companionship between husband and wife. All these are modern trends, and there appears to be a direct correlation between modernization of marriage and receiving such benefits of modern life as better health and medical care. This is evidence that not everything good belongs to "the good old days," and it contradicts the idea that modernization and value change has only dire consequences for marriage and the family.

PARENTHOOD: FOR AND AGAINST

Taken by Surprise Is No Blessing in Disguise

Until about 1970 most first births in the United States were unplanned. Even though the birth control pill has been available since the early 1960s, most women became pregnant for the first time accidentally when they were in their late teens or early twenties; in terms of timing, these pregnancies were not wholeheartedly welcome. This is not to say that all first children born to these women were unwanted, because wantedness is something that can grow out of a situation. The important thing to realize is that the entry into parenthood, a most significant transition in life, was until very recently a matter of accident or circumstance rather than a matter of choice or even informed consent for most American women.

Being a good parent is difficult enough without having parenthood sprung as a surprise. But in the past young couples seemed to accept it as normal, perhaps inevitable, and not something that they could expect to control absolutely. Now that has changed. With the advent of medically safe, legal abortion, the transition to parenthood has become a matter of choice for most women in this country. In the early days of legal abortion (in New York and several other states starting in 1970, in the nation as a whole starting in 1973) the bulk of abortion patients—about 70 percent—were first-time-pregnant young women, mostly unmarried, who were choosing to delay parenthood. Some Americans were shocked to see how many young women chose to avoid motherhood at a particular time in their lives. But this strong wish for nonparenthood was not a new feeling; rather, it was one that has been suppressed and only now can be publicly expressed and acted upon.

---

[2]Lois Pratt, 1976, *Family Structure and Effective Health Behavior.* Boston: Houghton Mifflin.

Previously women who were "in trouble" or "caught" by an unwanted pregnancy had no choice but to bear a child and make the best of unwanted parenthood, place the child for adoption, or risk life and health by seeking an illegal abortion (few women could afford to travel to Japan or Europe for a safe legal abortion). The result of such a situation was a shamefully high level of dangerous, self-induced, and criminal abortions in our society. In some public hospitals half of all gynecology beds were taken up by women with incomplete abortions—that is, abortions that were crudely attempted (sometimes self-induced), resulting in hemorrhage or infection. The resultant death rate of young women in this country was unusually high compared with other societies in which family planning, including safe medical abortion, was more widely available.

Prenatal Health

A related health issue is that of infant mortality and child health. Adequate prenatal (pregnancy) care—including good nutrition and avoidance of such hazards as radiation, German measles infection, or certain drugs (thalidomide most notoriously, but even cigarette smoking)—is associated with satisfactory outcome of birth and the prenatal period. Unwanted pregnancies usually are not as well cared for as intentional ones. If a woman did not attempt an abortion outright, she might nevertheless wantonly neglect or be indifferent to her own health. She might lack enthusiasm for the newborn baby or be too depressed to give it much love. As a result of such factors, the illness and death rate of young infants ran very high in this country until the early 1970s, when our perinatal health care began to match that of the other industrialized nations of the world.

For years our country took pride in having the best medical services in the world, yet its infant and maternal death rate ranked fifteenth or below. The reason for this was not so much lack of good obstetrical services as it was lack of family planning information and services and safe legal abortion. After abortion became legal and it became clear how many couples chose not to become parents, an added impetus developed for primary prevention of unwanted pregnancy—that is, sex education and safe methods of contraception. Only a few years before, it was entirely too controversial to suggest that high school and college students be taught all of the facts of life, including contraception and abortion. Now it is regarded as a legitimate and essential part of health education and human rights for individuals to know what their bodies can and cannot do, the risks entailed, and the public health avenues and medical resources needed to increase responsible freedom of choice for individuals and the community.

TAKING ACTION

Outline and discuss what you think should be taught about sex, family planning, and parenthood in the sixth, ninth, and twelfth grades.

Nonparenthood is the state in which we all begin; parenthood is an expected state for many of us. Until this decade motherhood was the normal status for American women of 21 or 22. More than half of those who would ever become parents already had their first child. In recent years, with the advent of effective choice through more widespread birth control, the pattern began to change. Suddenly young couples had the power to extend the period of nonparenthood to the point where becoming a parent was a matter of mature choice rather than routine accommodation or the acceptance of the inevitable. If more nonparents are present in the population, more options remain open. (Many people will delay marriage as well.) We do not know how many will choose nonparenthood as a permanent lifestyle, but surveys on college campuses in the early 1970s indicated that 10 to 15 percent were seriously considering it for themselves, about 10 times more than in any previous American population sample. This may reflect only a temporary disillusionment with established family forms. But with parenthood being delayed so much for so many, it is likely that a much larger proportion than ever before will adopt a permanent child-free lifestyle.

Do not assume that only those who are inadequate or who feel inadequate as parents will choose nonparenthood. The matter is not that simple. Unfortunately, some who are least well suited for parenthood are also least likely to give thought to the whole matter. They do many things haphazardly, and birth control is one of them; the result is often an unplanned family with inadequate parents. The records on child neglect and child abuse in our society offer testimony to this fact. Other people have children for what may be called the wrong reasons: to perpetuate one's name, to give oneself an identity, to please one's parents, to live vicariously through a child, to "solve" emotional problems, or to ensure against loneliness. Just as people can have children who are not well suited to parenthood, so can those who are good parent "material" decide nevertheless that they wish to fulfill other possibilities in life that simply cannot be done as well if conscientious parenthood is also undertaken.

There is no need to fear that "good" people will deselect themselves from parenthood to the point that only "bad" parents will be left. By "good" and "bad," we mean many different things, of course, but we can examine two: genes and care-giving. Much controversy still exists about the relative importance of nature and nurture, or heredity and environment. In a society that has failed to meet the needs of so many of its families, environmental factors must be considerable. It is particularly insidious to suggest that those segments of our population that have been most deprived socially and economically should be labeled unfit for parenthood. It would be more just and effective to bend our resources to enhance the social functioning, health, and care-giving capacity of more people, especially those long deprived of societal benefits.

As it happens, family planning as well as health services and other amenities have been lacking for many Americans. Poor people, when asked, almost always express a wish for fewer children than they expect to have and do have. Once we make health education and other benefits of modern society a matter of personal right, equitably available for enjoyment by all, we can expect parenthood to improve across the board, average family size to decrease, and nonparenthood to increase.

Genetic counseling is a particular matter of interest for persons who have a family history of a hereditary disease. As genetic technology improves, detection of carriers of genetic defects will be more applicable, as will genetic testing of the fetus prenatally in doubtful cases. It is good to be able to reduce the incidence of major genetic disorder. This is quite different, however, from trying to increase the average IQ of a population by genetic selection—a highly dubious proposition on scientific and humanitarian grounds. Until all children have good physical and mental environments from the beginning of life, we should be wary of exaggerating the genetic element.

Let us also be wary of generalizations about either parents or nonparents in terms of their qualities as human beings. People can be selfish and materialistic in their motivations to avoid child rearing. Just as much if not more, however, people can be selfish and materialistic in having children. The main thing to hope for is that the decision be made with as much care as with other contemporaneous decisions such as career choice, where to live, buying a car, or choosing a vacation spot.

Family Size The smallest family with children is, of course, the one-child family. Only about 5 percent of children are "onlies," but the proportion is growing; in Sweden about half the children have no siblings. For a time the only child was regarded as an unfortunate being. It was said that such a child must be either spoiled or deprived or both and would grow up to be selfish and unsociable. These stereotypes are not merely unproved, they are mostly false. It so happens that only children tend to do very well in the measures of success and adjustments that are available to us. There is no justification from studies on health, mental health, or achievement that another child should be introduced into the family only to improve the well-being of the first. In fact that would be misguided, because *a child is an end in itself* and should not be used as a means, a tool, for the benefit of anybody else, whether parent or sibling. If parents have a second child, it should be for reasons other than to provide company for the first.

It is easy to see why only children get much contact with adults, and this could explain why they master language at a rapid rate and do well both academically and emotionally. Of course, it is possible for parents to dote too much on an only child, to spoil him or her, to be overprotective and excessively anxious because it is "all they have." This kind of anxiety or overprotectiveness needs to be handled by counseling of the parent rather than by introducing additional children as "ballast."

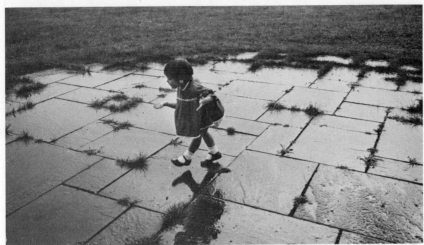

Inge Morath/Magnum Photos

Parents of an only child are able to have careers and to provide resources such as *quality* child-care and nursery school experiences to help socialize the youngster. Siblings are not always the best companions for each other anyway, so nursery school and preschool experiences are highly desirable in any family. In the future the one-child family will grow in popularity because it is a viable alternative between nonparenthood and a family of two or more, which may be all-consuming of the emotional and tangible resources of the parent.

With the two-child family we consider the spacing between births and the sex of offspring. Of course, an interval usually exists between marriage and the birth of the first child, a prebirth rather than a birth interval. That length of time ought to be enough for the couple to have a child-free period together to enjoy life and develop levels of understanding and intimacy that would be interrupted by the early advent of a third member. (Exceptions are couples who have lived together unmarried for appreciable periods and those marrying relatively late, such as in their mid-thirties.)

The birth interval following the first child has been much debated. Solid research does not exist to make the decision simple, nor should it be the same for everyone. Having children in rapid succession is undesirable because there should be certain recovery period for the womb and because there is a need for the parents to have sufficient time to invest in each child as it comes along. Probably an interval of three years should be considered. This gives the older child a chance for substantial ego development, including language, bowel and bladder control, walking, and the ability to differentiate him or herself as an individual before a sibling comes along. If functions such as talking and toilet training are barely achieved when a new sibling comes along, these skills in the older one may be set back, thus increasing conflict for that child and the parents at a time when there is already sufficient conflict over sibling rivalry.

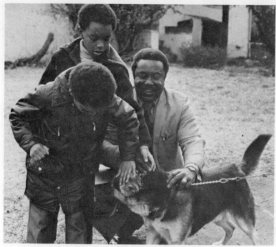

The two-child family is becoming increasingly common in this country.

Ann Chwatsky/Editorial Photocolor Archives

Some may worry that children three years apart won't be good playmates, but it can be argued that the older one in that case will be less threatened and can be more protective of the younger sibling than would be the case if there were only a year or two difference. Three years is not too great for many joint activities between siblings, but as mentioned earlier, siblings are not always the best companions for each other and should not have to be sole companions. Other sources of socialization are necessary.

Some people will want larger families than one or two children. This may be tempered if choice of sex of offspring is a possibility, and this may be the case very soon. Research on timing of insemination and other factors may lead us to the point where we can help couples determine the sex of offspring. We should not expect, however, to be able to make an absolute guarantee, and couples who are not willing to accept and cherish a child of a particular sex should probably not have children at all.

Those who want larger families but do not wish to reproduce, or cannot, have the option to adopt or provide foster care for children in need.

TAKING ACTION

Sample your class for birth-interval range and average. Is average interval following a boy baby more or less than that following girl baby? Why? Debate the advantages of different intervals based on "teams" with similar opinions. Do opinions correlate with experienced birth intervals? How much is based on wishful thinking or "the grass is greener on the other side"?

Adoption The situation regarding adoption has changed dramatically in recent years along with the decrease in unplanned births. In former years maternity homes (that is, homes for unwed mothers) were filled to capacity, and adoption agencies had plenty of very young and healthy infants for infertile couples. (Recently it has become possible for a single woman to adopt a child, but it occurs infrequently.) When abortion became legal, the situation changed rapidly. With the resulting shortage of unwanted infants, children who formerly would have been difficult to place in an adoptive home—those who are older and may have been in several foster homes, and those with handicaps or with mixed racial backgrounds—suddenly became adoptable because they represented the difference between parenthood and involuntary childlessness.

Whereas in the past infertile couples were in a "buyer's market," the market recently changed, in favor of the children, to a seller's market; that is, fewer children could be rejected if people wanted to be parents. This new situation alarmed those who viewed parenthood as an inalienable right. They were shocked at the impossibility of adopting a same-race, healthy, younger child. Imagine the dilemma, for instance, of a couple with strong religious or racial sentiments who want very much to be parents and because of infertility face a choice of nonparenthood or adopting a child of a different race. We have no sympathy for racial prejudice, but in this case many couples are thrust by chance (infertility) into the position of having to break down society's racist barriers in a most personal way.

Certainly for children the change was good news. Every child deserves an optimal upbringing, and by chance alone—by the biological accident of infertility—the social errors and injustices that cause some children to go without good homes (birth accidents or racial difference or poverty) were no longer the barriers that had inevitably existed.

There has been an emphasis all through history on the necessity and normality of biological parenthood, but happy adoptive parents say that, after the first few weeks of the child's arrival, he or she is no less "theirs" than any child in any home.

The point of the story is that psychological parenthood is the human part, whereas biological parenthood is the animal part. There has been an overemphasis on the process of birth, and even if it is a miraculous and memorable experience (although not positive for everyone), the idea that one must experience it in order to be fulfilled is an unfortunate exaggeration. The real fulfillment depends on what happens as the new human being is integrated into the human family, not what happens in the loins of the parents.

The future of parenthood, in a rapidly changing social scene such as we have described, is open to speculation. As voluntary nonparenthood becomes more accepted, the pressure on those who cannot reproduce, although they want to, should be somewhat reduced so that some of them will be able to adapt to their childless status with less grief than their childless forebearers suffered. In the larger world scene there are still many children who do not have benefits of being wanted, and transnational adoption remains a possibility to fill those homes that are too empty with children from homes that are too full. However, there are controversies and conflicts to be expected about national and racial pride on both sides of such a transaction. Should we adopt poor children from Asia in large numbers? How would we react to a proposal from Sweden or China to adopt our homeless or very poor children?

Figure 6-1

Family chart. Code: square = male, circle = female, d. = year deceased, two horizontal lines = marriage, two slanted lines = divorce, dotted lines = unknown to chart maker, X = deceased, arrow = person formulating chart.

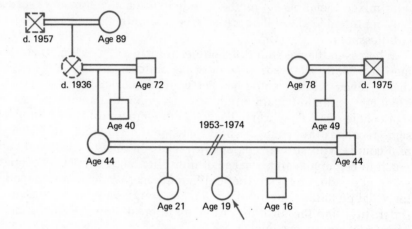

TAKING ACTION

Whole systems of family study and family therapy have grown up around the exploration with members of all three generations of the experiences, recollections, and current feelings of grandparents and children.

1. *As an exercise, prepare a family chart as shown in Figure 6-1. Such a chart will enable you to organize the study of your own family across three (or more) generations. It is surprising how few people take the trouble to inquire about their own personal family history, considering that in many cases the prime sources of information are lost—grandparents, uncles, and aunts—before we are well into adulthood and before our curiosity has been aroused.*

2. *Once a family chart is done, a study of a group, such as a class in college, can be made along several lines. A composite family chart can be made for a group identifying such things as average family size, average birth intervals, age of parents at marriage and at the birth of the first child, age of grandparents at marriage and at the birth of the first child, number of surviving grandparents, average age at death of those who had died, percentage of couples divorced in each generation, number of children involved per divorce, and so on. By comparing these figures across generations one can get an appreciation for social trends in a much more personal way.*

3. *Another experience of great importance is that of child care. Every person, whether or not he or she intends to become a parent, should be experienced in taking care of children. Every high school and college*

should have a nursery school attached to it so that child development can be a normal and practical experience in one's emergence into adulthood. Young children need care from more people than just their parents, and adolescents need experience of responsibility for children. Each student in the class should be qualified to give competent round-the-clock child care. This can be learned by apprenticing yourself to young parents, spending enough time so that they can trust you to be alone with their young child(ren) at increasing intervals up to the point where the couple can take a weekend vacation and confidently leave their children in your care. Students can work in pairs for such an exercise, especially where there is more than one child in the family.

The professions of child psychology and psychiatry and various professions dealing with problems of child development and family relations—special education, speech and hearing, rehabilitation, marriage and family counseling, financial counseling—are important but are relatively neglected in our society. There are far too few trained people in these fields to adequately care for all the children in need. As the number of children in need decreases due to better prenatal and pediatric care and family planning, we will finally make inroads on the overwhelming surplus of families in need.

HELPING TROUBLED FAMILIES

Wherever a child has a major psychological problem, it can be assumed that the parents have problems, not necessarily because they psychogenically created their child's difficulties, although sometimes this is the case. The child's difficulty itself is a strain on the family; children do have effects on parents too. Even the wisest and best-intentioned parents need outside help in coping with special difficulties. However, the helping professions have tended to focus on the child without giving adequate attention to the parents, who happen to be the primary caretakers.

The emergence of family therapy in mental health has helped in this regard, as has the strengthening of family practice as a medical specialty. The return to the old theme of "general practice" and the family doctor has also helped to emphasize the major importance of the family in taking care of individuals with health and other special problems.

TAKING ACTION

1. *As an exercise in this area, spend time in health clinics, paying particular attention to prevention and treatment of various family problems. Often there are opportunities to be helpful in situations where the very nature of the institution requires the processing of large numbers of people. This processing takes on a dehumanizing quality. The presence of students in pediatric settings, old age homes, and so on should be a boon to these institutions as well as to the psychological and social development of students.*

*2. Explore with individuals and married couples at different stages of life
their feelings about marriage and parenthood. This does not mean that
you become a therapist, but use the family graph and your sympathetic
interest to develop an appreciation for the joys and sorrows of married life
and parenthood or single life and nonparenthood. It would be well to
structure these efforts so that the person interviewed knows in advance
the duration of the interview and its purpose. It would also be desirable to
make the experience broader by talking with people who represent
different age groups and life statuses, including singles, divorced, gays,
and widowed people. Some respondents will permit interviews to be taped
for classroom use.*

DISCUSSION   It is hard to see how people can expect to go through life enjoying
significant relationships without periodic outside help or at least the
assistance of an objective and expert observer. This is not to argue that
everyone needs therapy. Many do, but many would probably escape
the need for remedial help if (like a dental or physical examination) a
"marital checkup" was available and if marriage—and other
nonmarriage—relationship enrichment programs existed.

Churches and synagogues offer some of these resources, but increasingly health resources and social service agencies are becoming involved. The latter are often treatment-oriented, established to cope
with sickness and social maladaptation. With a public health and
preventive awareness, such services will become more effective in a
positive way, thus promoting health and well-being, not merely treating or preventing illness.

It is ironic, perhaps, that we have so few experts in human relations,
relatively little instruction in these areas in our schools, and virtually
no standards for quality of human relationships that would serve as a
guide for individuals at various stages of life. Success in this area is a
mixture of art and science, of taking from our parents and teachers
whatever is helpful and leaving the rest—taking a chance on making
some mistakes in order to make some important discoveries of our own.

This chapter and the activities suggested should alert you to issues
that, although difficult, are better faced "a year too soon than an hour
too late"—to adapt a good adage about sex education. Moreover,
discussion among peers of both sexes, with family members, and with
respected elders is an opportunity to be enjoyed and treasured.

FOR FURTHER READING

Astin, Helen S., Parelman, Allison, and Fisher, Anne, eds., 1975. *Sex Roles: A
Research Bibliography.* Washington, D.C.: U.S. Department of Health,
Education and Welfare.

May, Jean T., ed., 1974. *Family Health Indicators.* Washington, D.C.: U.S.
Department of Health, Education and Welfare.

These are samples of annotated bibliographies issued from time to time by government organizations in the family field. To keep up with rapidly changing events and research findings, readers should be aware of at least four organizations and their journals:

National Council on Family Relations
1219 University Ave., S.E.
Minneapolis, Minn. 55414

American Home Economics Association
2010 Massachusetts Ave., N.W.
Washington, D.C. 20036

American Public Health Association
1015 18th St., N.W.
Washington, D.C. 20036

National Association for Mental Health
1800 N. Kent St., Rosslyn Station
Arlington, Va. 22209

Bernard, Jessie, 1972. *The Future of Marriage.* New York: World Publishing.

This large but very readable work reflects the lifetime of research of a renowned family sociologist. It includes historical perspective and interpretations of recent trends, with valuable insights into the probable evolution of marriage forms.

Lieberman, E. J., and Peck, Ellen, 1973. *Sex and Birth Control.* New York: Crowell.

A complete guide to contraception, abortion, and sterilization. This book also deals with the future of the family, population, sexual decision making, what is "normal" and what is "moral," and venereal disease. It also provides a list of places to turn for help.

Peck, Ellen, and Senderowitz, Judith, eds., 1974. *Pronatalism: The Myth of Mom and Apple Pie.* New York: Crowell.

The first book on the subject, this collection of essays examines the pervasive bias in society toward child rearing. Television, advertising, home economics textbooks, army rules and regulations, and the tax structure are among the influences analyzed. Actual effects of children upon marriage and other adult relationships are reviewed. Personal statements and viewpoints are also offered by parents and nonparents.

Smith, James R., and Smith, Lynn G., eds., 1974. *Beyond Monogamy.* Baltimore: The Johns Hopkins Press.

This collection of studies covers a broad range, from mate swapping to group marriage and communes. There is a chapter on infidelity by Jessie Bernard and one on sexuality in a zero-growth society by Alex Comfort. The book leans toward the less conventional alternatives to monogamous marriage, which have been given short shrift in most texts on marriage and the family.

223

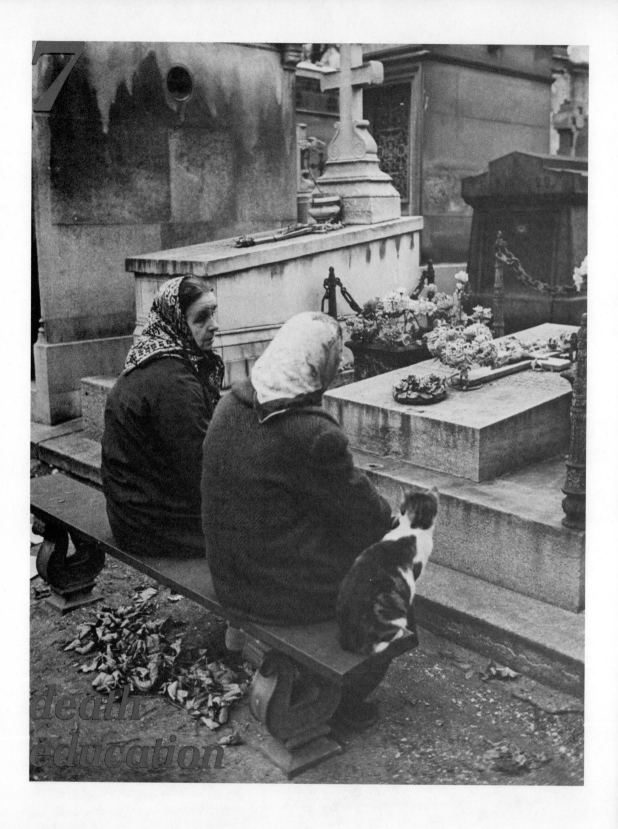

7

death
education

The study of death and dying is presented in the context of improving the quality of life for ourselves and future generations. For many the study of death serves as a stimulus to clarify values and provide a meaning for life and living.

Death can be viewed from four human foci: death of the self, death of the significant other, dying of the self, and dying of the significant other. The meaning of death is varied and does not always connote despair or terror; rather, it can mean release from pain, a new beginning, and a natural aspect of life akin to a deep sleep.

Death can be defined in different ways. We can die untimely, stupid, man-made deaths through homicide, war, mass starvation, and other holocausts—a fact suggesting action by health-educated persons. Death education is seen as playing a worthwhile role in helping people work through such issues as euthanasia and understanding grief, a normal developmental process related to significant loss.

The funeral industry is the institution designed for caring for the dead and providing an appropriate setting for mourning. In that regard it can be therapeutically helpful for the bereaved. However, since the funeral industry is a profit-oriented business, the consumer would be wise to "beware and become educated."

INQUIRY

1. What is *death* doing in a text on human health?
2. Why is it difficult to talk of death?
3. What is the meaning of death to you?
4. What is the euthanasia controversy?
5. What is the nature of grief and bereavement?
6. Is the funeral industry of value or is it a "rip-off"?

WHAT IS DEATH DOING IN A TEXT ON HUMAN HEALTH?

What do death and dying have to do with health and living? Human sexuality, ecology, emotional health, and disease are topics fit for health education—but death?

The following data are presented to support the argument that health, life, and death are all related to one another. Later, it will be shown that thanatology (the study of death and dying) may very well be considered among preventive, remedial, and optimal health aspects of health education.

How Death Can Affect Health and Living

1. The stress of death on the survivor can cause physical pathology or sickness and/or emotional problems. Suffering the death of a parent, brother or sister, close friend, or pet by a child can affect later healthy development. Studies have suggested that the unresolved grief of

children often gives rise to juvenile delinquency, alcoholism, and cancer in later life.

2. The first year after death can be a particularly vulnerable time for the surviving mate and children. Suicide and other forms of premature death (representing "giving up") often follow the death of a mate. One psychiatrist devised a system to simplify the prediction and recognition of stress-related illness (scale on p. 197).[1] He found that people run the risk of developing a major illness in the next two years when more than 300 points in any given year were accumulated as measured by his scale. The event worth 100 points and leading the stress parade was *death of a spouse.*

3. Most people in the hospital setting know when they are dying whether they are told or not. They pick up cues from the way they feel and from doctors, nurses, and visitors. When interviewed, the dying say they wish to discuss their imminent death, to put their affairs in order, and to die with some control over their final moments. Yet few discuss this vitally important last scene of one's life drama with the dying person (Shneidman, 1973).

4. There are growing indications that children 7 to 10 years old are trying to commit suicide by drinking household cleaners, medicines, and other poisons. Data support the conclusion that suicide among college students is accelerating at an unprecedented rate.

5. There is some evidence that children can be traumatized by death themes in fairy tales, television, and indirect and direct contact with homicide and war. Just why some individuals are more vulnerable to such traumatizing is not known.

6. We can die at any moment from any number of natural or man-made causes. There is no guarantee that we will reach the life expectancy of 68 years for a white male, 76 years for a white female, 62 for a nonwhite male, and 70 years for a nonwhite female (life expectancy at birth as of 1972).

**Preventive,
Remedial, and
Optimal Health
Aspects of
Death Education**

Death education forces us to realize that much death-related fear, anxiety, and misery are due to psychological and social factors. Death education is concerned with *preventing* and *remedying* those contingencies leading to *unhealthy* death and dying.

Once we look at our total environment and ways of interacting with other human beings from the viewpoint of the life-death interplay, we can work toward improving the quality of life. We look for whatever seems to enhance or destroy our quality of life as seen against the backdrop of death. Thus both health and death education are concerned with a third aspect of health which has been labeled *perfectivist health, high-level wellness, élan vital,* or an *exuberant spirit of*

[1]T. H. Holmes, 1975, *American Psychological Association Monitor* 4:8.

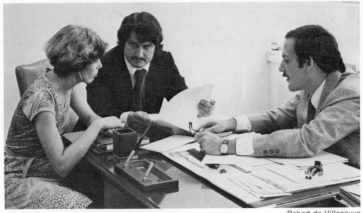

Robert de Villeneuve

well-being. We will use the term *optimal health* to indicate this superior state of well-being.

Although death education is a young field, research indicates that it can help students develop a personal philosophy about life and death. In the midst of life students reflect back upon life and ask the profound question, "If I were to die tomorrow, what can I say of my life?" Contemplation of death encourages evaluation of values and priorities. What is important in life for each of us? Death education only serves to accentuate, clarify, and magnify life's meaning.

Eventually, however, your wishes concerning death must be communicated to those closest to you. Perhaps a compromise must be reached. Better to talk it over than to bring hardship upon those who survive. For example, you may wish to be cremated after death, but your mate wishes something more traditional to remember you by— say, a headstone. What do you decide? As another example, you may wish no life-sustaining, "heroic" means used to prolong your life, but your mate has a contrary view. How is the ultimate decision reached? Death education suggests meeting the need for communication and understanding of the needs of the person who will die and the survivors.

Thus death is more than merely a biological event. It has social, psychological, and health-related consequences; to use Herman Feifel's (1959) phraseology, "Death is for all seasons."

Talking about death is difficult. Most of us shun any mention of it. Yet language is the vehicle by which we communicate. It is a medium by which we learn. One problem is that death-related language is often so anxiety-provoking that intellectual and perceptual functioning is inhibited.

What does the word *death* conjure up in your mind? Do you find yourself avoiding its mere mention? What of the words *dying, corpse,*

WHO CAN TALK OF DEATH?

227

funeral, burial, or *coffin*? Do they trip as lightly off the tongue as *joy, beauty, fun*? Research indicates that death words are generally rated as *negative* and *bad*, arouse the emotions, and can affect perception.

Anxiety level can also be affected by death language. Words have always elicited powerful emotions sometimes leading to aggressive or self-defeating behavior. Death words can arouse emotions leading to irrational behavior when we really do not know their precise meaning. Take the word "cancer." Often patients react to the news that they have cancer with a host of stereotypes, myths, and other anxiety-arousing fantasies. Cancer has many types, treatments, and prognoses. It has many different meanings. Thus trauma in cancer patients could be reduced if we were all systematically educated about it.

"Hard-core" death language is generally so stark that we prefer to use the *euphemisms* instead. One does not die but *passes away, goes to the great beyond,* or lies six feet under. One is not buried but *laid to rest.* In the military deaths are never reported, only *casualties.* Yesterday's cemetery is today's *garden of repose.* A funeral director does what an *undertaker* or *mortician* did years ago. In the funeral director's list of euphemistic language a corpse is *remains*, and a cremation results in *cremains.* Some gravediggers have petitioned to be known as *excavation engineers.*

Yet death is also a common topic of humor. Humor relieves tension. One writer has said, "If you know what people joke about, you can guess what worries them." Thus the humor and satirical magazine, *The National Lampoon* of January 1973 was devoted entirely to the topic of death. One article was entitled, *"23 Ways to Be Offensive at the Funeral of Someone You Didn't Like."* Some directions to "appropriate" behavior included:

1. Offer $10,000 to the person who can draw the best mustache on the deceased.
2. Congratulate the deceased's parents on outliving him.
3. Immediately after the eulogy, stand up and propose to the widow.

We laugh, smirk, or choke because the behaviors suggested are so outlandish and unacceptable according to our traditional ways. Such behaviors, if actually carried out, would be viewed as obscene. We normally eulogize and honor the dead and express the greatest consideration for survivors. Yet, we may laugh, perhaps, because the satire and humor relieve the anxiety of confronting the inevitability of our own death.

Death Language, Expectancy, and Role

Chapter 8 of this book stresses that the meaning given to health-related language greatly influences our behavior. Certainly in the area of death education we find many examples. For instance, look at your classmates and teacher. Focus on one with whom you are friendly and think about what makes your relationship enjoyable. Suppose, in the course of conversation, one day you reasonably ask, "How are you?" To which your friend responds, "Well, if you wish to know, I'm dying." What is your mental picture, your perception of your friend under this circumstance? Would you start treating him differently? Would you look for behavior that might indicate dying? Would you avoid that person in the future? Would you start treating him with "kid gloves"?

The relatively new field of medical sociology suggests that we have *expectancies* of the dying person and of the physician, nurse, family, and others in the dying person's social environment. Often social expectancies do not fit the actual behavior. When this occurs, one can expect conflict, anger, frustration, or a sense of helplessness. For example, we expect the dying person to be cooperative with nurse and physician and to act "sick." Physicians and nurses expect the dying person to die on time. To die before the predicted time would be indicative of poor medical practice ("Dr. Jones must have fouled up on Mr. Smith"). To die "late" might arouse too much anxiety and expense ("Good Lord, when will Henry go? It would be better for all of us.").

One young lady, diagnosed as having Hodgkin's disease (a form of cancer), went to a hospital for her prescribed therapy. She was feeling fine at the time, able to function well in her role of mother, student, housewife, and high school teacher. Her disease had not reached its advanced state, so her morale was quite high. She walked into the hospital, filled out the appropriate forms, and took a seat to await her turn for blood tests. Within moments a rather alarmed technician, concerned that she was uncomfortable, immediately ushered her into the laboratory in a wheelchair. After her tests, she was taken to her room still in the wheelchair where a nurse helped her to undress and retire to bed. She remarked, "I was feeling just dandy until they started treating me as though I was a pariah." Once our friend entered the hospital, she was required to play the *role of dying patient* to meet the *expectations* of the medical staff.

Death education makes us aware of death-related social expectations and roles. Death education suggests that we be ourselves and remain unaffected by such implied societal coercion. Are we to play "social games" even while we die? It would seem so.

Apprehensions about developing a dialogue on death with dying persons are usually unfounded. If the situation is structured so that people feel free to talk of death, they will do so almost eagerly. Their feelings may be expressed verbally or nonverbally (body language, paintings, and so on) (Kubler-Ross, 1969). It is as though the avoidance mechanism preventing talk over one's terminal condition has been removed. One nonthreatening, open-ended technique is to simply ask, "What is your diagnosis?" or "Why are you hospitalized?" or words to that effect. Thus one college student remarked matter-of-factly, "I have kidney disease and things look bad." Another still avoids the thought of his own death as he replies, "I shall be leaving the hospital

Communicating with the Dying Person

soon—I'm feeling better." One graduate student with cancer of the stomach visited many of our graduate classes in death education and noted simply but starkly, "I'm dying."

Usually the person knows of the situation especially if some time after diagnosis has elapsed. This person may "mix" knowledge of impending death with denial of its approach. Such ambivalence is common. If the dying person is still avoiding facing the fact of death, it may be best to honor this reaction. The time for confrontation will come.

On the other hand, the dying may wish to talk of a variety of pressing needs such as pain, quality of care, chance of recovery, and economic and other concerns related to family. There comes a time when the dying may wish to discuss their *future* and *style* of dying. There is the need to assure one of an *appropriate death* (Weisman, 1972), which includes allowing one to die in the way fitting for him or her. It means helping the dying find fullest possible meaning in their lives while it is still possible.

Occasions arise when an individual must be told of his or her approaching death in a gentle, sensitive way. A family may be dependent upon the person to leave his or her affairs in order. Psychologically, to die without benefit of saying "good-bye" or without the mutual expression of love and sadness may be counterproductive to a healthy dying or bereavement.

The helpful friend carefully structures the situation and chooses the appropriate time for conversation about death. If the relationship between the dying and friend is one of trust, the results may be most gratifying for all. The death-educated person knows of the language barrier and is able to penetrate it in appropriate ways.

TAKING ACTION

1. List the expectations *you have of physicians, clergy, and funeral directors. Next find students with parents who belong to one of those three occupations. Ask them to comment on observable behavioral differences when their parents are at home enjoying the family and at work. For example, do they use a different "voice"? How do clothes reinforce one's professional and social role? What behaviors change as a function of the role one assumes?*
2. *Since most of you have been sick at one time or another, discuss your own role on such occasions. What did you expect from parents and other care givers regarding compassion, comfort, having every need met, and the like? How realistic were you?*

WHAT IS THE MEANING OF DEATH?

The meaning we give death varies with *age, situation,* and *experience.* Death has other meanings than the terrifying, horrible, or bad. Herman Feifel, whom many consider to be the father of the modern thanatological movement, has observed that death is often viewed as a friend who brings an end to pain through peaceful sleep. He quotes Macbeth's comment on the murdered King Duncan, "After life's fitful fever, he sleeps well," and Heine, in the thought, "Death, it is the cool night" (Feifel, 1959). The American Revolutionary War hero, Ethan Allen, who when told by his parson that the angels were waiting for him, cocked open one eye as he lay dying and said, "Waiting, are they? Well, God damn them, let them wait!"

The Child's View of Death

Children too give death meaning. A neighbor's child associates death with fiery, tortuous hell, and at age nine admonishes himself for the fact that he is "sinful." A four-year-old girl tells her father matter-of-factly that he will die. He asks her, "Will I be in pain?"

"Of course not, silly."

"Will I be hungry or thirsty?"

"No, Daddy, you'll be dead."

"Will I miss my friends and you?" he asks.

"No, Daddy, you can't think—you're just dead!"

At an earlier age, around one and one-half years, death had a different meaning—indifference! A small child came upon a dead sparrow lying stiff on the sidewalk. With interest, she waddled up to it, squatted down, and with her forefinger touched it. With that she walked away and went about her business. *Death* and *dead* apparently had little aversive meaning for her at that age.

Generally, longitudinal or developmental research that follows a group of children for several years finds certain definable stages, all of which are subject to tremendous variation (see Nagy in Feifel, 1959).

Up to the age of five the child supposedly does not know of death but equates it with separation and departure from the significant other person, generally the mother. Closed eyes or sleep is equated with death. The dead are expected to live—to literally get up or become resurrected. The "dead" cops and robbers, and cowboys and Indians always rise only to die ignominiously again and again.

Death may be personified between ages five through nine. The "Bogeyman," "Grim Reaper," and "Man with the Scythe" are seen as real death people. Personification may take two forms. Either death is a separate person, like the "Bogeyman," or it is the dead. Thus the parent who admonishes a child to behave by threatening capture or punishment by the Bogeyman may be inflicting unusual punishment and instilling irrational fears.

After the age of nine, the reality of death is appreciated. It is final, irreversible, and completely democratic in its touch and sweep. It is the cessation of corporal life accompanied by decay and disintegration of the body.

Themes of inevitability and universality dominate, but the young child and adult often see death as but one aspect of a circle of lives and deaths akin to Buddhist philosophy. Maria Nagy (Feifel, 1959) asked a nine-year-old the question, "What is death?" The child answered, "I think it is a part of a person's life. Like school. Life has many parts. Only one part of it is earthly. As in school, we go on to a different class. To die means to begin a new life. Everyone has to die once, but the soul lives on."

The College Student's Meaning Given to Death

In research with University of Maryland students enrolled in a death education class the most frequent response to the question "What does death mean to you?" was "the end," "the final process of life," "cessation of earthly existence," "and unavoidable." When the same question was asked following the death education course, the responses were more varied. They included "the beginning of a life after death," "a transition," "a new beginning," "a joining of the spirit with a universal cosmic consciousness," "a kind of endless sleep, rest, and peace," "termination of this life but with survival of the spirit," and "don't know."

Based upon this and other information it seemed that the death education course affected some in developing what might be called an ecological view of death. Death was seen as a part of the natural life cycle perhaps reflected in the saying, "Without life there is no death, and without death there is no life." Even within our bodies most cells die only to be replaced by new generations. The budding plant representative of rebirth is nurtured in the loamy rich soil consisting of decaying organisms. Thus earth to earth, dust to dust, ashes to ashes . . . for all things there is a season . . . a season to be born and a season to die.

Many college students also associate death with *loss*. Loss of human relationships, time, consciousness, and opportunity to experience. The loss of unfulfilled expectations and plans is particularly significant to this group. Thus we find experimentation and curiosity over the theme of death. We stop at car accidents, as our pulse and heartbeat quicken. We tempt death and it thrills us. Deadly, stupid gambles with death such as "Russian roulette" and "chicken" are common during this period when many flirt with death.

To some students death is a stimulus to enhance human relationships, to communicate feelings to loved ones. "Love, laugh, and be merry for tomorrow we may die" could have been coined by a thanatologist. Contemplation of death has prompted many to enjoy life and cherish loved ones more.

Time factors include maturation and our perception of futurity (Kastenbaum and Aisenberg, 1972). Death, dying, life, and living all change in their meanings as we progress from infancy to old age to dying. Some gerontologists and developmentalists have effectively argued that our behavior is very much influenced not so much by chronological age (distance from birth) but rather one's nearness to death. The eminent psychoanalyst, Carl Jung, felt that the second half of life, from middle age onward, should be in preparation for death.

Our concept of *futurity* is linked with death. The college-age student generally is concerned with the here and now—the present and immediate future. As death approaches, past and future time takes on greater meaning for the older person. The noted gerontologist, Robert Butler, has described the *life review* in older persons.[2] It is the tendency to reminisce (which people do to some extent at all ages) and the attempt to resolve the conflicts of the past. It may also signify the need for one's past life to be applauded, verified, and made to seem worthwhile as death approaches. Perhaps death can be better accepted when life is perceived as having been meaningful.

Certainly *culture* or *environment* can affect the meaning given to death. In some societies it is the *dead* who are feared more than death itself. It is the ghost or spirit that can wreak havoc with crops and bring drought, or reduce the availability of game and fish. In other societies death is celebrated. The Day of the Dead is a time for festivity and a holiday in Mexico and Italy.

During World War II Japanese kamikaze military aircraft pilots dove their planes unflinchingly into enemy targets. To die in this manner, for the emperor and the motherland, meant reward in another happier existence. Such a death was *appropriate* for members of that particular culture.

In our society many Christians believe in some sort of personal afterlife. To the Hindu or Buddhist the thought of the individual regaining his earthly form and personality in heaven is considered egotistical arrogance.

Undoubtedly, such *situations* as having a good friend or loved one die or having a close call with death, such as surviving an accident or near drowning, can influence our own view of death. Students who are Vietnam veterans have seen the death and dying of their buddies and civilian populations. They have seen children shot and burned to death by napalm. Some cannot forget and try to rub the thought from their mind's eye through alcohol or other massive forms of denial. Others become active in antiwar movements. In either case, the situation of contact with death has profoundly affected behavior.

Focus of the Meaning Given to Death

Edwin Shneidman (1973) has commented that death is both a nonevent and an event. For the dead person, death is obviously a nonevent. The state of death cannot be experienced by the corpse. Yet death, nearly always, is an event of great importance in the life and living of *others*. The meaning we give death and dying can be affected by the meaning and value we give to our human relationships. Thus, death may have four human foci:

1. The death of myself
2. The dying of myself
3. The death of loved ones or "significant others"
4. The dying of loved ones or "significant others"

---

[2]R. Butler and M. Lewis, 1973, *Aging and Mental Health*. New York: Mosby.

The time, culture, and situational factors just discussed, of course, interact with the person-directed focus to represent a mosaic of meanings. For a 44-year-old man with a healthy, fine family, *his death* may have the following meanings: a stimulus to enjoy life, especially family friends, and profession; the end of existence and loss of human relationships; a stimulus to fashion a better world for his children and other children; a possibility that can occur at any time catching himself and his family more or less unprepared; and possible problems for his family after his death as they try to adapt to a mixed-up, sometimes hostile world.

For this man to give meaning to the death and dying of *others* closest to him—his children, his wife, parents, parents-in-law, close friends—the task is more difficult. The thought of those people, especially his wife and children, suffering and/or dying may have no uplifting, positive meaning whatever. Still, if they were suffering a fatal, painful condition, death might very well be a relief. One woman watched her own child die and then devoted her life to serving other dying children.

Some Problems of Dying

Some consider death to be the last developmental task of our lives. As with most rites of passage the problems involved are often complex. Dying is not a simple event. Fearful of oversimplification, we will list a few of the most urgent problems of dying:

1. There is a problem of *loneliness and isolation*. Studies have indicated that the dying are seen as aversive and are often avoided by hospital personnel. One study found that nurses tended to respond significantly more slowly to the calls of their dying patients than to those of their other patients. Another study in the 1960s found that a large proportion of college students tested in an experiment would not willingly allow a dying person to live in the immediate neighborhood and would be reluctant to give him employment in the field they both wished to enter.[3] The investigator, Richard Kalish, concluded that "If these data may be taken at face value, the social isolation of the dying is a very real occurrence."

2. *Relief of pain* is probably the most important immediate problem for the dying. Methadone, morphine, and other analgesics are available for numbing pain. While he was dying, journalist Stewart Alsop recommended heroin to reduce pain and scorned the argument that it is "addictive" on the grounds that the dying couldn't care less.

3. The dying need to know that their *life has been meaningful*. Most people benefit from having their life and human relationships justified and legitimized by others. In some societies old people are honored simply because they are old.

4. The dying and their survivors need to *communicate* so that practical everyday affairs may be put in order. Wives need to partici-

[3]R. Kalish, 1966, *Community Mental Health Journal* 2:152–155.

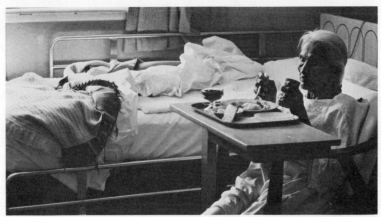

A terminal patient.

Michal Heron/Woodfin Camp

pate in all financial affairs so that they will know the location and contents of wills and other legal documents and how to manage financial affairs in the event of being left alone.

Needless to say, the dying as well as survivors need to say their good-byes and to comfort one another. The dying may well grieve too—both in preparation for their own death, the final separation, and the knowledge that their loved ones are dependent on them.

TAKING ACTION

1. *Divide the class into groups that will interview people at specified age levels from childhood to old age on the subject what do life, death, sickness, health, and growing old mean to you? How do the meanings differ for each age group? Compare your meanings with those found by others in the class. How did your subjects react to being questioned?*
2. *Write your own epitaph and obituary. What is the purpose in having you do such an exercise?*
3. *List what you fear of dying and death. To what degree are these particular fears based upon rationality or irrationality?*

DYING AND DEATH: WHAT ARE THEY AND WHAT HAPPENS?
Definition

Death can be pronounced only by a physician. Once death has been determined, the physician signs a death certificate, which remains on record with the local bureau of vital statistics. In the recent past the physician pronounced death when the *vital signs* and other indices of life were absent. These vital signs included absence of breathing, pulse, and blood pressure. Other indices of lifelessness were no movement, no reflexive response to painful stimuli, and inability to communicate or otherwise respond to stimuli.

Over the years the *methods* of assessing death have improved, and thus the probability of making a correct pronouncement has increased. In the days past the physician would hold a mirror under the individual's nose to detect breathing, listen for breathing or heartbeat, and feel for a pulse. Today we have a variety of electronic instruments, like the electroencephalogram (EEG) and electrocardiogram (EKG), which are being used to refine death assessment. These are considered helpful but imperfect as yet.

Iatrogenic (physician-induced) death used to be a fairly common occurrence. It was a saying of the nineteenth century that a deep swoon (faint or coma) and a fast physician brought forth an undertaker. Many a so-called corpse was buried—only to revive, much to his surprise. Prematurely buried individuals attempted to claw their way out of their casket only to die of suffocation. To alleviate this rather calamitous error, a flag or bell was placed with a cord leading through the casket so that a revived individual could summon help before suffocating.

Even today the honest physician will tell you that the pronouncement of death is still a statement of probability—probability that the individual will not revive. The ultimate sign of death is stiffening of the body (*rigor mortis*) and bodily decay. But with the widespread need for bodily organs for transplantation, more precise criteria and means of determining "death" are needed. It won't do to dismantle and destroy one person to help another.

For an organ to be useful to a recipient it must be viable. That is, the blood, which provides nutrients and removes waste products, must continue to circulate. Thus determination of death cannot be a prolonged process if transplanting is to be done at all.

With the discovery of "life-sustaining, resuscitative methods" like chemotherapy, electroshock, the mechanical lung respirator, and cardiac massage, the heart, for example, could be kept pumping and blood flowing almost indefinitely. Even though an individual could not maintain his own heartbeat and circulation independent of "machines," his physician could be legally liable if he "pulled the plug." "If the heart beats, the person is alive" according to the law. The law was not concerned with the means or conditions under which vital signs were maintained. Of course, physicians have stopped resuscitative procedures when they felt that the individual had no hope of ever again functioning in the ways we call "human"—that is, independently.

With the progress of transplantation surgery came the haunting fear that someone would be pronounced dead prematurely because of the need for a sought-after organ. A host of ethical questions have arisen: Are the same criteria of death used uniformly for different socioeconomic groups? Will the aged, the poor, minority groups, and those who were "different" be subject to ineffectual revival procedures in order to provide a healthy organ for someone else?

The New Definition of Death

A new definition of death has become necessary. Brain rather than heart functioning would seem the key criterion. In 1968 the Ad Hoc Committee of the Harvard Medical School to Examine the Definition of Brain Death suggested four criteria for determining irreversible coma—that is, death.

In essence, the criteria suggest that death be determined when an individual (1) is unreceptive and/or unresponsive to external stimuli, (2) does not move or breathe, (3) exhibits no reflexes to external stimulation, *and* (4) shows no cerebral function (as opposed to *total* brain functioning) over a period of time (after 24 hours the entire evaluation process is to be repeated).

Compared to the criteria of *absence of vital signs* the proposals of the Ad Hoc Committee is indeed a significant advance. It provides a *new meaning* (life and death are both centered in brain, specifically cerebral, function) as well as *operational methods* for determining death. It does not pretend to be the last word. For example, it notes that the EEG loses its validity in the case of hypothermia (very low body temperature) or reduced central nervous system functioning, such as after the ingestion of barbiturates.

While the focus of death has shifted from the heart to the cerebrum, all new definitions of death agree that the goal is to determine the death of the *integrated, total individual.*

Still there remains the further need for refinement of the definition. Cases have been reported where individuals have been resuscitated after death has been pronounced using the new criteria. H. Gillon, writing in *Science News* (January 11, 1969), tells of a 15-year-old boy who sustained severe brain injury. At the hospital "the doctors found that he was dead. . . . Nevertheless, the doctors were not prepared to issue the death certificate." Some intuition made them think that there was still hope. For *two weeks* the neurosurgeons kept the boy on drugs and artificial respiration despite a flat EEG. Oxygenated blood was kept circulating artificially in the brain so as to avoid brain injury. Within two months of the accident the boy was mentally and physically in excellent condition with a normal EEG.

Even with their faults we know today that modern determinations of death are far superior to the one-time assessment of vital signs. The problem is in getting physicians to adopt the new criteria and in gaining public acceptance.

Stages of Biological Dying

Dying is a predictable process with hues of individual variation. Some have said that we begin to die the moment after birth. A classic work of V. A. Negovskii defined the stages of biological dying and death as well as the methodology for all modern death reversal procedures.

After the cessation of *vital signs*, there is a *terminal pause*. It is a

> . . . *crucial moment for the metabolism . . . the interval after regular breathing has ceased and before agonal respiration has commenced. At this time the cortex (of the brain) is in a state of deep inhibition, and the regulation of the physiological functions is performed by the brainstem . . .* [4]

---

[4]V. A. Negovskii, 1962, *Resuscitation and Artificial Hypothermia.* New York: Consultants Bureau, pp. vi–vii.

The next phase is the *terminal stage*, consisting of the substages of *agony* and *clinical death*. During agony we find the last series of compensatory and adaptive reactions of the body, immediately preceding death.

The last stage of development of the terminal state is *clinical death*. Clinical death may still be reversed.

> At this time the cardiac activity and respiration have ceased; consciousness has usually been lost before this stage,. but life at some low level is still present in the body. . . . At present . . . clinical death is [seen] as a transitional state between life and death.[5]

The last stage is *biological death* or *irreversible coma*, which comes about 10 minutes after the loss of vital functions. In some cases revival is possible, as we have seen. Generally, however, the probability of reversal of coma (death) is greatest during the earlier rather than the later seconds and minutes of dying.

TAKING ACTION

Interview nurses or physicians in a hospital intensive care unit to determine their criteria of death. Are different criteria applied to different people on the basis of age, race, type of hospital (municipal or state versus proprietary)?

Psychological Reactions to the Dying and Death of Oneself

Dying follows a psychological pattern as well as a biological one. In fact dying might be viewed as a stressor with psychosocial consequences. Elisabeth Kubler-Ross interviewed dying patients and found that they often went through five stages, which interacted and overlapped with one another. In order these stages were denial and isolation, anger, bargaining, depression, and acceptance (Kubler-Ross, 1969). As with any human behavior the so-called stages are not static and invariate. Not all dying persons reach acceptance. In fact there is controversy over whether the great majority go through any well-defined five stages of dying.

Avery D. Weisman described three developmental stages of dying (Weisman, 1972). Stage I, *primary recognition*, covers the period from a person's first awareness that "something is wrong" to the time of definitive diagnosis. This stage is accompanied by *denial* and *postponement*.

According to retrospective reports patients often turn first to family and friends to complain about nonspecific symptoms, unusual fatigue, loss of appetite, and sleep disturbance. Only when one of the "seven danger signals of cancer" develops does the person go to a physician. Other manifestations of denial and postponement see the person resort

---

[5]Negovskii, p. 211.

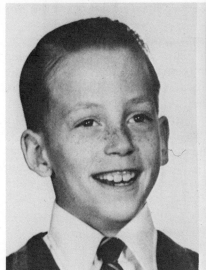
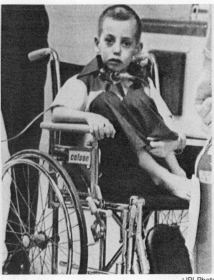

A young victim of brain cancer. The photograph on the right was taken five months after the photograph on the left.

UPI Photo

to "self-medication, optimistic rationalization, selective disregard, and avoidance of whatever might be a reminder of serious illness" (Weisman, 1972). Weisman calls this *first-order denial.*

Stage II, *established disease*, is typified by *mitigation* and *displacement* of concerns about death. One tries to lessen the impact of death often by displacement. Thus a person may feel that the recently diagnosed cancer is a result of "sin" or "God's punishment." Mitigating or reducing the sting of death often takes the form of reminiscing in nostalgic ways about the past.

Stage III, the *final decline*, which foreshadows death itself, presents problems of *countercontrol* and *cessation*. The decline into death compels the dying to relinquish control of himself or herself to some significant degree. *Cessation* is a psychological event marked by progressive loss of autonomy and consciousness. Cessation may occur long before death in some people. On the other hand, not all dying individuals experience cessation. It is possible to cease living as a responsible, conscious human being long before vital functioning actually stops. Weisman (1972) describes the transition from control to countercontrol in the person dying of a fatal illness:

> As a rule, the patient with a fatal illness must gradually yield choice and control to others. Cessation is indicated by a transition from control to counter-control. *Decency, dignity, and composure permit a dying patient to achieve this transition with minimal conflict and demoralization.*

But such a transition requires honest, open communication between the dying and significant others. Erik Erikson calls this *basic trust.* In attempts at meeting any new, stressful experiences, the guiding hand of a trusted friend can be helpful. While dying is essentially a lonely task,

239

other people can serve to instill confidence that hurdles along the way can be overcome.

For example, a consideration of great importance to the dying cancer patient is comfort and relief from pain. If basic trust and open communication exist, the patient's anxiety is often reduced. He can relinquish control of self if he knows that pain will be alleviated through analgesics such as morphine.

Disengagement theory[6] suggests that normal aging is a *mutual* withdrawal or "disengagement" between aging people and others in the social system to which they belong. The theory was in need of modification, however. Not all healthy and economically independent older people disengage from their friends, recreations, or former lifestyles. On the other hand, factors that are separate from aging—such as perceived or real poor health, poverty, isolation, social expectations, and so on—are associated with disengagement.

Richard Kalish, a pioneer in modern thanatology, has suggested that disengagement theory fell short of its mark because it did not consider the terminally ill.[7] Kalish's concept has been expanded by emphasizing the deterioration of physical and psychic energy as death approaches. Figure 7-1 shows the reduction in three arbitrarily selected levels of

Figure 7-1

Adaptation of the disengagement theory of the dying process (see text for explanation). (From D. Leviton, 1977, *Death Education and Counseling: An Aspect of Health Education.* New York: Wiley.)

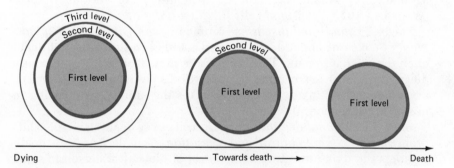

social interaction as death approaches. When healthy, we interact with various people, ranging from our peers in our classrooms or at work (third level), to aunts and uncles, nieces, and teammates (second level), to mate, child, parents, close friends, and (in the case of the dying) physicians, nurses, and others (first level). As dying progresses, only so much energy can be invested in human interaction. Levels of social interaction constrict and some are eliminated. The dying ration their human interaction to those who are *meaningful* and *significant*. The intrinsic and extrinsic motivations are so powerful that mutual engagement in these limited (first-order) interactions continues.

Of course, family members who perceive themselves as being the

---

[6]E. Cumming and W. Henry, 1961, *Growing Old.* New York: Basic Books.

[7]R. Kalish, 1972, *The Family Coordinator* 21:81–94.

"closest" to the dying may be terribly offended and hurt if the significant other turns out to be someone else. In the hospital environment the cleaning person, custodian, or nurse have often been chosen by the dying to fill this role. What are the factors contributing to the selection of the significant other person? Probably the ability to communicate openly, sensitively, and humanely is one. Empathy and kindness, and legitimizing the dying person's passing life are others.

The Final Moment: Panic or Peace?

Students always ask, "What is it like to die?" Of course, the answer transcends our experience, and thus the question is unanswerable. Perhaps the closest we can come to gaining insight is to listen to those people who have had a close call with death. We have all heard of them, or perhaps you have faced your own death by surviving a near drowning, a near or actual vehicular accident, or a serious physical illness. We learn from research on acute *life-threatening experiences* (LTE) that it is probably true that each man dies in a very personal way. Kubler-Ross insists that the moments before death are peaceful if not euphoric. Kubler-Ross summarized her insights gained from studying people who have recovered from "death" by saying:

1. The "dead" experience peace and wholeness. People who are blind experience sight. People who are filled with pain become pain-free.
2. They resent being brought to life but, after recovery, are exuberant about having a second chance.
3. Past a certain threshold, many are greeted by someone already dead—usually a loved one.
4. None is ever afraid to die again.

Another explanation considers the adaptive nature of the psyche to stress. We know that the organism fights dying to the point where central nervous system functioning becomes disorganized. Perhaps at this point of dying the psyche makes the crossing over from dying to death sanguine and euphoric. Psychologically, our brain protects us from pain. If pain becomes too great we faint or go into coma. Dying and systematic disorganization may very well be the organism's last adaptive, coping mechanism to death.

In investigating LTE as reported by college students, Kalish found that although 23 percent were fearful or in a state of panic, 77 percent of the respondents did not mention fear.[8] Alan Berman found in a later study that first reactions were panic, fear, concern about family, and friends and survivors.[9]

Long-term effects varied. In the Kalish study most reported increased caution, fear, or withdrawal. Berman's respondents wished to avoid

---

[8]R. Kalish, 1969, *Death and Bereavement*, A. H. Kutscher, ed. Springfield, Ill.: Thomas.

[9]A. Berman, 1975, *Suicide* 5:67–77.

death in the future. Some of the interviewees reported what might be termed self-actualizing experiences akin to that described by Kubler-Ross and others (Kastenbaum and Aisenberg, 1972).

THE EUTHANASIA CONTROVERSY

In classes in death education time is often spent on two ethical issues. The first topic is *war* and the second is *euthanasia* (from the Greek, meaning good or comfortable death). Our concern now is with the latter.

In contemplation of dying one wonders under what conditions it will occur. Will dying be painful, prolonged, and accentuated by technologies that may prolong suffering and diminish control of one's self?

On the other hand, will death come too soon if life-sustaining methods are withdrawn prematurely? Would the need for a body organ encourage the pronouncement of death before the fact? Might physicians "give up" too soon?

Is the specter of genocide present? Is it possible that certain "undesirable" groups of people will be valued less than others? In Nazi Germany, Jews and other non-Aryans were systematically killed on the pretext of genetic "inferiority." We have seen similarly baseless attitudes of superiority directed toward minority group members in our own society.

Today scientists talk of allowing entire nations to starve in the name of "triage" and the "lifeboat ethic"—a form of euthanasia. For the rationale offered is that in the long run those nations that cannot feed their populations are better off if their members are reduced. If birth control is not exploited, then "nature" will reduce population by starvation and disease. The prosperous nations would be better off feeding those nations that have a better chance of survival as a result of their aid. Thus populations in India and residents of the Sahel Belt in Africa are given low priority in terms of receiving food according to proponents of the "triage" theory. This approach may be seen as a form of euthanasia since others are pronouncing the style and means of death for others.

Our concern here is with individuals who might die in the hospital setting. We find that there are different types of euthanasia.

Types of Euthanasia

Four types of euthanasia have been described by theologian Joseph Fletcher:[10]

1. *Voluntary and direct.* The patient chooses his mode of death and carries it out. It is a form of suicide. A related question concerns effects of treatment or surgery in traditional medical ethics.

---

[10]J. Fletcher, 1973, *American Journal of Nursing* 73:670.

2. *Voluntary but indirect.* In this case the patient gives to *others* the *discretion* to end his life as and when the situation requires, if the patient is comatose or too dysfunctioned to make a formal decision.
3. *Direct but involuntary.* This is the traditional "mercy killing" done on the patient's behalf *without* his present or past request. It is in this form, as directly involuntary, that the problem has reached the courts in legal charges and indictments.
4. *Both indirect and voluntary.* This refers to the "letting the patient go" or "pulling the plug" tactic at the patient's request, which takes place daily in our hospitals.

Proeuthanasia Position

There is that individual who is physiologically alive—that is, vital functioning is normal—but for all intent and purposes is *psychologically* and *socially dead.* This person is the so-called "vegetable," one who might have suffered massive brain damage from an automobile accident or other cerebral trauma, or a microcephalic newborn, or a victim of massive neurologic deficit and lost cerebral capacity who continues to breathe. These are examples of people both "alive" and "dead." Such a person, Fletcher argues, is no longer a *human being*, no longer a person. It is this personal, humanness function that counts in defining "life" or *liveness.* Thus Fletcher raises two related ethical questions. First, "Is it harder to justify letting somebody die a slow and ugly death, dehumanized, than it is to justify helping him avoid it?"

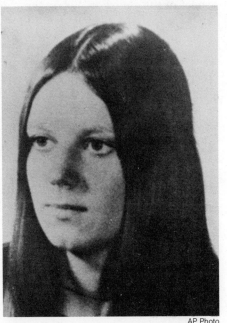

Karen Ann Quinlan, a young comatose woman kept alive by a respirator, was the subject of a euthanasia controversy.

AP Photo

243

Second, "Can we morally justify taking it into our own hands to hasten death for ourselves (suicide) or for others (mercy killing) out of reasons of compassion?"

Does the end justify the means? If the end sought is to release the patient from pointless misery and dehumanization, then the appropriate means are justified. But what justifies the end? According to Fletcher, human happiness and well-being represent the highest good. Thus euthanasia, suicide, or any other moral acts are right or wrong depending on the consequences aimed at, and the consequences are good or evil according to whether or how much they serve humane values.

Although the Nazis may have insisted that they were practicing euthanasia on Jews and others, they would be hard pressed to show how such behavior benefited the individual. On the other hand, administration of a lethal dose of a drug to kill an interminably suffering, miserable, dying individual might be the only humane means to attain the goal of relief and "well-being" for the individual.

Antieuthanasia Position

L. J. Weber argues that to group "pulling the plug" or "letting go" with "mercy killing" under the banner "euthanasia" is not morally acceptable.[11] The former type of death is compatible with the idea of not fighting death. It fits the statement of Pope Pius XII statement that the doctor should use ordinary but not *extraordinary* means to prolong life.

Mercy killing or "direct but involuntary euthanasia" shortens life regardless of how miserable. It emphasizes only the "personal" aspect of personality without recognizing that the soma or *physical* is an aspect of life also. For Weber, the "vegetable" is human until vital signs are no more. Anything less would lead to a dehumanizing of medicine.

We need to consider the ethics of "means" as well as "ends"—the nature as well as the purpose of the action. Weber maintains that man does not always know what is best for him. Medicine has always taken the position that the good of the patient is not always the same as the patient's desires.

What of the possibility of remission or the discovery of a new life-extending therapeutic approach? What if the individual had elected to die prior to this second chance?

The Nuremberg Trials

After World War II the Allies held the world-famous trials of Nazi war criminals in Nuremberg, Germany. The trial revealed the evidence of the systematic atrocities and murder practiced against large populations. According to Elliot (1972), "The idea of gassing people grew from the existing practice of 'euthanasia' in Nazi Germany, where thousands of aged and sick people had already been killed." The proeuthanasia side argues that Nuremberg taught that a person shall not have to bear

[11]L. J. Weber, 1973, *American Journal of Nursing* 73:1228.

man-inflicted suffering. Euthanasia, for this side, is a merciful release from incurable suffering and pain, the opposite of Nazi-like torture and undignified treatment of peoples.

But Nuremberg also provides a lesson to support the antieuthanasia side. When people can be killed by the state (or medicine) for any reason, then abuses will follow. Who can guarantee that the sick and the aged will not become expendable to be relieved from "suffering" by decree? And is it possible that those groups who are judged to be threatening to the state might also reap the "benefit of state-induced euthanasia"?

Both arguments are compelling. We would not extend the suffering of anyone, especially the dying. Yet we ask whether the state, physicians, or anyone can be trusted to judiciously administer such power. These are the problems that will have to be worked out by all members of society, including legislators, lawyers, physicians, theologians, ethicists, and you and me.

TAKING ACTION

1. Reprinted in Figure 7-2 is the "Living Will" developed by the Euthanasia Educational Council[12] with the hope that the wishes of the dying person will be observed by the significant surviving others, including physicians. It is not legally binding but only serves as a vehicle to transmit a person's wishes. Discuss the document. Would you sign it? Under what circumstances? Would you wish to review the document at certain time intervals? How do others in your family and immediate circle of friends react to the document? Take the document to your physician. Would the signer's wishes be honored? Under what circumstances?

2. Write your own Living Will. Considering the four types of euthanasia, which ones would or would not be acceptable to you? Under what conditions? Assuming that you can control the environment and mode of your dying, describe how you would wish to die. Considering your personal needs and the fact that others will survive you, write out in detail how you wish to die, how you wish your body disposed of, the type funeral service if any, and so on.

3. Role-play a euthanasia situation ("mercy killing"). Break up into groups of two. One person is dying and the other is a close friend, mate, or other relative. A possible scenario is in the hospital room of a dying person, who has almost no chance of recovery and who wishes to die. He or she calls upon you to help bring along death. Discuss your action, the conditions for the action, and the rationale or philosophy behind your action.

THE NATURE OF GRIEF AND BEREAVEMENT

Many students enroll in a death education course because they have had difficulty in coping with the death of someone close to them. One young woman wrote of one moment riding in a Volkswagen with a group of friends to attend a party. Another car veered through a red

---

[12]250 West 57th Street, New York, N.Y. 10019.

Figure 7-2
Euthanasia Education
Council's "Living Will."

TO MY FAMILY, MY PHYSICIAN, MY CLERGYMAN, MY LAWYER:

If the time comes when I can no longer take part in decisions for my own future, let this statement stand as the testament of my wishes:

If there is no reasonable expectation of my recovery from physicial or mental disability, I, _____, request that I be allowed to die and not be kept alive by artificial means or heroic measures. Death is as much a reality as birth, growth, maturity, and old age—it is the one certainty. I do not fear death as much as I fear the indignity of deterioration, dependence, and hopeless pain. I ask that drugs be mercifully administered to me for terminal suffering even if they hasten the moment of death.

This request is made after careful consideration. Although this document is not legally binding, you who care for me will, I hope, feel morally bound to follow its mandate. I recognize that it places a heavy burden of responsibility upon you, and it is with the intention of sharing that responsibility and of mitigating any feelings of guilt that this statement is made.

Signed _____

Date _____

Witnessed by:

_____

_____

light, smashing into the small car and killing the driver, her childhood sweetheart. In a flash a life was snuffed out by the stupid, irresponsible act of a drunken individual behind the wheel. Later she experienced nausea, a feeling of fear and trembling, choking sensation, waves of distress in the stomach, loss of appetite, and preoccupation with the thought of and face of her dead friend. She accused herself of being responsible for the death. "Why didn't I insist we stay home from the party?" "Why didn't we take my heavier car or go a different route?" are statements that give indication of the massive guilt and anger which she was experiencing. Our suffering student was experiencing an acute *grief* reaction.

Grief is an emotional state with both physical and psychological aspects associated with the awareness of *imminent* or *actual loss* (death) of a significant (beloved) someone or something. *Bereavement* might be considered as the socially sanctioned time period following death that allows for the expression of grief. Thus when someone close dies, another person may expectedly express grief. However, this bereaved individual may or may not *mourn*—that is, express his or her grief in socially prescribed ways.

Grief may precede or follow the death of someone or something special to us. A little girl may grieve and mourn for her rag doll when it is inadvertently discarded. Children suffer loss and should be allowed opportunity to mourn. The dissolution of the bond between the child or aged person and his pet by death can have unhealthy effects. Both call for the need to help the bereaved persons work through their grief.

Often *anticipatory grief* occurs *before* death. One woman suffered a stroke, which culminated in a vegetative existence for several years, finally ending in her death. Her two daughters heroically cared for her during that time, suffering her verbal and physical abuse resulting from her brain damage. When she finally died, they were relieved. They insisted on a funeral consisting of a closed casket and cremation. Other relatives were puzzled that they showed no visible signs of grief. Actually, they had worked through their grief during the five years of nursing their aged mother. Their feelings of guilt and anger had been expiated or reduced by their devotion to their mother and the realistic notion that they had done all that was humanly possible.

In the case of fatal leukemia in children, in which dying is generally prolonged, parents often will grieve and mourn prior to death. The *duration* and *quality* of the dying process seems to be two factors affecting whether grief precedes or follows death.

One's own imminent death can be mourned, of course. Perhaps the disengagement process discussed earlier is an aspect of grief.

It has been said that throughout life we suffer a myriad of "little, personal deaths" such as the death of a loved one, loss of a job, severe surgery and/or amputation, and loss of a romantic, loving relationship. Grief is the price paid for having made an investment of love in someone or something. Therefore any significant loss or separation significant to the individual can elicit a grief reaction.

The process of grief may be described as having two stages. With the realization of death or severe loss the individual suffers psychologically and somatically as he or she responds to this profound stress. Anger, shock, disbelief, guilt, despair, withdrawal, and loss of appetite are common during the *acute phase* of grief. Disorientation and disorganization are often noted in the recently bereaved.

The Process of Grief

It has been said that the body tries to heal itself. So does the psyche. With time and proper support the individual begins the process of reconstitution, of pulling oneself together to get on with living. Thus the Judaic tradition says that during the first seven days of mourning (Shiva) the bereaved are not to provide for themselves. Good neighbors or members of the congregation bring food for the table, care for the children, and otherwise attend to the routine of life. The Judaic mourning ritual seems to make therapeutic sense in view of what we know of the psychosomatic effects of grief.

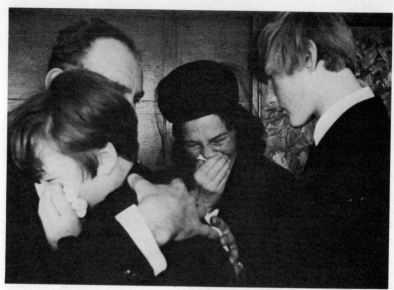

Magnum Photos

Disengagement is painful. Psychologically the bereaved wishes the dead to be alive. One wishes that death could be negated. But the reality principle forces the bereaved to accept the fact of death. The give and take between the desire to hold on and the necessity of letting go is manifested in the second phase, the *work of mourning*. It involves the cathartic, healthy effect of expressing the emotions, feelings, and attitudes one has toward the dead. Someone once said that both the dying and bereaved should be allowed and encouraged to cry, to scream in anger and sorrow, and to discharge all of one's suppressed grief. It includes talking about the dead: reminiscing over and psychologically justifying the human relationship. Eventually and gradually it includes reintegration into society.

Variations of Grief

Grief has many variations. One occurs along a *time* continuum.

We talked earlier of anticipatory grief. There is also *prolonged grief*. Some bereaved people will continue to grieve for years. Such behavior is probably a function of environment, the quality of relationship between the dead and the living, and other factors. An elderly woman was diagnosed as manifesting an "abnormal grief reaction." She had suffered the death of her husband some two years previously, but had continued to set a place for him at the dinner table ever since. She was known to carry on quite interesting conversations with "him" on the state of the world, national politics, and the arts. Her fantasizing was considered abnormal until someone with insight thought to investigate to see whether the woman might be lonely. She proved to be not only lonely but almost completely isolated as well. The introduction of friends and activities by way of senior citizen center activities and volunteer efforts gave new meaning to her life. She reported with humor that although she enjoys her new friends and activities, she does miss the stimulating conversations she had with her dead husband. Yet a change of her physical and social environment demonstrated that she was a victim of a lonely, meaningless existence rather than pathological mourning.

Grief may even be *delayed*. Following death some people report no immediate significant physical or emotional changes. A young man whose best friend had been killed in Vietnam in battle commented that it was only several weeks after the news of the death that he was struck with grief.

One expression of sorrow is *paralyzed inaction*. There is a feeling of deep fatigue and heaviness. To accomplish the simplest task is an ordeal. One is drained and severely depressed. Another finds sorrow actualized in a frenzy of *activity*. Thus we often find a bereaved individual working in a compulsive way. An immaculate house is cleaned again and again, a term paper is typed and retyped. Some physically oriented people work through their grief in a gymnasium by exercising to exhaustion.

Considering the profound effects of death upon our total functioning, it is not surprising to find that grief is associated with many physical and physiological problems (Parkes, 1972). Death of a loved one might be viewed as a stressor affecting the autonomic, hormonal, and immune systems of the body. Overall health status can be severely lowered during grief. It is important to maintain good nutrition and other aspects of health so that the defenses of the body are able to withstand the stresses placed upon it.

We know, for example, that during the first year following the death of a mate the number of deaths among surviving widows is significantly greater than among a matched control group who are not widows. Unresolved grief has even been associated with such later problems as cancer, alcoholism, juvenile delinquency, and suicide. Of course, not everyone who has endured the death of a loved one will resolve it in the ways mentioned. Human beings are much too complex for such generalizations to apply.

Role of Death Education and Grief Therapy

Grief and mourning are *normal* developmental correlates of loss, especially death. Death education can be of great service in helping one work through grief healthfully. Learning of the emotional and physical changes associated with grief can serve to allay fears and enhance the healing process. One student was relieved to learn that her anger directed toward the "bitch of a dead grandmother" was in no way abnormal. Those who did not treat us well in life do not always turn into angels upon their death, at least not in the minds of the living. The girl was asked, "Assuming your grandmother left much to be desired as a human being, what have you learned from your relationship with her that would make you a better person?" Her response demonstrated that she had learned improved self-control, tolerance, and the self-destructive nature of hating. She no longer felt suicidal or hyperaggressive.

Not only may death education serve to prepare the individual for the real-life trauma of grief when it occurs, but students report that they are able to be supportive of others coping with death. Thus those who have learned of grief become "grief counselors" and "crisis intervenors" in very special and real ways. Students themselves become the first line of defense in helping others with a variety of life crises and stresses.

THE HOUSE OF THE DEAD: THE FUNERAL INDUSTRY

Funeral ritual has been controlled and institutionalized in this country in large measure by the funeral industry. Originally the funeral service was an important function of religion. Today formal religion has conceded the care of the dead and the bereaved largely to the funeral establishment.

Today's funeral director operates a service-oriented business (Mitford, 1963). He or she is among other things a business person (some honest, some dishonest), a grief counselor (some good, some bad; some conscientious, some superficial or aloof), and the individual chiefly responsible for the disposal of the corpse. He or she will dispose of the corpse as requested for a fee. Unfortunately, the bereaved is usually in a weakened state and is therefore a vulnerable customer. One would not buy an automobile while weak and feeling depressed, or perhaps disoriented. Why should one be expected to deal effectively with arranging for a funeral service, where the financial costs are high, at a time when the level of cognitive functioning is generally impaired? Students of the funeral industry, many funeral directors, and their national organization emphasize the need for education so that funeral arrangements can be made while people are able to think and act rationally.

Following are some questions that students raise. The answers may be helpful to you.

1. *What is the funeral process?* It is a ritual designed to help the bereaved work through his or her grief in a socially sanctioned environment. The funerary business is part of our culture's "death establishment," to use Kastenbaum and Aisenberg's terminology (1972). The process may be informal or formal, but in our highly complex society it has become institutionalized.

After death has been pronounced and the death certificate signed by the physician, the funeral director picks up the body from the hospital morgue (refrigeration room). In the case of equivocal death or where the cause of death is questionable, an autopsy is usually required before the body is turned over to the undertaker. At the funeral home the body is prepared according to directions. There may or may not be embalming, open viewing, funeral service at the funeral home, cemetery service, and so on. The variations are many. One can request a short service followed by cremation or burial following a short service. One can request cremation ashes to be scattered in the yard or over the ocean. Whatever is requested will cost.

2. *How are fees determined?* In the *single-unit* method (the complete funeral) the price of the casket determines the price of the entire service. In other words, the services rendered are constant regardless of the type of casket ordered. A $300 or $3000 *service* is the same; the difference in price is in the "elegance" of the casket. Services usually include placing an announcement in the newspaper (obituary), transporting the corpse from the hospital to the funeral home, determining the funeral benefits applicable to the client from social security, veterans benefits, service organizations, flowers, use of the home for services and viewing, transportation to the cemetery, making arrangements with the cemetery, and so on.

The *biunit* method breaks down the funeral cost into the price of the casket and another sum for all other services and facilities. A third method breaks down pricing into separate costs for casket, services, and facilities, the so-called *triunit* method.

A recent *Federal Trade Commission Survey of Funeral Prices in the District of Columbia* found that the average cost of a regular adult funeral in Washington, D.C. was $1137 during the first nine months of 1973. *Minimum* prices for the complete funeral ranged from $210 to $900.

However, there are numerous other expenses above and beyond the cost of the so-called "complete funeral." First, some goods and services sold by the funeral director such as a burial vault or outer case, burial clothing, additional limousines, and a vehicle for conveying flowers. Second, there are costs connected with the burial or other disposition of the body. These include the cost of a cemetery plot and perpetual care, the fee for opening and closing the grave, and the cost of a grave liner or box, if a vault or outer case has not been purchased. Other costs might include those for a crypt or mausoleum space or the cost of cremation and sometimes an urn and columbarium niche. Third, there may be costs for memorialization such as for a marker or graveside monument.

Cornell Capa/Magnum Photos

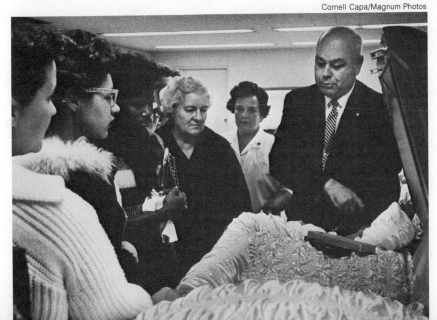

A funeral director pointing out the advantages of a luxury casket.

These and other costs suggest that the wise, death-educated consumer would do well to investigate the business end of the funeral before the emotional trauma of death obscures reason and the ability to discriminate between exploitive and fair prices.

3. *Are there legal misconceptions that can affect prices?* The Federal Trade Commission report said that in Washington, as in many other jurisdictions, there is no law requiring the consumer to purchase embalming, a casket for cremation, or a vault in ordinary circumstances. Embalming may be legally necessary in some *few* instances—for example, if death was caused by communicable disease or if the body is transported through a jurisdiction that requires that bodies shipped interstate be embalmed. In reality, zoning boards restrict burial to cemeteries. Their decision is usually based upon unwarranted fears of contamination and disease, the fact that most people wish no proximity to the dead, and the efforts of cemetery lobbying groups.

4. *Does the funeral director do any "good"?* Yes and no, and much in between. *Yes*, in that the funeral director is often the one to legitimize and encourage the expression of grief in the bereaved individual. Phyllis Silverman, an authority on widowhood, has described how immensely helpful many funeral directors are in their crisis intervention work with widows and widowers and bereaved children. Often they step in where others (clergy, friends, and relatives) fear or avoid going—to the aid and support of the bereaved. Some funeral directors go out of their way to help the bereaved make a judicious choice of services that can be afforded by the individual. There are funeral directors who have conducted death education classes in their establishments to better acquaint the public with all aspects of funerary practice, including the economic.

No, in that the funeral *system* by definition may be in need of reform. Considering that the body decays regardless of the type container in which it is placed suggests a low cost, simple casket and burial. Because of the business nature of the funeral system the buyer is seen as a "sale" and is often approached for "all that the traffic will bear."

No, in that many of the features such as the need for embalming and "open viewing" of the body are often sold as a necessary palliative for all who are mourning. Embalming and open viewings are profit items. No solid body of research supports the need for *universal* viewing of the dead as a means to improving emotional recovery. When one opts for an open viewing, many expenses are added to the final bill such as embalming, clothing, cosmetology, viewing room, flowers, and so on.

5. *Are there alternatives to the traditional funeral?* Yes. One alternative involves prearrangement of the funeral before a death actually occurs. This may not include actually paying for the funeral beforehand. A second alternative is cremation, which involves burning the body by intense heat so that only ashes remain. Funeral directors may try to sell an accompanying service similar to a "casket service." Some try to sell a special casket to hold the urn that holds the ashes. Many will allow a simple delivery of the body to the crematorium and return

the remains in a simple urn to you. It depends upon your needs and your ability to ask for what you wish. In many cases it means overcoming a sales pitch or induced guilt. For example, a funeral director may say, "I'm sure you would like to provide your generous and wonderful father with a more elaborate ceremony than just cremation and burial. . . ." It takes courage to say, "My father is dead, and this is precisely what I want. Now do it, please!"

Another alternative involves donating one's body or body organs to a medical school or to medical research. Many states have adopted the Anatomical Gift Act, which allows you to designate your body or organs to a physician, hospital, storage bank, or other medical institution. Figure 7-3 is a reproduction of an Anatomical Gift Form, which is

TO MY FAMILY AND PHYSICIAN:

It is my wish that upon my death, my body, or any part of it, be used for the benefit of mankind.

I therefore execute the following Deed of Gift, under the Anatomical Gift Act, and I request that in the making of any decision relating to my death, my intentions as expressed herein shall govern.

I am of sound mind and 18 years or more of age. I hereby make this anatomical gift to take effect upon my death. The marks in the appropriate places and words filled into the blanks below indicate my desires.

I give: my body _____; any needed organs or parts _____; the following organs or parts _____. I give these to the following person or institution: the physician in attendance at my death _____; the hospital in which I die _____; the following named physician, hospital, storage bank, or other medical institution _____; the following individual for treatment _____; for any purpose authorized by law _____; transplantation _____; therapy _____; research _____; medical education _____.

_____
Signature of donor

_____

Date _____   _____
Address of donor

Signed by donor in presence of following who sign as witnesses:

_____   _____

Figure 7-3
Anatomical Gift Form.

253

legally binding. You should investigate the recipient of your choice to determine whether they will pick up the body when notified of death, return ashes of the body if so desired, and so on.

Memorial societies, another alternative, are a relatively recent innovation and are established in well over 120 cities in Canada and the United States. Their headquarters[13] provides a valuable kit, which includes a *Manual of Death Education and Simple Burial*, a list of memorial societies, forms for making an anatomical gift, the Living Will, and other materials. Their role is twofold. First, they are interested in providing death education for the public. They are independent of the funeral industry and are working toward providing lower-priced, simple burial. Second, they are able to provide lower funeral costs to their membership. They seek funeral directors who will offer a "discount" for their members. Memorial societies are nonprofit organizations, of course.

In summation, one might safely say that some sort of *ritual* for the dead is beneficial for most in working through the very natural, transitional phase of life known as bereavement. A good funeral director can help the bereaved in so many ways. On the other hand, funeral directors are business people interested in the greatest possible profit. In this case, *caveat emptor* (let the buyer beware) remains a valuable guide to the consumer.

TAKING ACTION

1. *Visit a few funeral homes to "shop" and arrange your own funeral. Assume that you have a family who survives you. What did you learn by doing comparison shopping?*
2. *Interview a funeral director. What types of death are most difficult for him to handle emotionally? What training is required to become a funeral director?*
3. *Interview or invite a widow or widower to talk to your class to discuss the ways they had to adapt to their new status psychologically and socially. What very practical problems did they have to contend with?*

DISCUSSION Death education has been presented as a *preventive, remedial,* and *optimal health* aspect of health education. It is *preventive* in the sense that individuals can learn to prepare for the contingencies of life and death. To learn how the language of death might affect behavior and particularly our role as "sick," "dying," or "patient" might cause a more humane interaction between people and helping medical personnel. To learn of the child's view of death may help us rear our children to enjoy happier, healthier lives. To be able to subject death to the

---

[13]Continental Association of Funeral and Memorial Societies, 1828 L Street N.W., Washington, D.C. 20036.

scrutiny of clinical and scientific inquiry is a beginning leading to a better understanding of the origins of many of our anxieties and fears.

Police officers, nurses, physicians, soldiers, expectant parents, long-time parents, teachers, husbands and wives of the dying, clergy, librarians, social workers, physical and behavioral scientists, and others report that death education was *remedial* for them. Death education may contribute to what has been called *optimal health*.[14] The confrontation of the fact that we and our loved ones can die at any moment because of unnecessary man-made hazards can motivate reform to a higher order of social health. For example, many of us share the notion that war is unhealthy. This suggests that we adopt *action* that would eliminate war as a viable option for the resolution of world problems. It is possible that those who are always recommending war either avoid the possibility of their own death or *think* that they are safe due to their economic-political status.

If we look at air and water pollution, starvation, and similar problems in the context of contributing to your death or your child's death, then those problems become extremely important to us and move us toward taking action. In a sense death education suggests the need for community awareness and action concerning the *death-causing* factors in our society.

If death education can serve as a stimulus to improve the health of society, it has the potential of doing the same for the individual. Our contemplation and knowledge of death can help us fashion our lives and deaths as we see fit. It prods us to *choose* rationally how we will live and die. It encourages communication and solidarity between loved ones. Knowledge and communication are two of the components necessary for action toward change.

FOR FURTHER READING

Elliot, G., 1972. *Twentieth Century Book of the Dead.* New York: Scribners.

This book describes the mass deaths in our time. On the battlefields of both world wars, in the death camps of the 1930s and 1940s, in Vietnam, and in hundreds of local disasters, pogroms, and organized famines, some 110 million have died. A useful tome for reminding us of our propensity for producing untimely deaths.

Feifel, H., 1959. *The Meaning of Death.* New York: McGraw-Hill.

Dr. Feifel is the father of modern thanatology, and the book is still a major resource. Sections include theoretical outlooks on death, developmental orientation toward death, death concepts in religious and cultural fields, and clinical and experimental studies.

---

[14]H. Ratner, 1971, *Child and Family* 19:28.

Kastenbaum, R., and Aisenberg, R., 1972. *The Psychology of Death.* New York: Springer.

The authoritative text on psychosocial aspects of death. Encyclopedic in breadth, it is a necessary reference and text for the sophisticated student and researcher.

Kubler-Ross, E., 1969. *On Death and Dying.* New York: Macmillan.

This work has served as the single most powerful force in acquainting the lay public with the urgent need for the study of death and dying and for reforms in medical and nursing care of the dying.

Lifton, R., 1969. *Death in Life: Survivors of Hiroshima.* New York: Vintage Books.

Dr. Lifton interviewed 75 survivors of the atomic bomb blast at Hiroshima. His work provides support for the notion that death education should include consideration of the consequences of atomic war and the need to eliminate it as a means for resolving international conflict.

Mitford, J., 1963. *The American Way of Death.* New York: Simon and Schuster.

The classic analysis of malpractices in the funeral industry. It includes a directory of memorial societies, information on how to organize a memorial society, and information about eye banks and about donating bodies for medical science.

Parkes, C., 1972. *Bereavement: Studies of Grief in Adult Life.* New York: International Universities Press.

One of the best research-oriented studies on the varied, developmental effects of grief and bereavement.

Shneidman, D., 1973. *Deaths of Man.* New York: Quadrangle/New York Times Book Company.

The author defines and discusses "partial death," "postself," the "psychological autopsy," "megadeaths," "equivocal death," and other unique conceptualizations.

Weisman, A., 1972. *On Death and Denying.* New York: Behavioral Publications.

On the basis of clinical and psychometric data Dr. Weisman proposes that nearness to death and stages of refusal to accept the idea of dying are interrelated. This knowledge is most useful in understanding and helping the dying.

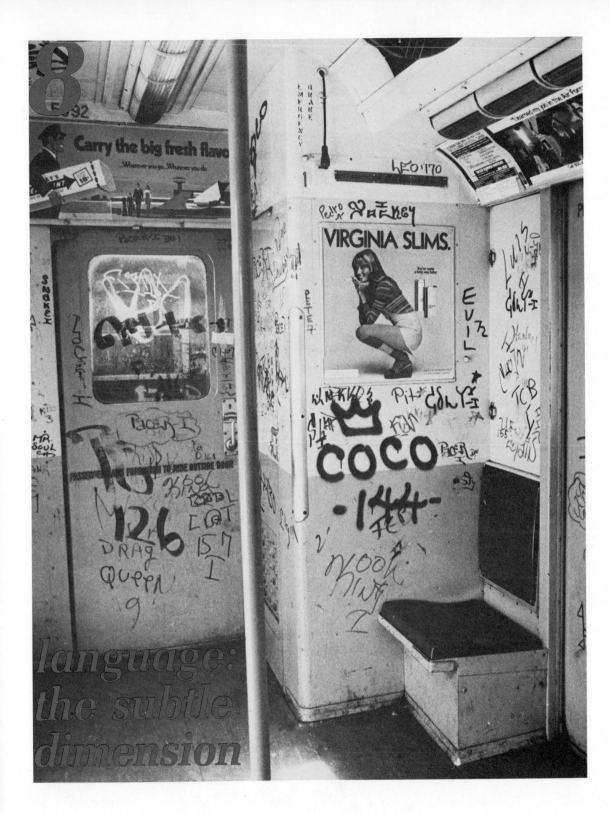

language:
the subtle
dimension

OVERVIEW

*This chapter is intended to demonstrate that language, though
generally unnoticed, is a major factor in human health—perhaps
on a par with microbiology, physiology, psychology, and
sociology. To illustrate this point, each chapter of this book is
examined briefly for language-related implications. It is seen,
among other things, that the emotional impact of particular words
(such as death, disease, and sex) affects health behavior,
including our ability to think clearly and objectively about the
particular subjects under consideration; that language problems
commonly interfere with good patient-doctor communication; that
to a considerable extent we talk ourselves into our physical and
emotional health status; that our social interactions and
adjustments are very much dependent upon how we talk to and
with others, including our mates, children, parents, co-workers;
that progress in some major areas of disease fighting is
hamstrung by language barriers; that labels rub off on people and
through labeling on the basis of condition ("cardiacs,"
"psychotics," "aphasics," "elderly") we tend to dehumanize them:
they become more the label than the human being. Suggestions
are made in the hope of focusing attention on language-health
problems, evaluating them, and taking steps to avoid them.*

INQUIRY

1. How does language sometimes interfere with medical treatment?
2. Can a girl be both "feminine" and physically fit? Athletic? Strong?
3. Might you like certain foods if they were called something else? (For example, shark, eel, turtle, squid, fish meal bread.)
4. Is much health product advertising designed to mislead if not actually untrue?
5. Can you talk yourself into and out of emotional health?
6. Are we failing to beat some major diseases because of the language barrier?

INTRODUCTION In recent decades more and more of the academic disciplines, ranging from English and speech to psychology, sociology, and anthropology, have been recognizing the important and sometimes crucial role of language in human behavior. Generally, health specialists have so far neglected the language dimension of their discipline. They have continued to view language as communication, which it is, but not as a prime factor influencing health behavior, which it also is. This chapter is concerned with illustrating how language plays a very important role in many aspects of human health behavior. It may also illustrate how, often unfortunately for us, it sometimes influences health behavior profoundly—without our being aware of it at all. Hopefully, considera-

tions presented here will lead to (1) greater awareness of the possible
role of language in human health, (2) less vulnerability to intentional
and unintentional linguistic tricks that may affect health, and (3)
progress in the healthful use of language in health-related matters.

Our approach here will be to look at each subject dealt with in this
book to try to identify significant language implications. It should
become clear why some claim that language is not only a major obstacle
in the way of communication about certain health matters including
disease fighting but is also a frequent cause of emotional (which
includes physiological) upset and disturbed social relations. What
evidence is there for such broad contentions?

Try the following for openers. According to experts, perhaps the
greatest obstacle preventing the conquest of VD is the *words* associated
with them. In the first place, nice people are not supposed to talk about
such nasty things, especially how transmission takes place, so educational campaigns founder. More fundamentally, even though parents
know that their children are aware of how babies are conceived, almost
none can bring themselves to use the words needed to educate them
about these diseases and their prevention. The situation is similar in
many schools—with the result that VD incidence is rising astronomi-
cally, particularly among teenagers.

With regard to emotional upset: just let someone *tell* you that you
made an ass of yourself; if you're a typical male, let someone tell you
that you think like a woman; or let someone give you some bad news,
for example, "There will be an important quiz on this material in five
minutes!" Then notice your physiological responses, which are a part
of your general upset. Notice that your upset is not "just in your head"
but throughout your body as well. Your heart rate and blood pressure
probably increased; your hands, feet, armpits, and forehead may have
begun to sweat; your mouth may have become dry; you may even have
begun to tremble; and your face may have changed color. Any such
changes were accompanied by various changes in your blood chemistry, all in response to a few words. If what was said to you was very
upsetting, there is a very good chance that your ability to *think*
declined. As emotional upset goes up beyond a certain point, thinking
ability tends to go down. This accounts for why people oftentimes fail
exams even when they really know the material. Moreover, if you
continue to say the things to yourself that were said to you: "I made an
ass of myself," "I think like a woman," "I'm a failure," "I'm abnormal,"
you can keep yourself in a state of upset and be miserable for extended
periods. As a matter of fact, large numbers of people go to doctors and
psychotherapists for help with psychosomatic (mind-body) disturbances based not really on what was said to them originally but on
persistent, faulty self-talk that keeps the message alive psychophysio-
logically. But more of this later.

Our emotional responses usually involve other people, and language
is an important factor in this social aspect of our health. In the

foregoing examples, it is easy to see social implications and how the language of another person triggered the emotional responses described. It is also apparent that the words of another person initiated the self-talk that gave rise to continued upset. The self-talk very likely became social in terms of comments about the individual whose statements were permitted to give rise to all of the commotion ("That bastard! What did he mean saying . . .").

As we will see, language affects health behavior in ways that range all the way from being labeled as having some diseases (people who have been cured of cancer often continue to suffer from job discrimination because of the boss's or other employees' dread of the word) to greatly influencing our health product buying practices (most dry cereals have very little nutritional value, but words like "vitamins" in advertising convince people that they do). Let us look through the key health topics covered in this book for a hint as to how language may be an important factor in each.

COMMON HEALTH PROBLEMS AND MEDICAL ADVICE

Evaluating our health and seeking medical advice are complicated by our ways of talking and feeling about our physical and mental health, about our bodies, and about doctors. People tend to be suspicious of their health status because from childhood we are often bombarded with statements suggesting how vulnerable we are to sickness: "If you eat that, you'll get sick," "If you don't eat, you'll be sick," "If you go without your coat, you'll get sick," and so on. One child who came down with paralytic polio was convinced that he felt "a little bad" because he had disobeyed his mother and played in the woods, behavior which she had told him would make him sick. Similar magic-mindedness is often seen when people become ill after drinking and automatically blame "drinking too much" because of deep-seated attitudes toward alcohol rather than because of any necessarily logical connection between the two.

We have a very special attitude towards germs, an attitude that is exploited regularly by the advertisers of soaps, deodorants, mouth washes, and so forth. We have been led to believe that our mouths, other body openings, and our skin are literally teeming with germs, against which we must struggle mightily. Not only are large industries supported by this message, but also it convinces many people that unless they scrub and douse themselves with products, they are unsanitary, dirty, smelly, and likely to be diseased.

In addition to the largely word-based apprehensions about our health, there are the very real hazards of the environment such as irritants in the air. The effects of these may be intensified by talking about them in alarmist terms. (The message may be delivered in nonalarmist terms, but self-talk of the hearer may then be alarmist.) For example, it may take only a comment about poor air quality to trigger nose and eye running, even though the irritants present may actually be lower than usual. In fact whole wards of asthma patients have been known to respond to falsified pollen reports and charts, breathing easily in "bad" air, and having attacks when the count was low. Thus the power of verbal suggestion is not to be underestimated with respect to our health status. Did you ever see what happens to people when several others take turns telling them how ill they look? It's almost bound to happen if the victim starts to panic, engaging in catastrophic self-talk about how awful he must indeed feel if he looks so bad.

Then there are the very real stress factors, with their body-mind repercussions in symptoms commonly associated with new and demanding circumstances. Starting college, getting a new job, going into military service, and so on are examples of common stressful experiences. The chapter on emotional health in this book is intended, among other things, to help young people adjust successfully to the demands of college. Failure to act upon such guidance can easily give rise to a variety of symptoms such as digestive upset, interruption of menstrual cycle, headaches, and feelings of tension and anxiety—all of which send people off to doctors for help.

Chapter 1 is concerned with medical advice. Let us begin this discussion by noting some ways in which going to a doctor can pose some interesting language-related problems.

When we do feel ill enough to seek medical help, we risk receiving inadequate care if certain common language factors are not taken into account.

The authority of the medical profession is so great that many people tend to take a doctor's word as gospel—perhaps without really understanding what the doctor has said. At the other extreme, some people rebel at the doctor's status and authority; they may refuse to do anything the doctor says or perhaps will not even go to one unless forced. Of course, both positions are unrealistic. Doctors are human beings with some specialized knowledge and skills, but they are fallible human beings nonetheless and possess every human right to make mistakes. There has never been a perfect doctor, teacher, mechanic, parent, house builder, or whatnot, and there never will be.

One of the problems with dealing with doctors is that they have a special jargon, just as every other profession has. Moreover, after many years of using medical terminology day in and day out, it becomes their language. Unfortunately, many doctors forget that most patients are not familiar with their special terminology; the patient is literally afraid to ask questions, so any really worthwhile communication breaks down. Not only might the patient not fully understand the doctor's comments or instructions, but the words might very well be misinterpreted. The result then is failure to do the recommended thing; even worse, the patient may do the wrong thing.

In some areas, a problem may exist because the doctor's training did not include the particular subject we are talking about: language. Although medical schools and postgraduate studies are now attempting to resolve this problem, the fact remains that there are definite blind spots in medical training, and thus many doctors are simply not prepared to handle some common problems. If this difficulty seems to be arising, ask questions just as you would feel free to ask an automobile mechanic, "Do you fix automatic transmissions?" If he doesn't, you go elsewhere.

Do you find it easy to present some symptoms but not others to doctors? It's not surprising if you do. Most people have a hierarchy of body parts. Where would you rank eyes and hands in comparison with crotch, genitals, and anus? From early childhood we tend to be taught that some parts of our bodies and the *words* associated with them are much less acceptable than others. Thus many people are reluctant to go to doctors because of certain symptoms, even though they may be extremely unpleasant, even painful or embarrassing. If they do go to a doctor, they clam up, finding it most difficult to use "dirty" words in front of such a respectable person. There is sometimes the further difficulty that the doctor knows or will use only the "correct" technical words for parts and functions. The patient may know only the "vulgar" language (that is, language of the people), so, of course, communication breaks down completely, and consequently medical effectiveness suffers.

Does it make sense to allow language to prevent the treatment of symptoms and waste money? Hardly. Perhaps it is time for us all to make friends with our bodies in their entirety and with the words we must use in order to communicate effectively about them. Perhaps in our dealings with children we can help eliminate this problem in the future by making sure that their body attitudes are positive and that body words function as facilitators, not stoppers, of vital communication.

It is perhaps especially important that women learn to be assertive, to speak up and ask questions in the medical situation. There is evidence that doctors do not tend to take as seriously the complaints of women as they do those of men. The inevitable result is that many serious conditions go undiagnosed and untreated, sometimes with very serious consequences.

Similarly, it has been found that some male psychotherapists are sexist with regard to their treatment of women who come to them. Their attitude is reflected in their language to clients, which suggests to them that their need is to learn to accept their inferior, nonassertive, second-sex status rather than attempt to grow as human beings. Sometimes they are led to believe that all they need is more frequent sexual servicing by a male. But then the doctor is the expert, the one trained to know his business. It takes real effort and determination on the woman's part to resist such pressure to conform to old stereotypes.

The intent here is not to be critical of medical or other therapists. Some are extremely sensitive to the importance of verbalization and understanding in their dealings with patients. Some never fail to find the time to talk so as to get, as nearly as possible, the full picture. However, since language considerations are not a routine part of medical training, such sensitivity cannot be counted on in doctors any more than in anyone else. It is ironic that most people get some training in public speaking, which relatively few of us are required to do, and almost no one gets training in *private* speaking, which we all do all of the time! Effective treatment cannot be left entirely to the doctors: there must be a two-way communication. Those going for help need to assume responsibility for providing all relevant information about their symptoms that they can. This often requires taking the time to jot down notes about when symptoms first appeared, under what circumstances, whether they have grown worse or changed, and so on. Moreover, they need to be ready and able to interact verbally with the doctor, answering *and asking* questions freely. After all, how is the doctor going to know you don't understand if you don't tell him or her, or if you say you understand when you don't? And finally, it means that patients should view themselves as consumers in the medical marketplace with every right to question, get second opinions, and shop around when not satisfied. The last chapter of this book on consumer education provides some detailed guidelines for you to consider following.

TAKING ACTION

1. *You can use the following instruments to evaluate key words in connection with each topic discussed in this chapter. Item A below will give you an idea of what people associate with certain health words. Item B will show how strongly people feel about these words.*

    A. Word association. *Instructions for administration: "I am going to say a word (or phrase). Please say (jot down) the first word that you think of in response to my word (or phrase)." For example, try the word "apple."*

    Note: If you give A to a group, you'll find that responses tend to fall into a few categories. Thus you can quickly see what predominant associations the group has with the particular word.

    B. Word cathexis. *Instructions: "Please rate the following words on a scale ranging from 1 to 5, going from very negative to very positive, depending on how strongly you feel about the word." For example, rate the words "apple" and "spinach," the words "tangy" and "yecch."*

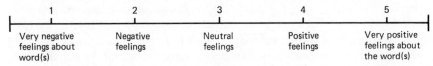

Figure 8-1
Word cathexis: a personal
reaction scale.

    Note: If you give B to a group, you can analyze each word as to how strongly people feel about it and compare words in terms of their average numerical values.

    Now select a number of words associated with this discussion, and try them out using word association and word cathexis techniques. Use such words as eyes, anus, hospital, injections, drill, sick, diagnosis, prescription, and so on. Not all class members will respond in the same way, but do patterns emerge for the group? Is there evidence that although people sometimes react mainly to some experience recalled by a word, much of the reaction is to the word itself?

2. *With at least one other person recall situations in which you have known language to facilitate or interfere with desired medical, dental, or other treatments. What exactly helped or went wrong? Why? How might problems have been avoided?*

3. *Discuss specific plans for getting the most out of future medical appointments.*

4. *Identify a person (perhaps yourself) who has an appointment to see a doctor. Rehearse preparation and verbal interaction with the doctor. After the session with the doctor, recap it with respect to how satisfactory it was. How would you rate the quality of communication that occurred? Is there full understanding of words and instructions? What should you do to train yourself to be a better consumer of medical services?*

NUTRITION AND WEIGHT CONTROL

A couple of extreme examples may help to establish that language can be very much a factor in our eating behavior. In one documented case a young African who was on a journey stopped for breakfast with a friend. When being served, he asked whether the meat was wild hen, because for him this food was taboo. A few years later the young man visited his friend again, and this time he was offered wild hen. But he refused, stating that he dared not eat it. Then his host laughed and asked why it should hurt him now when he had eaten it without harm on his last visit. When the traveler thus learned that he had been tricked and had unintentionally violated his tribal taboo, he began to shake with fear and was dead in less than a day. Note that the meat eaten long ago did not change. Only the verbal label had been changed. The great physiologist Walter Cannon, who described the above case, studied the well-documented phenomenon of voodoo death and concluded that words and other symbols of black magic are indeed capable of setting off such severe neurophysiological reactions associated with fear as to destroy the usual cortical control of emotional behavior and culminate in shock and death.

We have many "loaded" words associated with foods that are likely to affect us physically. For example, a rancher in Arizona enjoyed serving his guests sandwiches that they considered delicious—until he informed them that they were eating rattlesnake meat salad, not tuna fish as they had supposed. Upon hearing this, the guests typically became upset, nauseated, or began vomiting. Note that the substance in reality—the meat—did not make them sick. They thought it fine until a particular word was introduced, and the word made them sick.

Numerous food words are enough to turn the stomach of people, although what may trigger unpleasant reactions in one person may give rise to enjoyable gastric sensations in another—for example, squid, shark, eel, larvae, and asparagus. "Steak" is a dirty word to the confirmed vegetarian but quite the opposite to most others. Incidentally, "vegetarians" may not be exactly a dirty word to meat eaters, but it does suggest that the nonmeat eater is an oddball. This is true in spite of the fact that meat is not essential in the diet and that rejection of meat either from preference or conviction does not necessarily mean that there is something wrong psychologically. Spinach, which is supposed to be so valuable a food, is an upsetting word as well as food to many of the children forced to eat it. Incidentally, the word "spinach" is a nice example of how a label may not really describe what it is fastened to at all or may only partially describe it. Many a person has been surprised to find that not all spinach is the severely boiled, almost mushlike gob that is ladled onto the plate with its juice flowing over everything else. It may not even be recognized when served lightly steamed or raw in salads. Still it is likely to be damned by its name, and call forth a "yecch" if identified.

Some edible foods are unacceptable to whole groups of people even though they are enjoyed if they are not identified—horse meat, for example. Others have been referred to as "halo" foods; that is, foods that are considered so good that people sometimes view them as indispensable in the diet. Orange juice, milk, spinach, and lean meat are among these. "Whole grain" flour, "dark" bread, "golden" honey, and so on are near halo in status. In spite of the fact that these words make people feel good, none of them is really needed in the diet. Many if not most of the people of the world have managed to be reasonably healthy without any of them. Why? Because other foods that are available to them contain the same needed substances. Oranges are fine,

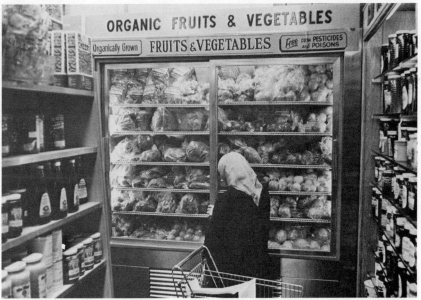

Advertising affects many of the choices consumers make in supermarkets.

Hugh Rogers/Monkmeyer

but don't worry if you don't like them or can't get any for a time. (This is an important point, because many people have gained the impression that their health will be affected if they miss their morning orange juice for a single day. As for milk, although babies need it, large numbers of adults of the world cannot tolerate it physiologically. We've made many people sick with our gifts of milk.)

As we shall note in the consumer education discussion, advertisers play with the halo words so as to increase sales even though there may be no substance behind the words. For example, "vitamin-enriched" sounds great, but such foods often contain insignificant amounts of vitamins indicated. "Brown" bread is likely to be nothing but some food dye or molasses added to ordinary white flour—not the staff of life it is represented to be. But we buy the words every day.

Sometimes the nutrition situation is confused by the fact that some foods are both halo and dirty words. For several decades now, people have been warned that sweets are not healthful, at least insofar as the teeth are concerned. Moreover, in recent years, a considerable amount of evidence has suggested that refined sugar in the quantities we consume may be harmful to us in a variety of ways. On the other hand, children are often enticed to eat by sweetening foods, and sweets are often used as rewards for obedience and other desired behavior. So to health-conscious parents and teachers, "sweets" and "sugar" are dirty words; but terms such as "sugar-coated" help companies sell products. Sugar is thus also a halo food—and word.

The area of weight control has its full share of attitude- and behavior-shaping words. Both "fat" and "skinny" are objectionable; "round" and "thin" are somewhat less so. "Solid" and "lean" are moving up on the favorable side, and so on to "beautiful hunk" and what not. But a little round is fat to some, just right to others. Unless you are recovering from an illness, you are likely to feel complimented if someone says, "You've lost weight," even though you know for a fact that your weight has not changed at all. (Note that as with the rattlesnake sandwiches mentioned earlier, nothing has changed in reality—your weight is just the same—but the *word* is changed, and you feel differently.)

People get into serious trouble with their weight when they begin to *talk* negatively to themselves about themselves. "I'm too fat" or "I'm too thin," followed by "Therefore, I'm no damned good." It is entirely possible that a factual statement to oneself about the weight situation makes sense: clothes may no longer fit, physical performance may be suffering, a modeling job may be threatened, or whatever. But none of these things has any bearing upon one's value as a person. The "I'm no damned good" kind of thing makes no sense whatever, even though societal attitudes conveyed via parents and others may suggest this. If the insufficient or excess weight is indeed self-defeating in some way, you can calmly set about making the necessary adjustments without going through self-deprecating, self-damning self-talk (which is likely to make you eat more if you're fat and vice versa).

One of the things complicating an approach to weight control that is not self-damning is the tendency to make a great to-do about children's weight as they grow up. Obviously, some children need to put on weight, for example, when growth and ability to be normally active having been endangered by starvation or disease. Similarly, some children are so overweight that their ability to function is restricted seriously. In both such cases the individual needs professional and parental *help*—not condemnation—in the interests of health and total life adjustment. However, the great majority of children are more rounded or more lean at different stages of their growing up, "chubbiness" (a clean for children, a dirty for adults) before puberty commonly giving place to leanness as the growth spurt of puberty takes place. Even with a good nutritional environment and ample physical activity, children will fluctuate between chubbier and leaner. Therefore there is simply no point in making a moral issue about normal developmental events. Unfortunately, many parents and others do make a moral issue of such things. Words like "fat" and "skinny" are then likely to become triggers capable of causing emotional reactions in the victim—feelings of ugliness and worthlessness as a person. Indeed, so widespread is the negative attitude toward "fatness" that the obese may be viewed as a minority group suffering from such things as college entrance and job discrimination. Feeling the social prejudice against them, they are likely to judge themselves inferior and blameworthy.

In brief, much of our popular attitude towards "fatness" is based not so much on its possible health implications—which are not at all fully understood with respect to degrees of fatness, and so forth—as on our reactions to the word itself.

TAKING ACTION

1. Using the word association and word cathexis scale techniques, evaluate various key words associated with the chapter on preventive eating. Compare various words such as "vitamin C" and "fat."
2. Compare with others: What foods that you have never eaten are upsetting to you if proposed as foods? Would you try squid, snails, shark, insects? Can you describe or label your favorite foods in such a way that they seem revolting (for example, "veal" is muscle from a sweet little calf that was clubbed to death or had its throat cut by a butcher who then bled it and . . .).
3. Discuss with others some of the words that were used on children (perhaps you) or adults who were considered too fat or too thin. Did such labeling help those individuals to alter their weight?

There are opposite, traditional attitudes toward the word "exercise." Therefore, on the one hand, it is a kind of "halo" word conjuring up notions of getting healthy, strong, fit, and perhaps living longer than

EXERCISE AND FITNESS

one otherwise might. On the other hand, "exercise" is a dirty word, perhaps conjuring up pictures of unpleasant exertions either self-imposed or more likely under orders of a gym teacher, army sergeant, or other authority. Although some people learn to like the word and speak happily of exercising or getting their workout, a great many will have nothing to do with it unless forced to, which tends to make the word still dirtier to them. There are the famous old sayings "Whenever I feel the urge to exercise, I lie down until that urge leaves me," and "I serve regularly as pallbearer for my friends who exercised." Morehouse and Walker (see Chapter 3) are doing much to improve the image of the word by removing some of the stress and conflict so often associated with it.

In schools and various organizations where exercising can be required, little effort is made to make the whole idea more attractive. Indeed, doing various exercises like taking laps or doing pushups may be a major form of punishment—hardly an arrangement likely to make people react favorably to those words or to consider exercising pleasurable. However, in nonrequired programs the major concern is to get people to want, or at least be willing, to exercise. One of the most common starting points is try to find more attractive words for it; "slimnastics" and "sexercises" are well-known examples.

To be slim and/or sexy are indeed attractive prospects in our society, and women in particular are lured to exercising by such words. Men are not under such pressure to be slim, and the mere fact of being male is supposed to confer sexual prowess. A degree of fatness in males is likely to have a favorable quality if labeled "husky" or some such. And in the male, bigness, if not accompanied by too much shortness, has suggested a degree of masculinity even if much of it is an amount of fatty tissue that would be considered unattractive in the female.

Now that more women are admitting to taking pleasure in looking at the sexy male figure and are availing themselves of the opportunity to look at muscular figures in *Playgirl* and other publications, it seems likely that increasing numbers of men will feel obliged to respond to slimnastic and sexercise appeals to "trim" up and be "fit."

A problem with the term "physical fitness" is that it doesn't refer to anything specific enough even for experts to agree on. This, of course, is a major problem with all kinds of abstract words. For example, nearly everyone is fond of such words as freedom, liberty, and morality; however, as with promiscuous, mentally ill, and evil, one is usually hard put to explain just what is meant by those words. One physical educator who is now in his seventies can still outdo all but the varsity-level athletes in his favorite track and swimming events. He believes that physical fitness means development to approximately our maximum potential, and he is famous for his training program which in his own case requires several hours of hard physical training every day. An equally famous physical educator has the opposite view. He takes it for granted that most people share his dislike for "exercising" and has therefore developed a popular fitness program that, he believes, will maintain a satisfactory functional fitness level with a few minutes of exercise and stretching per week.

Then there is the ambiguity of the term: "physical fitness" for what? Horseback riding, skiing, tennis, mountain climbing, modern or square dancing? People in good shape for football oftentimes simply cannot wrestle hard for three minutes. Some have argued that you are physically fit if you can handle emergencies that may occur. But what emergencies? One attractive definition is a level of fitness that makes it possible to handle an ordinary day's work and then have enough reserve to *enjoy* physical play afterward. This view received special attention when "physical play" was extended to include the sexual, and it was found by some that as the fitness program progressed, sexual responsiveness was reported improved.

One of the major problems associated with exercise and physical fitness programs has been the notion that they involved "masculinizing" of females. They have been supposed to make for ugly muscles, hefty appearance, gross and male mannerisms, and so on. Here was indeed a tangle of aversive words without tangible meaning. "Grossness" doesn't necessarily equal "masculine." Many male athletes are agile, polite, delicate at appropriate times, considerate, and so forth. Also, many top female athletes are obviously not "muscular," masculine, or any of the other things that women are not "supposed" to be.

How have those pushing physical fitness for girls and women been trying to change the popular negative attitudes? By offering more good programs for females and by trying to associate them with attractive words, pictures, and ideas: the "Physical Fitness Is Beautiful" song accompanied by pictures of attractive performers in action is only one of the ways. In like manner, "Black Is Beautiful" and "Gay Is Good" have at least made members of these groups feel better about themselves, and perhaps they have encouraged society generally to take a new look at them. In all such cases carefully chosen words are used in an effort to break down negative stereotypes—in this case negative attitudes toward being a muscular, masculine, female athlete. Instead, we see a healthy, attractive, active, physically fit girl or young woman.

Exercise and physical fitness have to do with physically moving and working the large and small muscles of the body long enough and hard enough to build or maintain strength, endurance, and flexibility. But our attitudes toward them and whether or not we will go to the trouble or take the time depends in part on the words we associate with them and how we *talk to ourselves* about them. Perhaps the things to do are: (1) evaluate the merits of being physically fit at some level appropriate to what we want to be able to do and (2) talk positively, not negatively, to ourselves and others about the activity program that we adopt for regular pursuit.

269

TAKING ACTION

1. *Use the word association and word cathexis techniques to evaluate key words in the foregoing discussion. Include such words as "exercise," "physical," "in shape," "soft," "sweat," "muscles," "fatigue," "jock," "female jock." Discuss your findings with the class. Compare responses of males with those of females.*
2. *Discuss with others some ways in which self-talk can facilitate or interfere with adopting and staying with an exercise program.*

EMOTIONAL AND "MENTAL" HEALTH

This book's chapter on emotional health is packed with examples of how language is an important factor in both emotional health and emotional disturbance. This is a forward-looking approach for a number of reasons, including the fact that it reminds us that a major tool for gaining or maintaining emotional health is readily available to us: our language, if we will learn to use it properly.

We discussed earlier the concept of private speaking as opposed to public speaking. Training in private speaking needs to include how to talk and *listen* to others, but it also needs to include lessons in self-talk, our ongoing dialogue with ourselves on every subject of interest to us. Chapter 4 of this book concentrates on these interpersonal and intra-personal kinds of language, and hopefully it will be an important step in the direction of correcting this glaring blind spot in our education.

The very terminology associated with mental health is loaded with pitfalls. Our National Institutes of Health, including the National Institute of Mental Health, are for the most part not really institutes of health at all but of disease: heart, cancer, and so on. "Mental health" as a term offers problems. For example, the word "mental" is difficult to define and suggests the old mind-body dichotomy, the idea that mind and body are two quite separate, basically unrelated, and even antagonistic things. One of them is high and lofty; the other, supposedly low, base, and perhaps animal. (Do you have any trouble guessing which was supposed to be which?) The term "emotional health" has certain distinct advantages. Most people agree that emotions involve the entire being, both the feelings in the body and psychological awareness of and about them. Moreover, people do not tend to react negatively to the term emotional health. It seems to suggest something like feeling good generally. On the other hand, the more popular term "mental health," which tends to make professional workers in that field feel very good, tends to trigger quite negative reactions in a great many, if not most, people. That is, thousands of people have been asked to respond with the first words that come to their minds when they hear the words "mental health." The vast majority have responded with words like "crazy," "nuthouse," "insane," "batty," and so on. Relatively few, and these were mostly professionals in the health field, responded with words like: "happy," "total health," and "well-being." So what the professionals perceive as something attractive and positive great numbers of other people perceive as darkly negative and suggestive of sickness and derangement. Might this not be a significant communication problem in this most important field?

It is not surprising that there is considerable confusion as to just what the terms "mental health" and "mental illness" mean. After all, much of what has been taught about mental health has been based on the study of more or less disturbed people. In fact one psychologist, Abraham Maslow, made history by studying the most symptom-free, mentally healthy people he could find. In this way he hoped to give new meaning to the concept of psychological health as opposed to illness.

However, in recent years an influential group led by psychiatrist Thomas Szasz has argued that mental illness as usually defined is a myth. That is, they claim that the medical model of illness cannot apply to the mind unless there is a demonstrable organic symptom such as one that might be caused by a blow, poisoning (as in severe alcoholism), disease (such as advanced syphilis), or brain tissue deterioration (as in senility). They argue that the great majority of disorders usually labeled mental illness are actually problems of adjustment, nonconformity, disagreeableness, or unusual ways of *talking* or behaving. Such behaviors are hardly "diseases," they claim, in the same sense that cancer and typhoid are. This matter of definition is no small thing, because many thousands of people have been in mental hospitals for many years—hospitals that are actually poor-quality jails—not on grounds of their having committed any crime but because they are "ill." Those in the Szasz camp insist that they are neither ill nor criminal, and they therefore are unjustly incarcerated, often for longer periods than are convicted criminals. Should this argument hold, the people involved will not have changed; only the language associated with them—their verbal label—will have changed. But they will be free. Indeed, a recent Supreme Court decision (1975) makes it illegal to forcibly hospitalize people without actual treatment unless they are dangerous to themselves or others. Families and society can no longer get rid of people because they are annoying or disconcertingly different on the grounds that they are mentally ill ("insane" is the legal word).

Homosexuality is a glaring example of societal labeling. For centuries homosexuality was defined as a sin, then it also became a serious crime, and finally it became, medically, a mental illness. Now, although homosexuality has not changed, through redefinition some churches welcome homosexuals or even have homosexual ministers; a number of states no longer have laws against it if practiced by consenting adults in private; and it was recently *defined* out of mental illness almost overnight by the American Psychiatric Association. Several million people were suddenly "cured" by words.

W. H. Auden called this the "age of anxiety." Evidently he was right, if one may judge by certain studies and the fact that hundreds of millions of dollars are spent each year on antianxiety pills. The question about all this anxiety is how to do something to improve those conditions which are at best unpleasant and at worst disabling. The drugs work for many people under certain circumstances. For example, in the past, when people were wheeled in and lined up in hospitals for operations, they usually showed evidence of more or less severe anxiety over what might be about to befall them. Now they are tranquilized in advance and usually can't make themselves feel very anxious even if they try. Most people would probably not want to change this situation or others in which anxiety serves no useful purpose. On the other hand, drugs do nothing to solve basic problems of living, and they may very well relieve us of anxieties that are useful warning signals that all is not well. In other words, if circumstances in a marriage, family, school, or job are giving rise to serious upset in people, mightn't it be better to accept the anxious feelings as a warning that some kind of action is needed—just as a toothache reminds us to go to a dentist? In many cases, to use tranquilizers is to float along in the problem situation while it very likely remains the same or grows worse. As Albert Ellis puts it: it's a question of *feeling* better versus *being* better. How to set about *being* better? Many psychotherapists tend to attack language itself, especially self-talk, as the medium whereby individuals constantly reinfect themselves, day after day, with self-defeating thoughts and feelings from the past. The medium (language) is literally the message: "Wouldn't it be awful if . . ." "I can't stand . . ." "He shouldn't treat me . . ." These are examples of the kinds of unrealistic phrases with which people stir themselves up and that guarantee worry, whining, self-upset, hostility, anxiety, and other self-defeating emotions and behaviors.

What we do and say makes some difference, whether we like it or not. A student, Frank, was reaching the boiling point because his roommate habitually left his clothing scattered about. He would mutter such phrases to himself as: "The bastard knows I hate . . ." "He shouldn't be such a slob . . ." "I can't stand living like . . ." Thus with words he often reignited and fanned his growing anger. He used words as his emotion accelerators and made horrors out of hassles. Fortunately, a friend raised a question: "Isn't it possible that he's so used to having his mother pick up after him that it just doesn't occur to him to do it?" Frank hadn't considered this possibility of nondeliberate nuisance making. He stopped needling himself with inflammatory self-talk, discovered in calm conversation that his companion was indeed not intentionally upsetting him, and worked out a plan whereby living together would be more agreeable to them both. Only then did he discover that his own late night reading with a bright light had been seriously disturbing his roommate's sleep.

Somewhat similarly, a wife complained that her husband did not care at all about her sexual desires. Indeed, he seemed very callous and indifferent. Had she ever *told* him of the problem? Well, no. But aren't men *supposed* to know about such things? When she was taught to be calmly assertive and talked to him about it, she was surprised to find that he thought she had lost all interest in sex. He had been reluctant to try to force lovemaking on her. Calm, open communication did indeed make a difference.

Increasingly, people of all ages are turning to professionally trained individuals for help in dealing with their emotions. Not only may thoroughly airing a problem provide relief, but also verbalizing it may provide insights helpful in healthful resolution of the problem. However, it is important to remember that counselors too are products of our tradition in which language conveys out of the past many irrational and inappropriate attitudes. Some of these have to do with such things as our sex roles, not how sex requires us to behave but how our sexual label of male or female raises expectations of how we *should* behave. It has been found that many counselors attempt to impose adjustment to traditional roles of male and especially female. Thus, as we noted earlier, the woman's normalness and femininity may be questioned if she deviates from the expected wife-mother role. "Woman," "wife," and "mother" are quite a combination of tradition-heavy labels. A woman may be very female in terms of sexual interest and may be an enthusiastic wife and mother, but she is basically a *person* and is increasingly insistent upon the primacy of her personness. She is certainly within her rights to challenge and resist anyone's efforts, including those of a counselor, to force adjustment to a partially outmoded label.

TAKING ACTION

1. Make a list of words and terms associated with the emotional health ("mental health") field. Using the word association and word cathexis techniques, test a group of people to evaluate their responses to these words. Discuss your findings with the class.
2. In the chapter on emotional health, a number of examples are given in which private talking and especially self-talk are identified as being crucial factors in striving for emotional health. Identify these, and discuss them in detail with a group. What applications can you see for life on the job and in the home?
3. Margaret Mead has commented that in this culture, just as failure emasculates men, success defeminizes women. Her contention tends to be true, but does failure necessarily emasculate men? And does success necessarily defeminize women? Discuss things (especially along lines of self-talk) that can be done to prevent these reactions to failure and success.

The words, even the medical words, related to sex are "loaded" emotionally and tend to be very upsetting to many people. This **SEXUALITY AND SEX EDUCATION** well-known fact would seem more significant than might be realized. As noted previously, as emotional upset increases beyond a point, thinking ability or functioning intelligence decreases. Thus if you are upset by sex words, you and everyone else are less intelligent when dealing with this subject than when dealing with other subjects. Many professional counselors, including doctors, lawyers, and clergy, are still uptight about sex words. What kind of solutions to problems can be hoped for when both the client and counselor are shaken by the words that have to be used to discuss sex-related events and behaviors? For example, in one recent case a young woman got better advice from her taxi driver than she had received from her doctor or her clergyman. He was not uptight about sex words; they were.

Thus it would seem that anyone wishing to go into any of the helping professions where sex-related matters arise has an obligation to escape the tyranny of sex words. Moreover, when people realize that many important human relationships such as those of husband and wife, lovers, and parent and child are impaired when sex-related words interfere with good communication—they too decide to fight off the tyranny of words. Some teachers have done such things as tape-record themselves saying "vulgar" words used by their pupils and then listen to themselves and repeat over and over the loaded words. Why? So as to be able to get over being upset by them. For what purpose? Because they wanted to be able to function intelligently in the presence of those words rather than to freeze up or become enraged and in either event behave less intelligently. After all, they came to realize that most of their children were not out to shock them. For many of them these were the only words that they knew, the "proper" Latin medical terminology being completely foreign to them. Instead of getting upset, these teachers set about teaching their pupils to know two sets of terminology, one for the neighborhood, one for on the job, and when to use each.

In addition to its possible effect on intelligence, language actually preprograms responses and behaviors in people. For example, it has been found that girls tend to have more trouble with menstrual discomfort and pain if they grew up in environments in which menstruation was talked about in very negative terms. In particular, girls growing up in fundamentalist faiths that associate menstruation with uncleanliness and perhaps sin are significantly more prone to menstrual disorders. Similarly with childbirth. Mothers who dwell upon the dreadfulness of their own or other mothers' pregnancies and deliveries are likely to produce daughters whose emotional state (body-mind) is poorly adjusted to pregnancy and childbearing.

Adjustment in marriage can be very much influenced by language. Innumerable men have been devastated to discover that the possession of a penis does not guarantee automatic knowledge of all things sexual. Many men have had to slink off unhappily because the illusion built of words prepared them little if at all for sex in the real world. For their part, women have traditionally been deprived of a usable sexual language, with the result that they consider it unladylike to express their sexual interests and preferences (if they have discovered any). To this day the language blackout even prevents many women from knowing what sexual parts they have. In particular, the clitoris, the sole known function of which is production of pleasure, had until recently gone virtually unnamed and undiscovered. Thus one of the potentially important things in marriage, sex, is all too often a profound disappointment because husband and wife are preprogrammed to *not* communicate effectively about it.

In addition, it has been found that girls' and women's emotional responses to "exhibitionists," child molesters, and even to rape depend in large measure on how they have been preprogrammed by language about them in advance as well as how such events are talked about if they happen. Exhibitionists are harmless (they're usually afraid to have closer contact with women), and the vast majority of child molesters are friends of the family, neighbors, or relatives who rarely do more than touch and fondle. (The disturbed molesters who injure and even kill children are a very real threat, but at least they are very rare, statistically speaking.) Thus if the behavior is usually harmless, it has to be the emotional charge of these words that gives rise to hysterical responses. Preprogramming again at work. Some women who do not catastrophize about the label are able to laugh at exhibitionists (thereby completely unnerving them) or just find them peculiar. Some mothers are able to keep their wits about them and thereby avoid causing emotional trauma in their "molested" daughters. Girls may be reassured and taught appropriate means of dealing with such situations instead.

In some ways rape is quite another matter because by definition it is

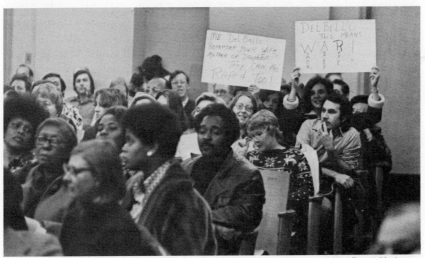

Town residents meeting to retain the local rape squad.

Mimi Forsyth/Monkmeyer

275

always an assault, very possibly violent, on another person's body. The word is so emotionally charged that some women cannot use or hear it without becoming upset and perhaps irrational, often to the detriment of any serious discussion attempted. Still, the fact remains that some women who are raped are terribly upset by the experience and have to undergo extended psychiatric treatment, while others who were just as terrified and badly hurt recover quickly from the upset and need no psychiatric support. How come? You've guessed it. Preprogramming, especially by language in past years, plus (1) whether or not influential persons like parents react with catastrophic language about how terrible things are, how she'll never be the same, and so on, and (2) whether the individual uses such catastrophic language on herself. To the extent that the girl (and others) can treat rape as they would nonsexual assault or traffic injury she can be expected to recover reasonably promptly from the emotional trauma.

On a David Susskind show a guest commented that although our society esteems sex very much, it also considers it in a very negative light; it considers it evil and rejects it. Susskind attacked the second point, maintaining that our attitude is positive, as illustrated by the prominent position that sex holds in entertainment. "That's part of my point," the guest answered. "But to complete making my point, answer me this: what is the subject of a *dirty* joke?" A long, very unusual silence followed. Everyone knows that dirty jokes are almost always sex jokes. Thus the very language of sex tends to encourage a negative attitude toward sex itself, as everyone learns more or less forcefully in childhood. Some people never learn to enjoy sex fully because of this association with the "dirty." ("It's sinful, dirty, revolting, and immoral—so save it for the one you marry.")

Attitudes toward the words of sex not only block communications between individuals but often bring professional enterprises to a halt. Some ministers, their followers, and certain far-right political groups would forbid even the use of medical sex terminology in schools. This restriction would not only effectively block all sex and VD education but all reproduction education in, for example, biology classes. Physicians have been reported for going beyond the sexless anatomy charts to teach nurses about the genitals. Medical practice has drawn to a halt because patients did not know what they were supposed to do in the specimen bottle and nurses could not bring themselves to say the word "piss," the only one the patients understood.

The "forbidden" sexual behaviors have dark labels that tend to block efforts to understand and evaluate them objectively. Masturbation, prostitution, and homosexuality are among the dark labels that tend to be aversive stimuli rather than verbal handles for the mind to take hold of. Efforts are being made these days by many people to take a closer look to see just what is actually under such labels. Masturbation, which used to be such a horrible word that it was almost never spoken and never appeared in print except in a few medical publications, is no longer seen as being so awful after all, either as a behavior or as a word. Whereas in the past people, especially women, would rather die than admit to masturbating, today they will commonly say in counseling sessions: "Of course, I have always enjoyed masturbating . . ." and the like. This has been a surprisingly rapid (and healthy) change associated with the last few years. And it is due to the insistence of scholars and other researchers on looking through the label. Often, even to their own surprise, they have found something far more positive than negative there.

"Prostitution" has always been an ugly word associated with an ugly social pathology. However, a second look is forcing the question of whether even this institution is all bad. After all, William Masters of the famous Masters and Johnson sex research team got his start studying cooperating prostitutes in St. Louis, He learned from them much that is now incorporated in his widely used approach to sex therapy. Prostitutes are now being used widely as "surrogate lovers" under the direction of sex therapists to help people solve serious sex problems. Moreover, many men and some women whose mates cannot or will not deal with them sexually meet their sexual needs by visiting prostitutes and enjoy a happy home life otherwise. In other words, in spite of the fact that some prostitutes roll, injure, rob, and even kill their tricks, others have contributed to medical science and therapy and even to marital happiness. Is the one dirty word "prostitution" adequate to cover all of these possible meanings?

As homosexuals have increasingly been coming "out of their closets," declaring themselves different only in terms of their sexual preference and demanding their civil as well as human rights, homosexuality has been becoming less of a dark label than it used to be. True, the word "gay" is often used to soften the impact of the older term. But the new look beyond the label has already led people to less frequently consider homosexuality a sin or even a sickness. Laws are rapidly being changed; as we have said, in many states homosexual acts between consenting adults are no longer illegal. Societal attitudes change slowly, but it seems that "homosexual" is on its way to becoming simply a word for sexual preference and not quite so much the dark, dirty label it has been in the past.

Social changes do occur, but our language often has a hard time keeping up with them—for example, patterns of behavior of males and females. How are you *supposed* to act as male or female? Are you really able to act like both the Virgin Mary and Raquel Welch? Like both Jesus and John Wayne if you're male? These days some people simply try to be themselves and act in ways appropriate to situations rather than trying at all times to be "masculine" or "feminine." Thus a male may sometimes be gentle and nurturing, and he may be relatively passive in sex; whereas a female may at times be bold and aggressive, and she may play the initiating and dominant role in sex—depending on the situation. The word *androgynous*, the combining of the Greek words

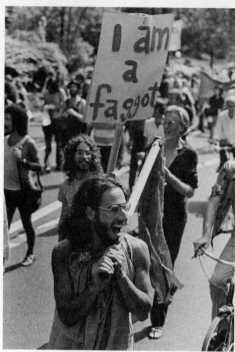

Jim Anderson/Woodfin Camp

for man and woman, is now commonly used to describe those individuals who are able to escape the strict sex role stereotype, combining appropriate qualities from traditional maleness and femaleness. This does not mean that male and female will become the same in behavior. Freed of imposed traditional stereotypes, perhaps some basic patterns of male and female behavior will emerge, and the words will take on new meaning.

Sports provide an interesting example of how the language of sex roles is having trouble keeping up with the times. In the last half century or so it has become increasingly respectable for women to participate in vigorous sports competition. But it is still not necessarily a compliment to be called a "female athlete." The term "tomboy" is still not entirely free of the suggestion that the girl is not really playing her role properly, even though indications are that these girls are especially healthy and relate especially well with males.

If a boy plays well, that is, hard and aggressively, he's "playing like a man." When a girl plays like that, what is she playing like? A woman coach was heard to say of her coed team before a final practice: "Today we separate the men from the boys." She immediately looked puzzled: "The sheep from the goats?" That wasn't quite right either, but the language simply did not provide her with a really appropriate way of saying what she meant. Girls from the women? The ladies?

And, finally, many sex-related words are understood quite different-ly by different people, with the result that people often think that they are communicating but really aren't. To some, "promiscuous" means "sleeping around"; to others it means *any* sexual activity outside of marriage—as in the case of the clergyman who insisted that an unmarried 65-year-old woman, who had had one brief affair when in her thirties, was and is promiscuous. If you ask a group of 30 people what they mean by promiscuous, you're likely to get at least six definitions, probably many more. Actually, the word means "indiscriminate," which is to say that it has reference not to the quantity of sex but the quality. For analogy: the promiscuous eater is the one who will eat just about anything.

To some, being "in love" is the highest human experience. To one physiologist it is a disease of the endocrine glands that is readily cured by marriage. To many, it is infatuation ("to be made foolish"). According to an old navy saying, it is a mental hard-on that is quickly cured by any good whore. But Shakespeare wrote: "But thy sweet love remembered such wealth brings/ That then I scorn to change my state with kings." How might people with such different views of the meaning of love communicate on the subject unless they do a lot of defining? They try all of the time to communicate and almost never bother with definitions.

Promiscuous, love, homosexual, sodomy, sex offender, masculine, feminine, and so on and on: these are all *words*. Let us begin by agreeing on some definitions or, perhaps better still, drop those words and describe behaviors.

TAKING ACTION

1. *Using the word association and word cathexis techniques, evaluate and compare some of the more common sex words. Compare responses to the Latin medical terms and their so-called "vulgar" equivalents. Discuss your findings.*
2. *Discuss some of the implications of having negative and highly emotional responses to these words. How might individuals such as teachers and nurses and parents learn to be less uptight and perhaps more rational in relation to these words?*

**PAIRING AND
BEARING**

Marriage, to get married, to be married: these are terms of considerable impact, positive and negative. Research has shown that of all groups studied, young wives are the happiest; perhaps not surprisingly young husbands do not trail far behind. Apparently, in spite of the increased independence of women and much antimarriage propaganda, marriage is still considered women's greatest achievement. They are euphoric and actually enjoy housework that most other people, including single women, consider drudgery. "Marriage," like "Christmas," symbolizes something that rarely or only briefly exists. Even when their own experiences with marriage have amounted to sheer disillusionment,

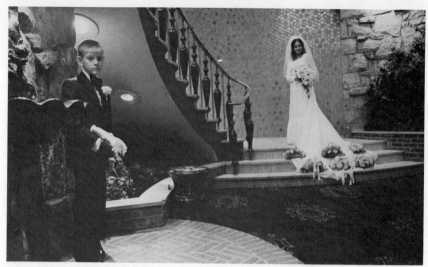

Joan Liftin/Woodfin Camp

mothers are exalted when their daughters marry, just as Christmas always raises high hopes. A woman shed tears of joy to learn that her brother had at last married. It mattered not at all that brother and his "girl" had been living together for several years and that marriage changed nothing whatsoever between them. Except that now the label was in place. Who ever heard of people *not* getting married and living happily together ever after?

We tend to speak of marriage as though it refers to a specific state, but actually, of course, a variety of marriage states have always existed and are now being recognized as options to choose among. Prince Charming and the Princess do sometimes marry and live in a largely friendly, even blissful, loving state all their years. More commonly marriage is something people are driven into by various traditional pressures, and after shocks of disillusionment they either separate or they gradually create some kind of enduring relationship that, for better or worse, is more inconvenient to leave than to tolerate. So, it hangs in there, officially as much a marriage as that of Prince Charming and the Princess. The word "marriage" seems hardly adequate for all of its possible meanings. Thus the words "husband" and "wife" are not entirely clean words. "My husband" often translates out to "that character (or bastard) I have to put up with." And Swinburne's lines are still famous because so many husbands can identify with them. His verse speaks of time changing "Loves into corpses or wives/ Making barren our lives." Some husbands call their wives their "brides" so as to avoid what they consider the derogatory term "wife."

Marriage has always tended to mean exclusive sexual rights to a person—even if you did not wish to or could not exercise those rights yourself. Of course, this meaning of marriage has been more binding upon women than men. However, the very first Kinsey report of 1948 made it perfectly clear that even this meaning of marriage did not jibe with reality for large numbers of women as well as men. The same is undoubtedly true today to an even greater extent. Still, to many people, marriage still means or is supposed to mean sexual exclusiveness. Such individuals can't take seriously the several other forms that marriage often openly takes today: open marriage, communal marriage, couples swinging with other couples and/or in orgies or involving another person in their sex lives, which may then involve simultaneous homosexual and heterosexual activity on the part of three or four individuals. These days people have to decide for themselves what, if anything, marriage is going to mean to them.

Patterns of verbal communication prior to and then during marriage deserve consideration. During courtship couples tend to be attentive to each other—a fact that is also true among animals. However, the courting female tends to carry attentiveness and responsiveness to an extreme. Everything the male says is fascinating and/or funny. So young Mr. Dull suddenly finds himself as fascinating as Clark Gable and as funny as Bob Hope. Not long after marriage, however, this illusion is shattered. Mr. Dull is Mr. Dull again, neither fascinating nor witty. He may now get the impression that the only thing fascinating or funny about him is his effort to act like a "he-man."

Rather typically in marriage, people are able to talk about almost anything, from how eggs are to be fried to how they should dress for dinner—except how, in detail, they like to play and be stimulated sexually. Every experienced sex counselor has been impressed by the extent to which the language barrier successfully blocks optimal sexual communication.

Also, rather typically, before marriage people tend to use language with care and consideration with their prospective mates. Not long after marriage, however, things change, and home becomes a verbal dumping ground where, since almost anything can be gotten away with, it is. Couples pick away at each other, ridicule appearances, attack personality traits, highlight and elaborate upon deficiencies, including those associated with body build, housekeeping or money-making ability—and sexual competence. In very sharp contrast, away from home, especially perhaps on the job, mates may be models of verbal decorum, especially when talking to His Eminence, the Boss.

Any thoughtful person can see that this tendency toward kid-gloves handling of the boss coupled with baseball-bat use of language in the home is foolish and self-defeating. Most people put in very little time with their bosses but spend hours daily, all night and weekends with mates. In other words, why foul your own nest with careless talk? Better talking within marriage will improve the image of the word.

Now for parenting. It used to be that a girl could justify her existence as well as feel quite good about herself by saying, "I plan to get married and have five children." These words described a socially approved kind of game plan for life, and they implied realization and fulfillment as a woman. Increasingly today people are taking a skeptical look at parenthood. The word has lost much of its luster, and numerous people are deciding against having children.

However, this is not to say that a more rational approach to parenthood is by any means universal. Numerous women undertake motherhood because their mothers want to be grandmothers, and/or because it proves their womanhood. Whether they work inside or outside the home, they often put in as little time as possible mothering. And even more irrationally, sometimes unmarried teenagers are having and keeping their children because as "mothers" they are *something*, someone of significance. They usually have no knowledge whatever of child rearing.

The word "childless" continues to carry a certain amount of stigma, so the term "child-free" has been coined to carry a favorable connotation. As a matter of fact, probably the major effort of the organization National Organization for Nonparents is to make becoming parents less a symbol of "fulfillment" and achievement and more a matter of careful choice and preparation. Thus it is actually a very prochild organization. It's for reserving parenthood for those who really want it.

An example of how far removed a word may be from its presumed meaning is in connection with the "machismo" attitude towards fatherhood. Everyone, including their wives had supposed that the true Latin male desires to have as many children as possible, thereby demonstrating manhood. A recent study showed this not so. Since people cannot talk about such matters, innumerable children have been produced in poverty to the despair of nearly everyone involved.

Leading mental health experts have traditionally claimed that having and rearing children is important if not crucial for the achieving of "mental health" and "maturity." Unfortunately, they have not defined these terms precisely, nor have they demonstrated the mechanism whereby parenting accomplishes these conditions. As a matter of fact, studies of happiness have shown that happy couples tend to be less happy when they have children. Demands on both parents are enormous, there is far less time and money for recreation and self-betterment activities, and sex life is likely to decline markedly and even vanish for appreciable periods. When children come on the scene, conflicts, desertions, suicides, and other symptoms of severe stress appear. All this is not intended to argue against having children. Obviously, human survival requires them. It is merely to argue that "having children" has lost much of its traditional usefulness to couples and tends instead to mean trouble. Perhaps it would be well if instead of "having children" being a compulsive response to getting married, getting married would merely reinforce earlier care in *not* begetting children unless and until real desire for parenthood is demonstrated by careful preparation for it.

When people do have children, they frequently demonstrate such lack of knowledge of child health and developmental needs—if not neglect and abuse—that some form of "licensing" for parenthood has been proposed. Everyone seems for the concept: parenthood is a difficult job and requires qualifications. But *licensing*? Another word had better be found or the concept may never be acceptable.

The words "unwanted," "illegitimate," and "adopted" have often been a source of distress to children and young people. Some parents deliberately tell their children they were unwanted (contraception failed or some such) as a put-down. The child could laugh at this or be indifferent, but many let the word make them feel lonely and depressed. Interestingly, individuals have suddenly found out that their parents weren't married or that they were adopted—and they have been terribly upset, even though their circumstances in reality were not changed at all. Recall the rattlesnake meat sandwich story at the beginning of this chapter? This "illegitimate" and "adopted" business is the same kind of thing. All that's changed is the words, but how upset some people become!

TAKING ACTION

1. *Use the word association and word cathexis techniques to evaluate key words in the foregoing discussion. For example, compare the words "wife" and "husband." Do you find evidence that some "good" words such as "wife" are also to some extent "dirty" words?*
2. *On the basis of small group discussion, propose some specific ways in which language pitfalls might be avoided and language might be a constructive factor in family relationships.*

DEATH AND RELATED MATTERS

In our society "getting old" and "dying" are just about the ultimate in dirty words. It is therefore not surprising that, as with sex, numerous efforts are made to talk around the whole subject (circumlocution) or to somehow sweeten it up by using a (hopefully) less offensive or objectionable word. "Old" becomes "elderly." One doesn't die but "passes on," "expires," "steps out," or even "kicks the bucket." Sometimes it is most difficult to work out a verbal compromise that is satisfactory. Old age becomes "the golden years," but the euphemism does not really make them golden, and it sometimes becomes rather patronizing: "We've called you something special. Now go away." In response to being relegated to second- or even tenth-class citizenship, older people have been organizing. Their term "Gray Panthers" conveys their vigorous, activist intentions, and it neatly avoids conveying anything of a doddering, feeble, or senile kind.

There are many other examples of how words may alter feelings with respect to aging and how emotions may be bounced back and forth by words. A graying man went for a haircut. The barber said, "Your hair is getting quite gray," but added, "How dignified looking!" The customer

283

had immediately begun to feel depressed over the word "gray" but quickly perked up at the word "dignified." The barber then noted, "Your hair is down over your ears." "What a messy slob I've become," the man muttered to himself. But the barber went on, "The *casual* look is certainly becoming to you." Needless to say, the man immediately felt better about himself—entirely because the barber was astute enough to say the right words. Men who in fact are young may become upset if called old even as in "old man," meaning old chap or friend. Young women tend to be even more sensitive.

Billions of dollars are spent each year by people frantically trying to remain young while growing older. However, the definition of old is vague or uncertain to say the least. Some women consider themselves growing dangerously old if unmarried by 22; others may think they are too old to start having babies at 30. When 27- to 30-year-olds speak of getting old, they usually mean that they are no longer a wonderful 18 (which may not have seemed so wonderful at the time).

At age 55 many women are still keeping up the battle to look 18. Americans simply do not let their women age gracefully, comfortably, or naturally, and few try. The need to try to look 18 for the next 40 years is not usually felt so urgently by men. A certain amount of wrinkling and graying in the male can easily have favorable words associated with it: maturity and dignity among them. Whereas an older woman may look good *in spite* of aging, a man may look good *because* of it. If women put on weight as they grow older, their clothing conceals little of this. They are getting "broad in the beam," turning into "all ass," and so on. Derogatory words of these kinds are less often used on men, even though clothiers report that the girth size of American men has definitely gone up appreciably in recent years. Not only do men's clothing tend to minimize fat appearance, but what the heck? Big is a good word for a male. So he is husky.

At the beauty parlor

Abigail Heyman/Magnum Photos

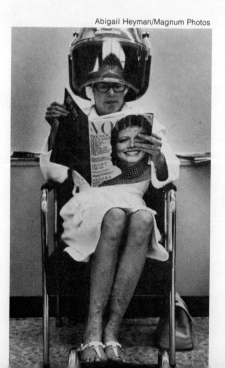

On the other hand, aging carries a special onus for the male. For example, a young woman said, "It makes me furious to hear that a child has been molested by a dirty old man!" The other women present agreed heartily. But someone said, "How about by a dirty *young* man? Or by a *clean* old man?" She was taken completely aback by these questions and had to admit that a child involved would probably be equally affected without regard to the age or cleanliness of the molester. In fact, she was forced to admit that she didn't know just what she meant by the term "dirty old man," except that it was evil. Sexual interest on the part of older males seems especially obscene and revolting to many people unless the male happens to be wealthy. Sexual interest on the part of older women is likely to be viewed as silly. However, studies in recent years have shown that the asexuality attributed to older people is a fiction created by a societal attitude, and it is conveyed and kept alive by language.

Some researchers on aging have been impressed at how *talking about* elderly persons influences behavior toward them.[1] For example, they are talked about as though they were all one sex except for clothing, and they had all better behave sexlessly. Husbands and wives are commonly separated in homes for older people. A special language tends to be adopted by attendants when addressing the residents: language ordinarily reserved for small children. Terms like "sweetie," "honey," and "dearie" are commonplace, and they are "naughty" boys or girls if they wet or soil themselves or drool. The old are expected to play a particular role, to be entirely cooperative and submissive. Being defined "old," it seems justified to treat them as infants, without modesty, sex, or privacy.[2]

In point of fact, probably the great majority of these people are perfectly capable of leading active, enjoyable, largely self-sufficient lives but are devastated psychologically by the requirement to act "old"—that is, worthless, out of it, infantile, and so on. As every student of human behavior knows, our identities, who and what we are or think we are, how others see and define us, are greatly affected by language.

The words "dead" and "died" tend to have magical effects on people's emotions, in part because most of us have never come to terms with our own mortality or that of others of importance to us. For example, upon learning that their father or mother has died, people tend to feel obliged to provide expensive funerals—in spite of the fact that father or mother may have been a royal pain personally, economically, socially, and so on. Moreover, the deceased may have made childhood an unpleasant experience. Still, he or she *died* or is *dead* and therefore this irrational emotional and financial extravaganza. But what does it really mean? Among other things, it means that the

---

[1]H. Maas and J. Kuypers, 1975, *From Thirty to Seventy.* San Francisco: Jossey-Bass.
[2]S. R. Curtin, 1972, *Nobody Ever Died of Old Age.* Boston: Little, Brown.

survivors are using words on themselves that arouse feelings of guilt. Why guilt? Because of the feeling that the dead one was inadequately served or respected while alive, so we'd better make up for that now. Sometimes guilt is based on the suspicion that the older person died because of our imperfect performance; so in effect we killed him or her. Again, irrational self-talk, which plays into the hands of the funeral business.

There is clearly such a need for realistic death education and counseling that will help people come to terms with death and the emotions that this word gives rise to. As we pointed out in Chapter 7, death education is for the enhancement of life. Also, greater awareness of what is really involved in aging and being old—awareness gained from actually working and playing with older people—helps us to deal with real people the way they are and not with their usually meaningless but derogatory label: old.

TAKING ACTION

1. *Use the word association and word cathexis techniques to evaluate words related to age, death, and dying, and bereavement. Discuss implications of your findings.*
2. *Prepare an argument to the effect that circumlocutions and "soft selling" aging and death are wise and beneficial practices. Prepare a rebuttal.*
3. *Spend some time with older people, and note, among other things, how they talk and are talked to.*

ECOLOGY AND ENVIRONMENT

The word *ecology* comes from the Greek root meaning housekeeping. In its modern application it refers to the study and maintenance of man's living place, namely, "spaceship earth." What a good word—with its implications for knowing our environment well enough to know how to maintain a nice, healthful, unpolluted, attractive place in which to live. "Ecology" is a good but also a bad word. It warns us that we have to stop doing some of the things that give us the income to buy color TV sets, steak, and gasoline. Our environment can't stand the beating we're giving it and still remain a household we can live in. But this beating is the source of much of our wealth. Health versus wealth. So ecology, as a possible threat to production and prosperity, is also a dirty word to some.

Many in the health versus wealth (production, prosperity) debate attempt to put everything on a simple good-versus-evil basis, and, of course, words are carefully selected to drive home arguments. Ecologists are sometimes tossed in a bag with revolutionaries, eggheads, and communists. On the other hand, the more naive environmentalists see industry and big business as totally evil forces, hell-bent on destroying the environment and thus the world; they do not take into account the highly constructive contributions of many industries and businesses to

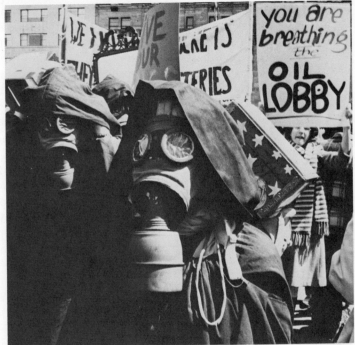

Bruce Anspach/EPA Newsphoto

human health and welfare. In other words, people tend to react to the generalizations, the good versus bad words without regard to the gradations between.

"Affluence" has traditionally been a "good" word, representing a condition available to most if they would but work hard enough (or choose wealthy parents or strike gold). To be called affluent is no longer necessarily a compliment, and to be an "affluent American" is something of an accusation: one who is destroying the world's resources faster than anyone else. For an extreme example, compare the energy consumption of a wealthy child with that, say, of a ghetto or Sioux Indian child. The poor city or Indian child gets very little, travels little, in general does little that consumes energy or damages the environment—but incidentally may be very happy. But the affluent child, just by virtue of being part of a group that has much, travels and enjoys "the good things of life," consumes enormously—but incidentally may be very unhappy. ("Incidentally" was added to the last two sentences as a reminder that affluence, even when considered a good word, has not really necessarily meant a good state of affairs. Similarly, an affluent city is not necessarily a healthful one to live in.)

Circumstances are much different today from what they used to be, but language has often failed to keep up and in some important ways. Such expressions as "throw it away" and "dump it out" made perfectly good sense in a sparsely settled rural area when one could simply step outside and throw refuse away from the house or carry trash a few

287

yards to the gulch for dumping. Or when almost anything could be
discarded into bodies of water. In those days there were so few people,
and so relatively little to dump, that the environment seemed able to
absorb anything individuals wished to discard with no ill effect.

How things have changed! But the language of disposing of things
hasn't. People who "litter" are usually not antisocial. They simply
assume that the environment will somehow absorb what they throw
away, be it cans, bottles, or the tons of trash and industrial wastes cities
produce every day. Similarly, "dumping it" did not used to mean
despoiling an entire creek, river, lake, waterway, or part—some claim
even all—of an ocean. Nor did "dumping" wastes into the air via
campfires, bonfires, even village trash burnings mean anything like
what gets dumped into the air today by things not dreamed of when the
terms for getting rid of wastes were invented. But the terms evidently
still help give people the feeling that the old ways are still appropriate.
Perhaps the major unsolved problem in the use of nuclear power plants
is where to dump the highly dangerous radioactive waste products that
they produce.

Many American women still feel the need to have many children to
demonstrate worth as a woman. Still our birthrate has been dropping
as the childbearing tradition seems to be losing its force. Not so in many
if not most parts of the world where women are taught to see as their
purpose in life the production of children, especially sons. So the
birthrate there continues to accelerate in spite of strenuous efforts of
many leaders and the cooperation of literate, urban dwellers. Plans for
social progress in much of the world is most gravely threatened by the
language-carried plague of overpopulation and its attendant miseries of
starvation, crowding, out-of-control pollution, disease, and upheaval.

The ancient Biblical passage giving man God's permission to exploit
the lands and seas and His demand that man be fruitful are words that
have been carried a bit far. In fact, human survival may well depend on
the growing acceptance of the spirit of another, less known, Biblical
injunction instructing man (God talked almost exclusively to men) to
husband the environment—that is, tend to and nurture it.

TAKING ACTION

1. Use the word association and word cathexis techniques to evaluate words
   associated with environment and ecology, including "conservationists,"
   "industry," "energy companies," and "populations."
2. Have each class member ask five adults to react to words concerned with
   the population problem such as "overpopulation," "family planning,"
   "birth control," "contraception," and "hunger." Pool your findings for
   discussion. Is education or economic level a factor in responses?

RECREATIONAL DRUGS: ALCOHOL AND MARIJUANA

There is not much of a problem in dealing with cigarette smoking,
healthwise; it's all bad. No controversy really. The industry thrives, as

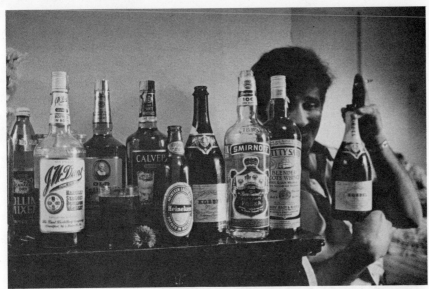

Jim Anderson/Woodfin Camp

we shall note later, by playing word and picture games to seduce. But it can present no evidence of beneficial or even neutral effects on health from smoking.

In contrast, although there are some well-known personal and social ill effects of alcohol and dependency-forming drugs, beneficial effects can also be claimed for them, as Belzer notes in Chapter 10. In spite of the best efforts of those in the Temperance League tradition (Leaguers used to preach to the young: "First comes a cigarette. Then a drink. The next step is prostitution!") most people are ambiguous in their feelings about alcoholic beverages: they're both against and for them. Similarly, few informed people react to the word "pot" as though it were the work of the devil. Even the hard drugs sometimes have some good things that can be said about them, particularly as medication for specific conditions. In other words, as with "sex" and "aggression," we tend to react both positively and negatively to alcohol and drugs—and thereby greatly complicate matters.

Just as men who visit prostitutes regularly often have the nastiest things to say about women and sex, heavy drinkers often denounce liquor in the strongest terms. A drinker's mishaps are almost certainly blamed upon his drinking—sometimes justifiably (as when driving the wrong way on a one-way street and killing people) but sometimes not. For example, as we noted earlier, when people become ill after drinking, they tend to blame the booze. But objective evaluation may show that an equal number of nondrinkers became ill. Similarly, when a drinker dies, drinking is likely to be blamed—even though he or she may have outlived most of his or her contemporaries. Still, it is quite possible to drink oneself to death just as it is likely that some nondrinkers would have lived longer if they had taken to drink, moderately. The language of drinking is indeed complicated.

289

The feelings associated with drug words are so strong that it is difficult to look at the subject calmly and objectively. Also complicating the drug scene is the fact that, as with alcohol, it is supported by an enormously rich and powerful industry—which, unlike the alcoholic beverages industry, is forced to function underground, profitably and tax-free, as in prohibition days with alcohol. The schools are again handed the impossible job of straightening things out: make the kids lose interest in sex, smoking, booze, and drugs!

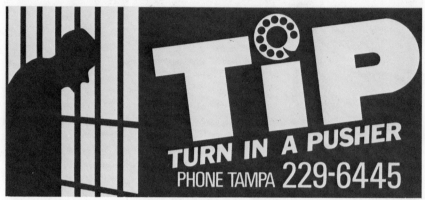

Virtually all research on drugs is suspect because of the likely bias of the researchers to begin with. The words involved are critical factors in all this because they trigger such strong emotional reactions that depress intellectual functioning and reduce most arguments to meaningless exercises. "Drug addict," "dope fiend," and "opium den" have been alarming people quite brainlessly like the words "Dracula" and "Frankenstein" for a great many years. A whole array of recent popular terms have similarly aroused state legislations to pass drug laws that are frequently more punitive than those for acts of physical violence. "Pot" and "grass" sound rather innocent, so maybe marijuana isn't so bad after all. (The intent here is not to make a case for or against the use of drugs but to point out something of the extent to which language is a major but usually unnoticed factor in the entire controversy.) Cigarettes do more harm to health than any of the hot-issue drugs, but since we have only minor negative reactions to the words "cigarettes" and "smoking," cigarette sales climb each year.

Medical opinion reflects the conflict and uncertainty concerning drug use. Being conservatively inclined, probably the majority of doctors would recommend against drug use (even though many doctors are users and some personally addicted). However, some recommend marijuana over alcohol, and many are happy to participate in their offsprings' pot parties.

1. *Use the word association and word cathexis techniques to evaluate "alcohol", "marijuana," and other drugs of interest (perhaps including "aspirin" and "caffeine"). Compare reactions to the "correct" terms with slang equivalents, for example, "booze," "firewater," "pot," and "grass."*
2. *Discuss the extent to which you feel that controversy in this area is based on objective knowledge of the recreational drugs versus emotional reactions to them and the words associated with them. Have emotional reactions implications for our laws?*

People are ordinarily conditioned in childhood to react to crises in a certain way. Some crisis reactions are physiological with nonverbal language expressions, including gestures, facial contortions, and gross bodily movements. Verbal language reactions figure largely in the total response, and they are the chief ones that determine the long-range reactions and the communicating of them to others. We have already described how girls are preprogrammed with respect to reacting to such crises as rape, and how alarmist and catastrophizing language at the time of crisis can intensify and prolong emotional reactions.

**CRISIS
INTERVENTION AND
EMERGENCY
MENTAL HEALTH**

Perhaps it would seem that when crises occur, we are virtually condemned to heightening our emotional responses to them via verbal preprogramming and catastrophizing. But must we make bad situations worse with our words, especially self-talk, about them? Of course not. Chapter 11 of this book is full of concrete examples for going into appropriate action, including verbal action. The first instruction to crisis workers is *"be calm"*—which implies the use of a certain kind of self-talk. Certainly such workers can render themselves useless or worse by using emotion-arousing language on themselves or others. Chapter 4 contains many examples of how we may be coached and coach ourselves to deal with emotionally charged situations. Thus if we will, we can train ourselves to handle crises in our own lives and to become rational models for others, especially our own children.

The death of a family member or friend can be extremely difficult to handle. Nothing said here is intended to suggest that it is best not to care when people die—not to have feelings or grieve. Of course, we do care and, depending on the person, may be deeply grieved. It is often saddening not to see a close friend for a week, let alone never again. However, the point of this discussion is: what are rational versus irrational ways of talking to ourselves and others when someone dies?

Death of close ones invites catastrophizing talk. In fact people tend to feel that unless they go to extremes, they are not showing appropriate grief and may very well feel guilty if they don't. Thus what often passes for healthy ventilating of grief is actually pouring verbal gasoline on the flames of genuine feelings.

Consider the following contrasting examples focusing on self-talk, whatever its source, following the death of someone close. (The death-related crises are merely used as models, direct applications to other, less drastic crises being evident.) The tire of a passing car was punctured, forcing the car out of control onto the walkway where it killed a small child. The mother, close at hand, witnessed the entire event. She rushed to her child, found it dead beyond question, and collapsed unconscious. The subsequent month was pure hell for her. But in time her underlying philosophy began to have its effect: no one is guaranteed a life of any particular duration, and therefore people die at all ages. Her child's life had been mostly a very happy one, and therefore it could be called a good life. Her own life was terribly shaken, but she decided not to die (of course, she had been drawn to suicide); that is, she decided to live a worthwhile life, seeking involvement and enjoyment. Although at times intensely sad and even torn apart emotionally by recall of what had happened, before long she was indeed on her way to becoming her former, usually happy, self.

As a contrasting example, a child suddenly vanished through the supposedly safe ice near the edge of a lake. His mother's most desperate efforts failed to save him. A hellish period followed during which she had fantasies of the tragedy by day and dreams of it at night. She called upon God praying for the magical return of her child; sometimes she cursed God for taking him away. She constantly said such things to herself as "I can't stand it," "I can't bear it," "This is awful," "I can't go on," and so forth. There evidently was nothing in her philosophy that had prepared her for death, which to her seemed invented for her child alone. She entered a prolonged state of incapacitating depression, which she considered was appropriate to her and reflected the attitude of fate toward her. She wanted no relief from it. Mirroring what others said of her, she said to herself, "I am a bereaved mother who will never get over her grief." Daily reinfection with words.

It is difficult for many to evaluate objectively such episodes as the foregoing because of human sympathy for the mothers involved. However, some important points may be noted. The two women experienced approximately the same thing, responded to it similarly at first with human, motherly feelings; however, they parted company, emotionally speaking. Their self-talk was the most significant factor.

These two extreme examples may serve as contrasting models of how people react to crises. Most people would probably agree that the first mother's response was healthier. Is it possible to increase chances that your response to crisis situations will be of this kind? Of course, it is. Think about some by analyzing what elements are involved in healthful responses and then rehearse responses to specific crisis situations that people are likely to encounter.

TAKING ACTION

1. *Use the word association and word cathexis techniques to evaluate words associated with crisis intervention and emergency mental health.*

2. *Discuss ways in which (a) language usage may increase emotional reactions to crises and thereby aggravate the situation, and (b) language usage may not aggravate but even may improve otherwise upsetting, even dangerous, situations. Talk with or have a first-aid expert visit class. To what extent does first aid take into account language considerations similar to those of emergency mental health?*

DISEASE

The language of illness and of the people and things associated with it is potent in many ways. Few people consider the word "disease" itself a positive word. (Possible exceptions: some people who profit from it and some in biological warfare.) Obviously, it means disruption of ongoing events and undertakings and very likely pain and economic loss—not to mention possible loss of life. So the word itself has become loaded, a negative stimulus that, like "sex" and "death," gives rise to circumlocutions, that is, efforts to get around it with "nicer" words such as "ill," "indisposed," and even "sick." We tend to have a "condition" rather than a disease. There are other important considerations associated with the words of disease.

Unlike sufferers from acute diseases, those with chronic (long-lasting) diseases often acquire the label of their disease. Thus the victim not only has to deal with the illness but with the onus of the label as well. He or she is a "leper," "quadraplegic," "cardiac," "epileptic," "alcoholic," "aphasic," "psychotic," and so on. The point is that to an incredible degree, as these victims become "symptomized," they become dehumanized. The saying "Labels tend both to create and to conceal the *individual* under them" has striking application to the chronically ill. For not only do doctors, nurses, family, and others tend to treat the person as a set of symptoms, but also the patient soon tends to recreate himself in terms of the illness. Granted, the survivor of a severe heart attack may not be any more able to pursue his normal activities than the badly injured survivor of an automobile crash. But the heart patient is much more likely to begin being perceived and living like a "cardiac" than the accident victim to spend the rest of his or her life acting like an accident victim.

Societal prejudice against the chronically ill and even the recovered is often severe. Only in recent years has it become fairly respectable to admit to having such diseases as tuberculosis and cancer (these used to be dirty words and avoided by the polite as the sex-related diseases continue to be.) If you're an "epileptic," even with seizures well controlled, can you get a job? Are you the same as other people in other regards? Similarly, if a person has had cancer or has controlled cancer that will in no way interfere with job competence, job prospects are reduced. Fat people—fatness is considered a disease by some doctors—are less likely to get into college or land jobs in spite of ability. Moreover, because they are unlikely to respond to treatment in hospitals and thereby are a threat to the doctor's function as a doctor, they tend to be disliked and are given derogatory labels. The dehumanization effect is painfully evident.

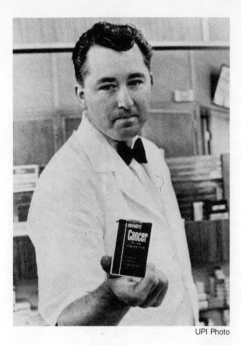

Pharmacy owner promoting his "brand" of cigarettes.

UPI Photo

There are many other ways in which the language of disease affects patients and others. Victims of heart attacks may be so terrified of the term "heart disease" that they will refuse to participate in prescribed exercise programs carefully planned to bring them back to near-normal functioning. They may quite needlessly call a halt to all sexual activity and other forms of physical play because of their associations with the dreaded words. As with the word "cancer," the very words "heart disease" may give rise to emotional states in patients that may complicate treatment and hinder recovery.

Diseases and other medical conditions tend to affect attitudes and behaviors in various ways. Pregnancy gives rise to unusual verbal responses by many, including family members and even strangers on the street. The word may trigger totally different reactions depending on whether the woman is said to be married. Nurses as well as people outside the hospital setting do not tend to talk with or about married and unmarried mothers in the same way. People undergoing "abortions" and "sterilizations" tend to be upsetting even to many hospital personnel, who express themselves accordingly.

Incidentally, we may note an interesting contrast between two disabilities: blindness and deafness. Whereas blindness tends to arouse the sympathies and desire to be helpful in most people, deafness tends to annoy. More accurately, deafness as such does not annoy people, but the deaf person's failure to follow instructions, answer questions, or otherwise respond to spoken language typically gives rise to impatience and anger. Thus, the adjustments of the deaf are enormously complicated, and feelings of persecution are often quite justified.

We have mentioned elsewhere that homosexuality has until recently been defined a disease but that millions of people have been "cured" of that disease by the verbal redefinition of the American Psychiatric Association. In contrast, a study involving genetic screening and counseling for sickle cell anemia in a Greek community was declared a failure in spite of the fact that the people learned a great deal about the disease. It seems that there was no controlling of the labeling of potential carriers. In spite of lack of danger, parents advised their children against marrying carriers, who were generally stigmatized and embarrassed. To all intent they were needlessly defined into illness by their label, just as homosexuals were defined out of it by majority vote.

TAKING ACTION

1. *Use the word association and word cathexis techniques to evaluate words associated with disease. Discuss your findings.*
2. *Observe ways in which sick people are talked to. Might people, especially perhaps children, be motivated to be sick sometimes because of the way they are treated, including verbally, when sick?*
3. *Discuss some benefits that might result when famous people openly discuss their own or others' diseases.*

Much of consumer education has to do with trying to teach the public how to defend itself against the advertising techniques of commercial concerns. However, the field of health education has a great deal to learn from Madison Avenue that would be applicable to "selling" the public good health concepts. Many of these techniques involve the skillful use of language, and they have to do with such things as associating attractive words with desirable health attitudes and practices, repetition of messages, and reinforcing "good" behavior.

CONSUMER EDUCATION

For an unusual example, in one U.S. county, an effort was made to increase the use of contraception for population control—not by the usual propaganda techniques of trying to push people into the desired behaviors with blasts of arguments and slogans. Instead, modern selling techniques were used. Among other things, the campaign went to the public with personalized appeals to arouse interest and to challenge. Women were made to see some personal advantages in using contraception; verbal reinforcement was right there when they responded. In other words, there was enticement and reinforcement for "good" behavior. Typical of good advertising, the campaign was expensive, but it evidently made a large "profit" in terms of reducing unwanted pregnancy, abortions, and forced marriages.

So much for the positive. The consuming public needs all possible help in evaluating selling techniques, whether for selling products or prejudicial laws or policies. Years of experience have shown that there is simply no limit to which some sellers will go to sell—no matter how unsafe, useless, or unhealthful the product. It has always been so; *caveat emptor* is a very old saying indeed.

There is no end to the verbal and nonverbal (pictorial) ways used to entice people to buy. Incredible amounts of money are spent each year to get the appropriate selling words and other symbols tied to the particular product. The word "liberation" is attractive, so it somehow gets associated with a tea. An entire sales campaign was based on the word "clean," even though the product in question was anything but clean and healthful—cigarettes. Very recently in Alabama, "Ulcer RX," a "remedy" for ulcers turned out to be almost pure, powdered cow dung. A style of eyeglasses sold extraordinarily well in spite of serious deficiencies because they were called "Executive," and men liked the idea of looking like executives. Everyone likes the word "free," so it is surefire and is used endlessly. A popular beer is "Lively-Lusty." Obviously, the trick is to put the attractive words and/or picture together with the product; by association the product becomes attractive. Can you imagine a new car being labeled "Rat," "Snake," "Spider," "Fink," or "Weasel"? "Bug" is a rare exception.

Speaking of weasel, "weaseling" is a standard advertising technique used to avoid direct misrepresentation and thereby violation of the law. (According to Webster, a weasel word is "a word used in order to evade or retreat from a direct or forthright statement or position.") As Paul Stevens says in his book *I Can Sell You Anything*, "When you have a weasel word, you automatically hear the implication. Not the real meaning, but the meaning *it* wants *you* to hear."[3] His book has much to say about how language is used to manipulate buying behavior. For example, the ad does not say that so and so puts you to sleep; it would have to work like a prescription sleep drug to do that. Weaseling makes the ad say: so and so will *help* you go to sleep. In other words, advertisers don't have to substantiate their claims since they make you, the consumer, hear things that aren't really said. Thus by saying a product *helps* do something, they give the unsophisticated the impression that the product *does* what is being talked about. We have all heard: "Helps keep you young," "Helps prevent cavities," "Helps fight . . .," "Helps you look . . .," "Helps you feel . . .." Stevens considers "help" a major four-letter, dirty word. But then how about "like," as in "It's like getting one bar [of soap] free" and "Cleans like a white tornado." The advertiser makes you believe that the product is more than it is by likening it to something else!

Another common weasel word to beware of in advertising is "virtually," which means "in effect but not in fact." We hear: "Virtually trouble-free" and "Virtually never needs service." For accuracy, these phrases need to be translated "Not in fact trouble-free . . .," "Not in fact never needs service . . ."

If the advertiser can't say *cures* or *fixes* or some other specific

---

[3]Paul Stevens, 1972, *I Can Sell You Anything.* New York: Ballantine Books.

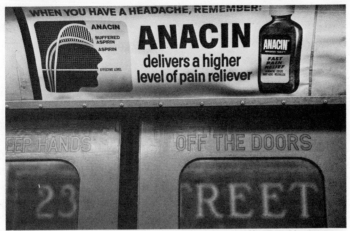

Alex Webb/Magnum Photos

positive word, he'll say "acts like" or "works against," which is weaseling so as to slide in a false impression. He hasn't really said anything that could be nailed down. Similarly with "can be," "up to," and "as much as." Anything *can be* almost anything; *up to*, as in "cured up to eight weeks," can mean actually one hour; and "*as much as* 40 miles per gallon" suggests that a possibility is the reality. Never does he come out with: "This it will do. You can count on it."

Adjectives are key tools of advertisers. Sometimes carefully chosen words can help sell a worthwhile product. For example, *additive-free*, whole-grain, or sugar-free may sway you to spend a few more cents for a considerably better brand, nutritionally speaking. However, the less health value products have the more heavily laden their advertising tends to be with adjectives—adjectives that are selected with the greatest of care to compensate for actual deficiencies. "Vitamin-rich," "enriched," and "high protein" are among the words lavished on dry breakfast cereals, the main nutritional value of which is likely to be in whatever milk and fruit are added to them.

Almost anything can be sold if it is dressed up attractively, and language is a major means of dressing things up. A large industry is devoted to doing this dressing up for selling, no matter what the product. We all need to be aware of this fact and to insist on looking directly at the product without its verbal and other decorations.

TAKING ACTION

1. *Use the word association and word cathexis techniques to evaluate words associated with consumer education.*
2. *Discuss some ways in which some promotional techniques of product manufacturers might be helpful in health education.*
3. *Collect for display examples of how advertisers use language as one means of manipulating prospective buyers.*

297

DISCUSSION   In this chapter we have identified very briefly some of the ways in which language is a factor in some major areas of human health. Since we use language all of the time, we tend to take it for granted like the air we breathe, usually not noticing the extent to which it often goes beyond being a means of communicating. When we do stop to take notice, we tend to be astounded at the extent to which words themselves affect our feelings and health behavior. Sometimes, as in the areas of sex, death, and disease, our words not only arouse strong feelings but actually impede and even cripple or break off communication. Still our language is so much a part of us that we rarely scrutinize it for its meanings and effects on us; nor do we often try to educate ourselves to guard against the possibly damaging effects of words or evaluate and use words in ways that will contribute to our health. Hopefully, after considering what has been said here, you will be more sensitive to the role of language in relation to human health.

Several basic points have appeared and reappeared in the course of the foregoing discussion of language in relation to the topics dealt with in this book. One of these has been our tendency to react to words as though they were actual things, often either all "good" or all "bad." Thus in a group of people who know virtually nothing about ecology, some react very favorably to "ecology" and some very unfavorably, depending upon emotional associations with the word. Another basic point has been that words that upset us emotionally tend also to lower the level of our available intelligence. For example, discussions of sex are often pretty emotional and brainless when they involve people who are uptight about sex words.

Other key points: beware of verbal labels, for they rub off on people and tend to dehumanize and to both hide and create the individuals under them; better interpersonal relationships require that we pay more attention than we do to skills of *private* speaking; our emotional health, including our ability to deal with the ups and downs of reality, require that we pay attention to our "self-talk"—our ways of talking to ourselves about and thereby directing our feelings about what happens to us; and that we be wary of the language tricks people play when they want to sell us products that may influence our health. May you heed carefully the subtle dimension of health.

FOR FURTHER READING

Chase, S., 1938, 1966. *The Tyranny of Words.* New York: Harcourt.

This old classic in the field outlines the nature and seriousness of the tyranny.

Ellis, A., 1973. *Humanistic Psychotherapy: The Rational-Emotive Approach.* New York: Julian Press.

This book is a leading example of how psychologists are tending to look to language as a major factor in emotional health, emotional ill health, and psychological therapy.

Eschholz, P. A., Rosa, A. F., and Clark, V. P., 1974. *Language Awareness.* New York: St. Martin's Press.

Several chapters deal with subjects of specific relevance to this book, for example, "The Semantics of Patient-Dentist Relations," "Burger Heaven," "The Language of the Hospital and Its Effects on the Patients," and "Nobody Ever Died of Old Age."

ETC.: A Review of General Semantics.

This is the journal concerned most specifically with analyzing the role of language in human behavior. Occasionally an article deals with a particular health-related topic, for example, "Labeling and the Mental Health Enigma" (June 1973), "Introduction to How to Live With a Neurotic," "Suicide, Semantics and Self," and "Rape Is a Four-Letter Word" (March 1975).

Johnson, W. R., and Belzer, E. G., 1973. *Human Sexual Behavior and Sex Education.* 3d ed. Philadelphia: Lea & Febiger.

"The Language Barrier" elaborates upon ways in which language interferes with progress in the sexual area. "The Polar Icecap of Human Relations" emphasizes the often complicating role of language in marriage relationships.

Minteer, C., 1970. *Understanding in a World of Words.* San Francisco: International Society for General Semantics.

A basic introduction to the subject, with many implications for health behavior.

part three

our health
and society

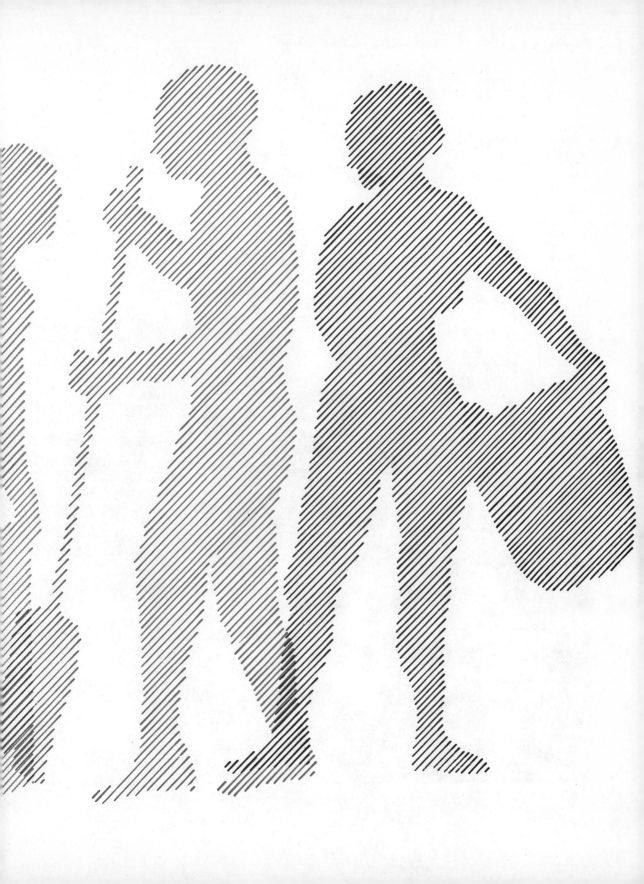

9

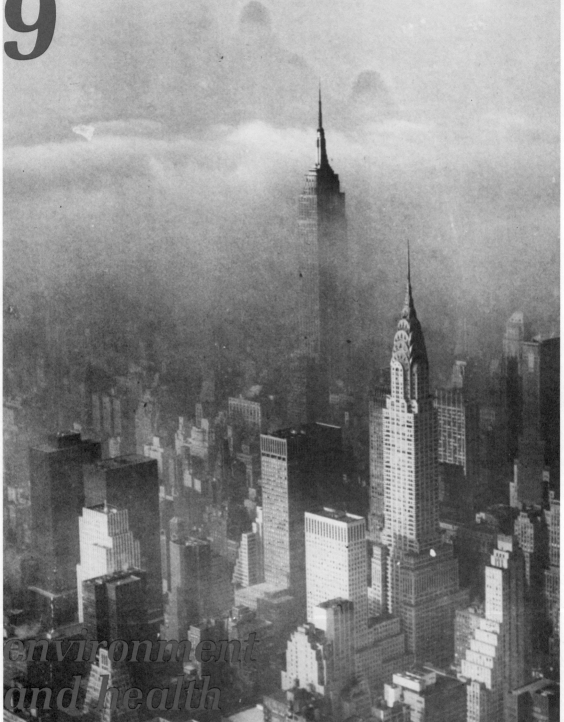

environment
and health

*Every human society possesses a two-way relationship with the
environment that it occupies. Its members modify the natural
environment, whether by hunting and gathering activities, the
pursuit of agriculture, or the complex activities of urban-industrial
life. This environment—in part the product of man himself—also
influences the well-being of the human population that occupies
it. Its particular characteristics expose and predispose the
population to various forms of disease: infectious, nutritional, and
even psychosomatic. In fact we may characterize any human
society by the pattern of disease that it shows. Primitive societies
of rural, underdeveloped parts of the world occupy environments
that predispose their members to a variety of infectious and
parasitic diseases and to certain severe forms of malnutrition. In
modern industrialized societies advances in public health and
nutrition have reduced many of these to rare occurrences. In their
place, however, a new set of diseases closely related to the
urban-industrial environment has appeared: diseases related to
environmental pollution, stress-induced patterns of ill health and
social pathology, and a growing number of rapidly evolving viral
diseases that continually challenge the technology of modern
medicine. Educated members of society must understand the
nature of these challenges and be aware of how their lifestyle and
choice of living and working environments may influence their
health. In addition, they bear the responsibility for exerting
influence at local, national, and international levels for improved
conditions of environmental health.*

INQUIRY

1. How can I minimize detrimental effects of environmental pollution on
   my future health by my choice of a place to live?
2. How should conditions of my working environment be designed to
   provide adequate protection for my physical health?
3. To what extent may the crowding and frequency of interpersonal
   contact in modern urban life influence my physical and mental
   health?
4. How do the conditions of modern society influence the type and
   severity of infectious diseases to which I will likely be exposed?
5. How can I exert an influence for improvement in local conditions
   relating to environmental health?
6. What sorts of programs are necessary at national and international
   levels to safeguard and improve conditions related to human health,
   and how can I exert influence to bring about these programs?

INTRODUCTION

Since we live in one of today's urbanized and industrialized societies,
it is easy for us to conclude that the advances of modern civilization
have made man more and more independent of the natural world. We

see sophisticated technology applied to many aspects of our well-being: comfortable homes and offices, stimulating educational opportunities, and effective treatment of disease and injury. Yet humans remain biological entities subject to diseases and parasites, nutritional disorders, and mental disturbances resulting from factors in the environment. Environmental ties have not been cut; instead they have become increasingly numerous and complicated. The creation of comfortable living and working conditions requires the consumption of materials and energy, with resultant waste discharges into the environment. Access to challenging jobs, cultural opportunities, and education often incurs certain costs imposed by life in crowded, impersonal urban environments. The effectiveness of modern medicines is, at the same time, a powerful agent for evolutionary change in the disease organisms against which they are used.

We exist within an environmental system—the human ecosystem—of which we are but one of many interacting components. We will examine some of the relationships within the human ecosystem that bear on our health. In so doing we will consider both how factors of the environment influence us and how in turn we may modify these influences.

THE ENVIRONMENT AND HEALTH OF THE INDIVIDUAL

Health-related factors of the environment are of several types. Some are of a chemical and physical nature: pollutant chemicals, noise, and ionizing radiation, for example. Others, such as crowding and interpersonal contact, are psychosocial in nature. Still others, influencing the incidence of infectious, parasitic, and nutritional disease in human populations, are epidemiological influences of the environment.

The Chemical and Physical Environment

Nowhere is humanity's modification of the chemical and physical environment more apparent than in the atmosphere. Our impacts on the atmosphere range from local effects, which we term "air pollution," to regional and global effects, which represent "weather and climate modification." Air pollution now constitutes one of the most serious environmental challenges to human health. Long-term impacts on the global atmosphere present potentially serious future threats.

Air pollution is largely the result of combustion processes. Combustion is responsible for somewhere between 200 and 225 million tons of pollutants that enter the atmosphere of the United States each year (Table 9-1). The largest single source of combustion pollutants is the transportation complex, primarily cars, trucks, trains, and airplanes. Manufacturing and electric power generation are next in importance. The heating of homes and other buildings and the burning of refuse are also significant sources.

If this total amount of air pollution was spread evenly over the entire continental area of the United States, the average concentration would be very low, no more than about 1.5 ppm (parts per million) at any one

Pollutant Group	TOTAL POLLUTANTS (10^6 tons)		PERCENTAGE OF U.S. POLLUTANTS FROM VARIOUS SOURCES				
	World	U.S.	Transportation	Space Heating and Electric Power	Industry and Manufacturing	Solid Waste Disposal	Other Open Burning
Carbon monoxide	280	100	63.8	1.9	9.6	7.8	16.9
Sulfur oxides	146	37	2.4	73.5	22.0	0.3	1.8
Hydrocarbons	88	32	51.9	2.2	14.4	5.0	26.5
Nitrogen oxides	53	21	39.3	48.5	1.0	2.9	8.3
Particulates	110	28	4.3	31.4	26.5	3.9	33.9
Total	667	214	42.4	21.0	14.0	5.2	17.4

time. But, of course, this is not the case; the bulk of this pollution is released over the highly urbanized 1 percent of the land surface upon which 50 percent of the population lives. To compound the problem, certain atmospheric conditions act to slow the dispersion of these pollutants and retain them close to the ground surface. These conditions, termed temperature inversions (Figure 9-1), involve the develop-

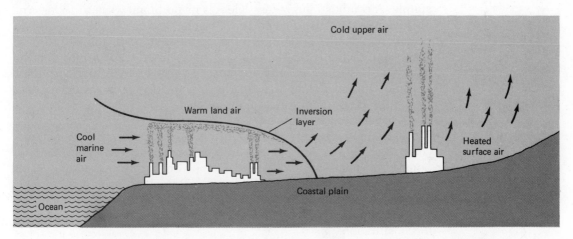

Figure 9-1

Development of a temperature inversion in a coastal area due to daytime heating of the land surface and landward movement of a cool marine air layer.

ment of a cool, surface layer of air overlain by a layer of warm air. Temperature inversions develop for a variety of reasons. In coastal areas during the day heating of the land surface produces warming of the associated air, causing it to expand and rise. As a consequence, cooler marine air tends to flow inland, close to the ground surface, to replace the rising, warmer air. Temperature inversions are not limited to coastal areas, however. In any valley or basin, inversions tend to develop during the night because heat loss is greatest from the land surface, due to infrared heat radiation to space, and the cooling of the air is thus greatest next to the surface. This is enhanced by the fact that the cooler, heavier air produced in this manner tends to flow, by gravity, into low-lying valley and basin areas. Most of our large urban areas are, of course, located in valleys or basins or along coastlines, and therefore temperature inversions are very frequent in occurrence (Table 9-2). In the Temperate Zone, especially during the winter, the stagna-

Table 9-2	FREQUENCY OF OCCURRENCE OF TEMPERATURE INVERSIONS IN VARIOUS U.S. CITIES			
	PERCENT OF DAYS ON WHICH INVERSIONS OCCUR			
City	Winter	Spring	Summer	Fall
Los Angeles	56	30	19	44
St. Louis	37	27	34	44
New York	14	16	19	26

tion of cold fronts may also create prolonged inversions, during which cold air brought in by frontal movements underlies warmer air.

The mechanism by which temperature inversions trap pollutants is simple. A combustion process releases its pollutant wastes in a mass of air that has also been heated by the same process. As this air mass is heated, it expands. Upon its release, therefore, it tends to rise and, as it rises, cool gradually. It will continue to rise until it encounters a layer of air that is warmer and lighter than it is—a layer existing as a result of a temperature inversion. If such a layer is present, it consequently acts as a "lid" to rising masses of polluted air.

The materials introduced into the air by combustion and other processes are extremely diverse in nature. Almost every element and compound known finds its way into the atmosphere in some quantity. Some of the materials involved are in the form of tiny particulates, such as soot and ash. The finest of these are colloidal in size and are termed aerosols. Other substances enter the air in vapor form. Once in the air, they may engage in chemical reactions, adding still further complexity to the situation.

Two major syndromes of air pollution have been recognized, based on the interaction between the predominant types of primary pollutants and the characteristic climatic conditions of the region involved. These syndromes, named after the cities in which they were first recognized, are known as London and Los Angeles smogs. In both cases a set of primary pollutants, the materials released into the air by combustion, and a set of secondary pollutants, those formed by chemical reactions in the air, can be identified.

London smog first appeared in the 1600s, when coal was introduced for heating purposes in the city of London. It is the principal type of smog in urban-industrial areas where large quantities of coal and high-sulfur petroleum fuels are used or where smelting of large quantities of metal ores is carried out. The primary pollutants of importance are sulfur dioxide (SO_2) and particulates (soot and ash). In the urban areas involved—the major industrial cities of the midwestern and northeastern United States, for example—the inversions that trap these pollutants are frequent during the winter, when these primary pollutants often become associated with cold fogs.

Under these conditions a set of rather simple chemical reactions occurs. Sulfur dioxide is slowly oxidized to sulfur trioxide (SO_3). This reaction seems to be catalyzed by metals such as manganese, iron, and copper, which may be present as the constituents of particulate pollutants, and also occurs more rapidly in solution in water. Thus the tiny droplets of fog, many of which are formed by condensation about microscopic particulate nuclei, act as excellent reaction laboratories. The resulting sulfur trioxide reacts with water within seconds to produce sulfuric acid (H_2SO_4), which is the major irritating and damaging secondary pollutant in London smog. The reducing, corrosive action of London smog is evident in its action on metals, limestone and marble statues, and the human lung.

Los Angeles smog differs in its primary pollutants, the climate to which they become exposed, and the reactions they undergo. Unburned hydrocarbons, nitrogen oxides, and carbon monoxide (CO) are the major primary pollutants—a set of materials reflecting an urban way of life for which the automobile and freeway have become symbolic. Most of these pollutants are colorless, odorless, and, except for carbon monoxide, relatively harmless. In the atmosphere and under the influence of bright sunlight they undergo a remarkably complex, and as yet incompletely understood, set of reactions. The energy source for these reactions is the ultraviolet component of solar radiation; hence Los Angeles smog develops during the day and disappears at night (Figure 9-2). The secondarily produced chemicals include nitrogen dioxide (NO_2), which is a vile-smelling, irritating, brownish gas, together with a number of peroxidized substances. The simplest of these is ozone (O_3); one of the more complex is a substance known as peroxyacetyl nitrate, or PAN, which is a complex organic compound formed by reactions involving free oxygen, nitrogen compounds, and unburned hydrocarbons. These secondary substances form the toxic and irritating constituents of Los Angeles smog. Their action is like that of a hydrogen peroxide bleach—one of oxidation rather than reduction. One of their oxidizing effects involves tiny, clear oil droplets in the atmosphere; oxidation converts them into opaque droplets. These, together with the brownish nitrogen dioxide, are major components of the typical smog haze associated with this type of air pollution.

Of course, the air pollution complex of any large city is a combination of these two types, varying in their proportion and changing in relative importance seasonally. Both, however, contribute to problems of human health.

Figure 9-2

Pattern of change in concentration of various primary and secondary pollutants during the diurnal photochemical smog cycle of a typical July day in Los Angeles.

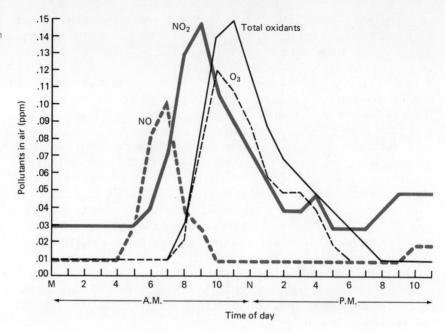

Attention was first drawn to the human health dangers of air pollution by a number of acute episodes of London smog that caused major increases in human mortality rates. In London during a five-day period in December 1952, when strong inversion conditions maintained an intense "pea soup" fog and smog condition, the mortality rate for the city exceeded that normal for the season by about 4000 persons. Similarly, in Donora, Pennsylvania, a steel-mill town in the Monongahela Valley south of Pittsburgh, 17 persons died during a smog episode in October 1948, and one-third of the city population became ill. Considering that the total population of Donora was only 14,000, this is one of the most severe mortality episodes ever to occur. More recently excess mortalities of between 150 and 200 have been recorded during inversion periods in November 1953 and November 1967 in New York City. The evidence in these cases suggests that smog conditions tend to produce early mortality of individuals with severe respiratory or cardiovascular conditions.

More recently studies in Los Angeles have suggested an association between carbon monoxide levels and "excess mortality," that is, mortality rates above levels normal for the season. The overall mortality rate in Los Angeles usually rises during the winter, in spite of the fact that the secondary photochemical components of smog are lower during this season. Carbon monoxide levels are higher in the winter, however, reaching average levels of 20 ppm on occasion. At this level the oxygen-carrying capacity of the blood is reduced by about 3 percent due to combination of carbon monoxide with blood hemoglobin. The fact that this is an average effect means that in certain parts of the city the effect is much higher. Obviously, any factor that reduces the capacity of the blood to carry oxygen will increase the strain on the cardiovascular system. Analyses have suggested that these high levels of carbon monoxide may lead to an excess mortality of about 11 persons per day for the city of Los Angeles.

Air pollution of both London and Los Angeles types contributes to increased incidence of nonspecific upper respiratory diseases caused by viral and bacterial agents. These diseases include the common cold and various streptococcal infections of the nose and throat. In simple terms this increase appears to be due to the fact that pollutants irritate respiratory membranes, making them more susceptible to establishment of disease agents.

More seriously, air pollution is related to increased incidence of several chronic diseases of the lower respiratory tract, including chronic bronchitis, chronic constrictive ventilatory disease, and pulmonary emphysema. To understand these diseases, we should review the basic microstructure of the lungs. The trachea, which carries air from the posterior part of the mouth cavity into the chest, divides to form two bronchi, one of which leads to each lung. These bronchi divide and redivide, eventually forming tiny, elastic, thin-walled tubules called *bronchioles*. These bronchioles end in a cluster of microscopic alveoli, which are blind air sacs that, when magnified, appear like a tightly clustered bunch of grapes (Figure 9-3). The alveoli are lined by a single layer of epidermal cells that separates the air of the alveolar sac from a surrounding network of capillary blood vessels. This is the actual site of gas exchange in the lungs. The total surface of these alveoli is great: half the area of a football field is the figure often quoted. This vast area is essential for providing the quantitative rate of gas exchange that a fully active individual requires.

Chronic bronchitis is a condition of continuous or frequent inflammation of the bronchial tubes and bronchioles. This inflammation produces swelling and overproduction of mucus by the lining of the tubes. Eventually it destroys the ciliated surface of the tubes that normally functions to remove mucus and dirt from deep in the lungs. The smaller tubes of the bronchial system may become constricted, or even blocked by mucus, and the individual suffers from frequent coughing and shortness of breath.

Chronic constrictive ventilatory disease is related in nature. Here, however, the major symptom is progressive constriction of the smaller bronchial tubes and bronchioles as long-continued irritation causes scar and connective tissue to be deposited in their walls. The more these tubes become constricted the more difficult it becomes to breathe.

Pulmonary emphysema is still another related form of deterioration of the terminal parts of the pulmonary system. Here the typical pattern of deterioration involves the bronchioles and alveoli. Prolonged inflammation of the walls of the bronchioles leads to their thickening with fibrous connective tissue and their loss of elasticity. Resulting difficulties of airflow into and out of the alveoli lead to ruptures in the membranes of the alveolar sacs and bronchioles. The long-term result is

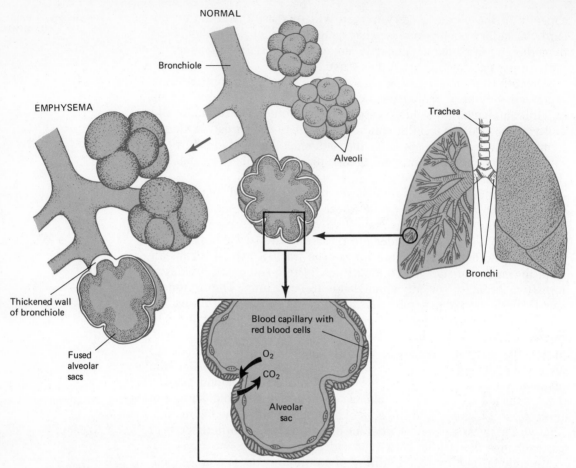

NORMAL

Bronchiole

Alveoli

EMPHYSEMA

Trachea

Thickened wall
of bronchiole

Fused
alveolar
sacs

Bronchi

Blood capillary with
red blood cells

O_2

CO_2

Alveolar
sac

Figure 9-3

The general alveolar
structure of the lungs and
the basic changes in
microstructure occurring
in pulmonary
emphysema.

progressive fusion of individual alveolar sacs into larger units with a smaller total surface area. In addition, accumulation of fluid in these larger cavities tends to occur, further restricting their gas exchange capacity.

All of these degenerative changes, by their reduction of efficiency of gas exchange, put increased strain on the heart. A greater amount of blood has to be pumped through the lungs to achieve the same amount of gas exchange.

Emphysema is a disease that can be triggered by various types of chronic irritation due to allergenic substances, smoking, or exposure to air pollutants such as sulfur compounds and photochemical oxidants. It can be fatal, and in urban areas it is being recognized as an increasingly important cause of death (Figure 9-4). In 1950, for example, the death rate in California for emphysema was only 1.5 per 100,000 per year. By 1957 this rate had climbed to 5.8, and by 1967 it had reached 15 per 100,000 per year. Thus a tenfold increase occurred over the same 17-year period that saw Los Angeles smog increase from a minor to a major feature of the California urban environment.

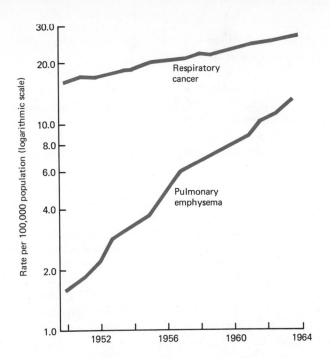

Figure 9-4
Pattern of recent change in death rates in California for respiratory cancer and pulmonary emphysema.

Still more serious, however, is the rapidly mounting evidence of association of air pollution and respiratory cancer. This evidence, statistical and circumstantial, comes from a variety of sources and is substantial. One of these sources is human migration studies. The incidence of respiratory cancer can be determined, for example, for individuals born in England but emigrating at an early age to New Zealand. If we compare their rate to that of a carefully matched group that was born and continued to live in England, we find that the cancer rate for the emigrating group is lower. In a similar fashion, groups of Norwegians that emigrated to the United States show higher lung cancer rates than those staying in Norway, but lower rates than do individuals of Norwegian stock born in the United States.

Other comparisons show differences in cancer rates for rural and urban populations. Rates increase progressively from rural areas to urban areas of larger and larger size (Figure 9-5). For urban areas with

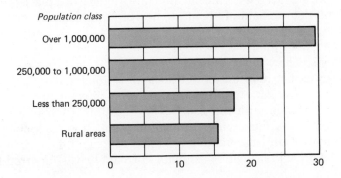

Figure 9-5
Annual mortality rates for respiratory cancer per 100,000 white males in U.S. cities of varying size.

populations of over 1 million, lung cancer rates are nearly doubled those of rural areas, a difference much greater than that attributable to smoking or occupational differences.

Along this gradient of increasing cancer rates, some of the specific carcinogenic chemicals are now being identified. In an area of south central Los Angeles, for example, a unique pattern of lung cancer frequently was recently uncovered. Investigators determined that in a zone 3 to 4 miles east and west of the Long Beach Freeway the incidence of lung cancer was about 40 percent higher in males than for the Los Angeles Basin as a whole. However, this pattern seemed to be absent among females.

Since this part of Los Angeles is an industrial area, it was at first thought that the higher rates might reflect differences in the socioeconomic composition of the population, or be the result of occupational exposure. When statistical comparisons were restricted to low-income segments of the population of the affected area and similar components of the population outside the zone, however, the higher incidence of cancer in this portion of the city was still shown. Likewise, since the area has many petrochemical industries, comparisons were made between cancer rates for workers in petrochemical plants and those working in other types of industry. Again, the results showed no difference.

What was found, however, was that the air environment of this part of the city is different. In particular it has concentrations of certain aromatic hydrocarbons that are considerably higher than those in other areas. The chemical benzopyrene, a substance known to be tumor-inducing in experimental animals, is about five times as concentrated here as in other parts of Los Angeles. The conclusion of this study is that the higher mortality from lung cancer among males may very well be the result of a synergism—a reinforcing interaction—between smoking and neighborhood air pollution. In other words, smoking, which is heavier and more frequent among males, may interact with air pollution factors to induce lung cancer at an unexpectedly high rate.

Still other studies have suggested a link between air pollution and cardiovascular disease. In Nashville, Tennessee, for example, the mortality rate from cardiovascular disease has been found to be 10 to 20 percent higher in portions of the city with highly polluted air.

Thus we are faced with the fact that one's choice of a place to live is a significant determinant of his future health. We are also faced with the fact that health-related air pollution effects have an enormous cost associated with them. Economists have attempted to assess some of these costs. They did this by drawing together data on quantitative relationships between air pollution and various major diseases and combining these data with information on medical expenses and lost income associated with the diseases in question. Their index of total disease cost was the saving that would result from reduction of air pollution levels in large urban areas to 50 percent of their 1970 values. In other words, their figures estimate the actual costs incurred by this "top" 50 percent of existing air pollution in this country.

In effect, a reduction of air pollution of this magnitude would be equivalent to lowering of pollution levels of all cities to those prevailing in cities with relatively clean air, a degree of improvement that seems well within our technological capability. For chronic bronchitis and related diseases, such a reduction would lead to a 25 to 50 percent decline in disease incidence, an improvement with a dollar value of between $250 million and $500 million annually. For lung cancer, a disease reduction of 15 percent, and a saving of $33 million are estimated. For all other respiratory diseases, a 25 percent reduction is also projected, with savings of about $1222 million.

In addition, it is expected that reduced air pollution would lead to reductions in cardiovascular disease and certain other forms of cancer—esophageal, stomach, and bladder—that also show statistical association with air pollution. A conservative estimate is that a 50 percent air pollution reduction would reduce cardiovascular disease by 10 percent, giving a savings of $468 million annually. Likewise, a 15 percent reduction of these other forms of cancer related to air pollution is likely, with savings of $390 million each year.

The total of all of these projected savings—the extra costs of the top 50 percent of the urban air pollution now existing—is in the neighborhood of $2.4 billion to $2.6 billion annually. Per capita, this equals $1200 to $1300 annually for each man, woman, and child in the United States. To the dollar value of these expenses incurred and income lost, of course, must be added considerable physical suffering and mental anguish. Unfortunately, the magnitude of this human damage resulting from air pollution has yet to be reflected in programs designed to improve the urban environment.

At the global end of the spectrum of humans' modification of the atmospheric environment, the impact has yet to become one directly hazardous to our health. Measurable changes in the concentration of CO_2 in the atmosphere and of its content of particulates—increases in both cases—have resulted from both industrial and agricultural activities. The long-term significance of these effects is very difficult to predict, as is any modification of atmospheric relationships. At present, however, the most serious challenge to human health appears to relate to stratospheric pollution and to effects of various pollutants on the ozone "layer" of the outer stratosphere. This layer, formed and maintained by the decomposition of molecular oxygen by ultraviolet light energy and the reaction of the resulting free oxygen atoms with oxygen molecules to form ozone, serves to filter out about 99 percent of the ultraviolet radiation reaching the outer atmosphere. With a reduction in the density of the ozone shield, a number of alarming possibilities exist. The most likely of these is an increase in the incidence of skin cancer. Further estimates are that a 5 percent ozone reduction, translated into a 10 percent ultraviolet radiation increase, would produce from 20,000 to 60,000 additional cases of skin cancer per year in the United States. (Most of these are curable if treated promptly.)

Two significant threats to the ozone layer seem to exist: introduction of nitrogen oxides into the stratosphere by supersonic jet aircraft and the increase in halomethanes ("Freon" and related materials) in the atmosphere. The high-compression engines of aircraft, like those of automobiles, release nigrogen oxides in their exhaust. One of these oxides, nitric oxide, tends to react with ozone, destroying the latter. The net result is a depletion of ozone. Recent estimates have suggested that a fleet of 500 planes might produce an ozone reduction averaging 16 percent in the northern hemisphere and 8 percent in the southern hemisphere. This in turn would bring about a serious increase in skin cancer and probably other health problems as well.

Halomethanes are compounds of carbon, chlorine, and fluorine. The most common halomethanes are used commonly as an aerosol spray propellant and as a refrigerant. In both cases, the reason for use of these materials is their high volatility and low chemical reactivity. Both are essentially inert, insoluble in water, and unaffected by biological processes. Thus the fate of all of these substances is ultimately to enter the atmosphere. Nearly 1 million metric tons of these chemicals were produced in 1974, added to 5 million tons produced in previous years. They have become worldwide in distribution in the atmosphere, although in greatest concentrations over large urban areas. In the upper stratosphere, to which they ultimately ascend, they are subject to photolytic decomposition by ultraviolet radiation, producing, among other things, free chlorine atoms. These atoms apparently act as a catalyst for ozone decomposition. Current estimates are that the quantities of halomethanes now in the atmosphere may lead to a reduction of at least 5 percent in the ozone layer by 1990. Although there is still a great deal of uncertainty about the seriousness of these threats to the ozone layer, these examples nevertheless serve to illustrate that humankind's chemical impact on the environment can have very serious global consequences.

In addition, modern technology is creating and stimulating environmental cycles involving a great variety of toxic materials, including heavy metals, radioactive substances, pesticides, and many others. Moving through the biosphere in complex pathways, many of them become concentrated in a fashion that directs them toward humans. Some, such as food additives and the constituents of household products of various types, are intended specifically for intake and body contact.

Over the years we have tended to concentrate certain natural but poisonous metals in our living environment. These metals include lead, mercury, cadmium, arsenic, copper, zinc, nickel, chromium, and beryllium. Our understanding of the lead problem is perhaps better than that of several of the other metals. Globally about 3.5 million tons of lead are mined annually. Until recently nearly one-tenth of this amount was used for gasoline additives that were eventually burned and released into the air. This use is, of course, declining now. Lead is also introduced into the atmosphere by smelting operations, industrial activity, and combustion in general. We can estimate the extent to which people have increased the rate of introduction of lead into the atmosphere by looking at concentrations of lead in ice layers of different ages in the Greenland ice cap (Figure 9-6). Evidence from this

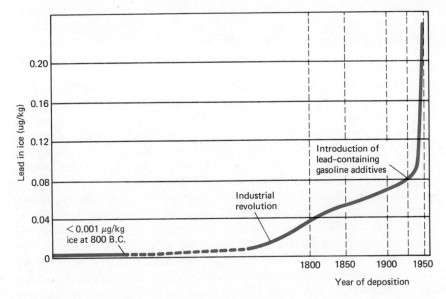

Figure 9-6
Changes in the rate of deposition of lead in the Greenland icecap in relation to major patterns of human activity.

source shows that the present rate of deposition is 500 or more times greater than it was in 800 B.C. This deposition rate took a large jump in the early 1940s when gasoline additives came into use. Other estimates suggest that the total lead input to the oceans, due to fallout increases from the atmosphere and waste disposal to aquatic systems, has increased to 27 or so times its original rate.

As a human health problem, lead pollution is most severe in urban areas. Lead may enter the human body in two ways: through the digestive tract and through the lungs. Particularly in ghetto areas of large cities, dietary intake by small children may reach very high levels because they often eat flakes of old lead-based paint. Thus critical levels may easily be exceeded. Lead also enters the body through the lungs, with small particles being retained in the lungs. Larger particles trapped by the mucous membranes of respiratory passages, may eventually pass into the digestive tract. For urban residents, ingestion through the lungs is roughly equal to lead intake via the digestive tract.

Symptoms of classical lead poisoning begin to occur at a level in the blood of less than one-tenth part per million, and this critical level may well be exceeded by many persons, especially those working in high-exposure areas such as parking lots or those living near smelters. Lead poisoning leads to anemia, chronic kidney disease, and serious

315

effects on the central nervous system. It has been recently estimated that perhaps 50,000 children in the United States suffer significant brain damage and mental retardation from blood lead levels approaching those at which acute poisoning begins.

The rate of fallout deposition of mercury in the Greenland ice cap has roughly doubled over the past 2000 years. This doubling has resulted from industrial and fuel-combustion activities like those involving lead. Evidence also shows that it has resulted from a general disturbance of the earth's surface—farming, road construction, overgrazing, and so on—that allows mercury compounds to pass more freely into the air.

At present these general effects do not seem to be cause for general alarm. In comparison to the quantities of mercury present in environmental systems such as the oceans, the doubled input quantities are exceedingly small. In all probability the high mercury levels in certain marine fish, such as tuna, reflect natural levels of mercury in seawater, together with the tendency of this material to be concentrated along food chains, which will be discussed shortly.

In local portions of the terrestrial, freshwater, and coastal marine environment, however, mercury pollution can become a serious human hazard. After its release, regardless of chemical form, mercury is usually converted by bacterial action to a form known as *methyl mercury*. Methyl mercury is taken up, concentrated, and retained by many living organisms. Several major instances of mercury poisoning of persons eating fish or shellfish contaminated in this manner have been reported. The most widely publicized of these occurred in Minimata City, Japan, where more than 100 persons died after eating seafood contaminated by industrial waste discharges. Grains treated with mercurial fungicides have poisoned people via grain or meat. The most recent of these cases occurred in Iraq in 1972 and led to the hospitalization of 6530 persons and the death of at least 459.

Mercury exerts very severe effects on the nervous system, including the loss of feeling, coordination, speech, vision, and hearing. Severe cases lead to blindness, coma, and eventually death. It is apparent that the potential hazards of mercury pollution justify the precautions taken in testing food products and in reducing the overall "leakage" of mercury into the environment from human activities.

A number of other heavy metals, such as cadmium and arsenic, are also highly toxic to humans. Several are capable of being methylated in a manner similar to mercury, thus favoring their uptake and retention by living organisms. It is clear that careful monitoring of all elements of this sort must be carried out.

A second major group of biologically active materials of major environmental concern comprises the various radioisotopes, which tend to undergo spontaneous decomposition into atoms of stable isotopes or even atoms of another element. In the course of this decomposition they release atomic radiation that can produce biological damage. The extent of such damage depends upon several factors: the strength of the radiation source, the types of radiation emitted, and the distance of the receiving object from the source of radiation.

The radioisotopes that actually or potentially enter the environment come essentially from two sources: nuclear explosions and reactor waste discharges. In quantitative terms the nuclear explosions resulting from atmospheric weapons testing have been the more important to date. The radioisotopes released in these explosions are numerous, but in largest measure they consist of what are called *fission products* or leftover fragments of uranium or plutonium atoms. The more common and biologically important of these fission products are strontium 90, iodine 131, and cesium 137. Moreover, in the course of atomic reactions the atoms of a great many elements, such as carbon and phosphorus, may be bombarded by neutrons in such a way that their atomic structure is modified to create radioisotopes of these elements.

Some of these radioisotopes belong to elements that are basic components of living systems. Iodine, for example, is an essential constituent of the thyroid hormone of vertebrate animals. Iodine 131 is thus readily taken up by such animals, including humans, and is in fact concentrated greatly in the course of this uptake. Other radioisotopes are taken in not because they are identical to required elements but because they are similar enough in chemistry to be subject to the same metabolic uptake processes. Strontium, for example, is chemically similar to calcium and is taken up and stored in bone tissues and milk by the same biochemical processes involved in calcium metabolism. Cesium is chemically similar to potassium and is carried along the same metabolic pathways as is potassium.

The effects of ionizing radiation upon organisms depend upon the size and complexity of the organism in question. The larger and more complex the body of an organism the more sensitive it is to radiation damage. Humans are thus more highly vulnerable to the effects of environmental radiation than, for example, insects or bacteria are. Sensitivity also varies with the stage in the reproductive cycle. The most sensitive stages are those of the early part of the reproductive process: egg and sperm cells, the fertilized egg, and the early embryo. Any disruption of organization at these early stages is in essence magnified during embryological development and growth and thus may lead to severe or fatal effects at a later point. Effects of this sort—abnormalities of development—are *teratogenic*. One of the other effects that radiation may have is that of disturbance of gene structure, the production of gene mutations, or *mutagenesis*. Most mutations are, of course, detrimental or even lethal in nature; only a few result in improvement in the characteristic controlled by the particular gene. Ionizing radiation may also act as a cancer-inducing agent. There is increasing evidence, for example, that alpha radiation from radioisotopes of lead and polonium in tobacco is a contributing factor to lung cancer in smokers.

Although no human health hazard appears to be involved due to present levels of environmental contamination by radioactive materials, it is apparent that were extensive contamination to occur, many routes exist to lead radioactive materials to man. Here we should note that current atomic reactors, as well as those of the so-called "breeder reactor" generation, operate by controlled fission reactions. A great deal of concern has arisen about the possibilities of reactor accidents, accompanied by the release of radioactive materials in large amounts. It may be the case that sufficient precautions can be implemented to reduce this danger to an acceptable risk. However, all such reactors produce large quantities of exceedingly dangerous radioactive wastes. Disposal of these materials into the environment is totally unacceptable, and the only alternative is one of their storage in a location from which they do not reenter active portions of the biosphere for thousands of years. That such a storage system is feasible is yet to be satisfactorily demonstrated. In the meantime reactor wastes are being temporarily stored in structures that must be constantly monitored for leakage—a manner of storage that is unsatisfactory in the long run.

In addition to the modification of geochemical cycles of these natural and seminatural materials, people are creating new environmental cycles of synthetic, highly stable materials such as the chlorinated hydrocarbon pesticides. Many of these materials were distributed worldwide through systems of air and water circulation before their dangers and in some cases their environmental presence were realized. Many of the substances in question, particularly the pesticide chemicals, are utilized because they possess powerful biological activity, and their patterns of use involve their deliberate release into the environment.

It was through the case of DDT that one of the significant features of environmental movement of many of these environmental pollutants was discovered. This mechanism, known as *food chain magnification*, has subsequently been demonstrated for substances as diverse as mercury, cadmium, strontium 90, cesium 137, iodine 131, chlorinated hydrocarbon pesticides in general, and the polychlorinated biphenyls, a group of industrial chemicals. Any accumulated pollutant substance in tissues of the food organism may be concentrated—magnified—in the body of the feeding species. For mercury and DDT the concentration process appears to be due to high solubility of these materials in fats, which are universal constituents of living systems. For radioisotopes the mechanism is simply their identity with or similarity to required nutrient elements.

Concern on the part of conservationists has tended to focus on the effects of these chemicals upon endangered species of wildlife. In these cases, however, what has been shown is that detrimental biochemical effects are usually exerted particularly on physiological processes associated with reproduction. These basic processes are quite similar to those involved in human reproduction. Furthermore, many of the materials involved have been experimentally shown to have mutagenic, teratogenic, or carcinogenic action. Thus these wildlife problems may actually be "distant early warnings" of more serious threats to human health.

Another area of significant concern in relation to human exposure to chemical substances is that of food additives. These are discussed in Chapter 2.

Concern has recently arisen over the presence of minute amounts of dangerous chemicals in treated drinking water supplies of many cities. It appears that chlorination of water may at times lead to the production of small amounts of carbon tetrachloride, which may constitute a contaminant of significant danger. Traces of various other materials, including pesticides, have also been found in some areas. In other areas, where persons are dependent upon well water, contamination with nitrate has occasionally caused health problems. Nitrates, generally entering ground water sources due to fertilizer use, may be converted to nitrites in the human digestive tract. Nitrite in turn, when absorbed into the bloodstream, tends to combine with hemoglobin, reducing its oxygen-carrying capacity. A number of human deaths, especially among infants, have occurred as a result. Thus careful surveillance of the chemicals present in water, as well as food, is a continuing necessity.

One of the most serious physical factors in the working environment is noise. Evidence indicates that it causes hearing loss, interferes with such important functions as braking an automobile, has an adverse delayed reaction upon subsequent efforts to learn and enjoy recreational activities, and encourages the emergence of aggression and asocial attitudes. Many jobs place workers in an environment of greater than average noise level. In the United States population it has been observed that the pitch range of hearing becomes restricted with age, particularly at higher pitches, and that the loss tends to be sex-related—greater in males than in females.

How extensive is hearing loss? Careful studies show that, first of all, no threshold for damaging noise levels exists. Second, they show that in most cases the hearing losses resulting from occupational exposure are the result of inner ear damage rather than middle ear disturbances. High-intensity noise appears to damage the hair cells of the organ of Corti, destroying them in regions of this organ that are responsible for sensing particular pitch ranges. Of course, certain occupations in construction and industry expose people to deafening sound levels. However, recently it has been discovered that many rock musicians have experienced appreciable hearing losses. In addition, there is mounting evidence that prolonged exposure to noise levels even under 100 decibels, corresponding to those created by many common items of machinery and various vehicles, may also lead to a degree of impairment of hearing (Figure 9-7).

Since 1972 the U.S. Environmental Protection Agency has been

Figure 9-7
Decibel levels associated
with representative types
of environmental noise.

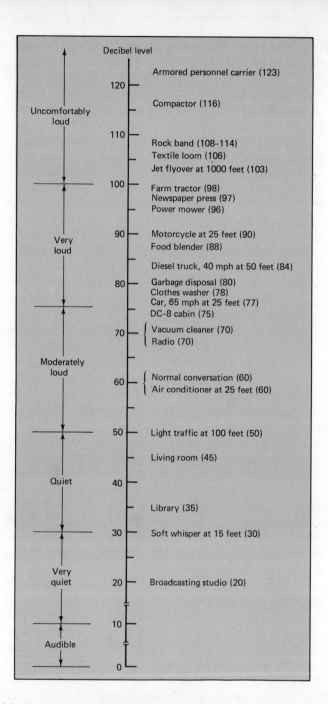

Decibel level

Armored personnel carrier (123)

120

Compactor (116)

Uncomfortably
loud

110

Rock band (108–114)
Textile loom (106)
Jet flyover at 1000 feet (103)

100

Farm tractor (98)
Newspaper press (97)
Power mower (96)

90

Motorcycle at 25 feet (90)
Food blender (88)

Very
loud

Diesel truck, 40 mph at 50 feet (84)

80

Garbage disposal (80)
Clothes washer (78)
Car, 65 mph at 25 feet (77)
DC-8 cabin (75)

70

Vacuum cleaner (70)
Radio (70)

Moderately
loud

60

Normal conversation (60)
Air conditioner at 25 feet (60)

50

Light traffic at 100 feet (50)

Living room (45)

Quiet

40

Library (35)

30

Soft whisper at 15 feet (30)

Very
quiet

20

Broadcasting studio (20)

10

Audible

0

responsible for coordination of federal activities relating to occupational noise research and regulation. The 1972 Noise Control Act that established this authority also sets noise limit standards on certain types of machinery and provides financial assistance for equipment purchases and other activities relating to industrial and community noise control programs.

Heat is another factor of the occupational environment that is physical in nature. Exposure to high temperatures in the work environment may result in a variety of clinical problems, ranging from heat rash to heat stroke. Heat rash, an irritating inflammation of the skin surface, may become severe enough to interfere with sleep and may also interfere with normal sweating responses, leading to more severe effects. High temperatures also produce dehydration and excessive loss of body salts, and these in turn may promote abnormal muscle cramping, cardiovascular upset due to reduced blood volume, and heat stroke. Unless body fluid and electrolyte balance can be reestablished quickly, permanent damage to the kidneys, liver, and central nervous system may occur; in extreme cases death may result.

Exposure to various forms of radiation—infrared, ultraviolet, and atomic—is still another physical characteristic of certain occupational environments, including welding, food sterilization with mercury-vapor lamps, and the use of X-ray machines and fluoroscopes. Radiation injury may range from superficial burns to various types of cancer due to effects upon basic cellular physiology.

Occupational hazards of chemical nature are extraordinarily diverse. Of the many thousands of chemical substances utilized in business and industry, however, only a few hundred have been studied in the detail necessary to allow formulation of meaningful exposure guidelines. Certain chemical substances, such as pesticides, are designed specifically to be toxic; the trend in this industry is toward more and more powerful poisons. However, the simple fact that industry continues to utilize increasingly novel, complex, and nondegradable chemical substances and to develop more and more sophisticated milling and processing operations that release these materials as fine dusts and vapors means a greater hazard to the unprotected worker. Farmers are exposed to herbicides, fungicides, insecticides, and fertilizers, just as construction workers are exposed to synthetic insulating, fireproofing, surface-protecting, and structural materials. These things contain chemicals that are injurious to the skin, damage the lungs, or affect other body systems. Any specific substance may have one or more of these effects. Injury may range from mild irritation to most severe bodily damage.

The first problem in occupational health—understanding the nature and severity of effects of physical and chemical agents on human health—is an extremely complex and incompletely understood relationship in itself. Beyond this, however, lie the problem areas of establishment of tolerance standards for the occupational environment, developing the technological means of maintaining conditions within tolerance limits, and enforcing the implementation of safe conditions. This has historically been an area in which industry and government have been slow to act. Furthermore, in contrast to the philosophy employed in the setting of standards for drugs and medicines, where the objective has been to employ the minimum quantity necessary, occupational exposure limits have been set to correspond to the highest levels to which it has been thought reasonable to expose the worker.

The magnitude of this health problem is suggested by an official report in 1972 that at least 390,000 new cases of disabling occupational disease were occurring in the United States each year, with perhaps as many as 100,000 deaths annually due to these diseases. Under the Occupational Safety and Health Act of 1970 the Secretary of Labor was required to develop standards of occupational exposure such that "no employee will suffer diminished health, functional capacity, or life expectancy as a result of his work experience." But progress toward this goal is left to the private industries involved! The medical and supervisory personnel are employees themselves and are frequently under strong pressure not to press for expensive programs of health or safety unless outside influences demand them.

TAKING ACTION

1. From the local department of public health obtain air pollution data for various localities within your metropolitan area (or the one nearest your area). Determine the relation of these levels to federal or state Clean Air Standards. Examine the relationship between pollution levels, regional topography, and urban-industrial centers, and identify the portion of the metropolitan area that has the most favorable air environment.
2. Examine recent Environmental Protection Agency data on municipal drinking water contaminants for your area, determine what substances are present, and investigate their potential health implications (favorable as well as unfavorable).
3. Arrange for use of a decibel meter (from the physics or engineering department of your school) to determine sound intensity levels at a rock concert or dance. Compare the results to scales showing sound intensities of various sources.
4. Visit an agricultural chemicals warehouse. Determine the commonly used chemical pesticides, and summarize data on the toxicity and the use precautions for these chemicals.
5. Obtain a copy of the ventilation and other standards that must be met by industries and chemical laboratories using toxic materials in your state. Visit the chemistry laboratories on your campus, and determine whether or not the appropriate standards are in fact met.
6. Arrange to visit a plant in which some form of occupational hazard is present. Request that the management explain and illustrate the use of protection equipment by employees.

The Psychosocial Environment

Environments differ not only in their physical and chemical nature but also in factors such as human population density, frequency of interpersonal contacts, and access to various cultural, educational, and recreational components. Thus it is pertinent to inquire about the impact of the psychosocial environment upon both the mental and physical health of the individual.

Studies of the psychosocial environment have concentrated on two

features: environmental "richness" and environmental "crowded-
ness," or the density and frequency of interindividual contact. In
studying these problems much of the experimental work has obviously
had to be done with laboratory animals. The extrapolation of the results
of these studies to humans must be done carefully and be reinforced by
detailed case history and statistical studies on human populations.

With a variety of laboratory animals, including primates, it has been
shown that individuals reared to adulthood in impoverished
environments—restricted in opportunity for contact with other individuals and simple in physical structure—tend to be more aggressive
and emotionally reactive than do individuals reared in enriched
environments. For some animals, such as laboratory rats, these behavioral observations can be correlated with biochemical and structural
differences in the central nervous system. Rats reared in enriched
environments possess higher ratios of RNA (ribonucleic acid, the
nucleic acid that "translates" stored gene information into protein
structure) to DNA (deoxyribonucleic acid, the "storer" of information
in the gene). This feature is best developed in those portions of the
brain dealing with memory. Enriched-environment rats also possess
better developed synaptic junctions, which are the contact points
between nerve cells where impulses pass from one cell to the other.
Thus for laboratory animals it appears that enrichment of early environment produces specific changes that influence adult brain function
in important ways. Of course, the human brain has major differences
from the brains of even the other primate species on which such studies
have been conducted. In addition, such other variables as sex, nutrition, and genetic makeup influence the development of the human
brain. Nevertheless, there is growing evidence that the availability of a
diversified physical and social environment may be important to full
development of the human brain.

Regarding the effects of population crowding, it has been observed
that in many ways the centers of highest urban population density are
generally centers of urban pathology as well. The highest levels of
certain diseases, both nutritional and infectious, and the greatest
incidence of what may be called "social pathologies"—mental illness,
family disintegration, crime—generally occur in urban inner-city areas.
Does crowding, in addition to ethnic, economic, and social factors,
contribute to this "inner-city syndrome"?

As for environmental "richness," many studies of the effects of
crowding have been carried out with experimental animal populations.
A number of studies of primate population under wild or seminatural
conditions, with varying population densities, have also been conducted. These studies show that differing densities are strongly correlated
with differences in behavior, physiology, and population dynamics.
With increased crowding, normal mechanisms of territoriality or
dominance relationship often become inadequate, and aggressive behavior typically increases. Normal sexual behavior becomes disturbed,
and various deviations from standard male-female interactions appear.

Maternal behavior is disturbed and pursued in abnormal fashion. Nests may be invaded by strangers or deserted by the parents and young animals deserted, attacked, or cannibalized. Under extreme densities, still other patterns of unusual behavior may appear. Individuals may group together in abnormal clusters—a sort of "pathological togetherness." Other individuals may withdraw from normal interactions and become unresponsive to stimuli.

In these crowded experimental populations physical health deteriorates as well. Fighting leads to wounds, and wounds lead to an increased incidence of infections. Major disturbance of the endocrine system, called the *general adaptation syndrome*, often appears. The increased frequency of aggressive contacts produces a constant drain on the adrenal cortex, the organ producing hormones that mediate the physiological response of the body to stress. Consequently, the pituitary modifies its activity, producing more adrenal cortex stimulating hormone (ACTH) and lesser quantities of hormones normally acting to stimulate reproductive organs. One result of this is impairment of reproductive physiology and thus reduction of birthrates. Ultimately, exhaustion of the entire stress-related system of physiology may occur, and individuals may enter chronic shock, become comatose, and eventually die.

Although these animal symptoms superficially correspond to components of the inner-city syndrome, there is a real question as to whether or not human "social pathologies" are a result of crowding, or whether crowding itself is simply another unpleasant condition caused by the same factors that produce these other social and psychological problems.

There is no doubt that the inner-city population densities are high or that "crowding," the perceived, uncomfortable feeling related to high densities, is felt by many urban residents. In any large city an individual sees and interacts with a large number of people daily, many of whom he has never seen or interacted with before. For example, it has been estimated that within a 10-minute walk of a given point in Manhattan one may encounter 220,000 persons, almost all of whom would necessarily be strangers even to someone who had worked in the area all his life.

To determine the influence of crowding itself is difficult. Recently a group of sociologists from Vanderbilt University attempted to do this, using data from the Chicago metropolitan area. Chicago was chosen because of the availability of various types of data on population density, housing characteristics, and social pathologies for 75 community areas varying widely in all characteristics. The social pathologies chosen for examination in relation to crowding were five: (1) fertility, expressed as the birthrate for women between 15 and 44 years of age; (2) ineffective parental care, measured as the number of public assistance recipients under 18 years of age; (3) aggressive behavior, considered to correspond to the juvenile delinquency rate; (4) mental disease, expressed as the rate of admission to mental hospitals; and (5) the

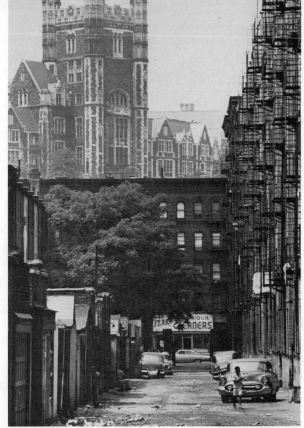

James Mitchell/Magnum Photos

mortality rate. Actually, for the studies undertaken, one of the 75 community areas, the downtown "Loop" region, was excluded. This was done because the levels of social pathology are much higher than elsewhere, and because these may reflect factors that attract people already having problems to this particular area. For example, the rate of admissions of residents of this area to mental hospitals equals 3757 per 100,000 population per year, a value about 5 times that of the next highest area and over 10 times the average for the city as a whole.

The objective of the statistical analysis of the data was to determine whether or not indices of population density were significantly related to social pathologies when ethnic and economic factors were in essence canceled out. Population density was considered in terms of several components. The total population per acre was divided into four categories: number of persons per room, number of rooms per housing unit, number of housing units per building, and number of buildings per acre. This was done because of the obvious fact that a high population density in a rich area of high-rise, luxury apartments means something different in terms of crowding than it does in a two-story tenement neighborhood with the same density per acre.

The statistical analyses revealed that density, in terms of these four components, showed significant correlation with all social pathologies. These latter factors, not surprisingly, accounted for a greater fraction of the variability in social pathologies than did population density, but an apparent influence of density itself was present.

Further analysis suggested that density was what might be termed an "intervening" factor. In other words, density is itself a product other socioeconomic factors, but it then exerts a causal effect of its own on social pathologies. It is "intervening" in nature because it acts to convert these socioeconomic influences into human behavioral and physiological terms.

We should recognize that studies of this sort are preliminary in nature and that repeated, detailed studies that are even more sophisticated are needed to accurately determine the influence of crowding on human health and well-being. We should also recognize that humans show a remarkably great ability to adapt to crowded environments, as evidenced by conditions in many cities of Asia. But we must also recognize that crowding, as perceived by the individuals in a given situation, may be an environmental factor significantly related to human health.

TAKING ACTION

1. *Discuss in a small group your observations of human behavior with respect to population density. What would seem to be an optimal density? Under what conditions? Have you seen people adapt well to light and heavy densities?*
2. *Design and conduct a population cage experiment in which factors such as birthrates, aggressiveness, survival to weaning, abnormal behavior, and mortality rates can be followed for one or more rodent populations as they increase in density.*
3. *Obtain statistics on various social pathologies for different portions of your metropolitan area or for various cities of different size near your area. Identify the variables, including density, that may be related to these pathologies.*

The Epidemiological Environment

Like many of the problems of human health that we have already discussed, the pattern of infectious and nutritional disease is a complex and historically changing one. The historically changing aspect of disease occurrence is the result not only of man's deliberate attempts toward control but of his unconscious modifications of the environment in which disease occurs—and also, in certain cases, of evolutionary change in human resistance and disease virulence.

Infectious disease may be viewed as a stage in the evolution of a symbiotic relationship between the human body and a second organism. The biological "goal" of each participant in this interaction is that of maximizing the genetic contribution of itself to future generations of its own species. To do this it must maximize its efficiency of utilizing the immediate environment, producing through this efficiency a maximum number of successful offspring. If it destroys its environment, it destroys itself, and the goal of maximizing its contribution to future generations is not realized. A highly virulent disease organism that rapidly kills its host is thus poorly adjusted to a symbiotic relationship. When the host dies, the disease organism is less likely to be perpetuated than might have been the case had the host lived longer.

A typical symbiotic relationship is illustrated by the colon bacterium *Escherichia coli*. This is a normal, nonpathogenic inhabitant of the human digestive tract—most of the time. This organism has certain valuable functions: it discourages the establishment of certain other bacterial species and produces quantities of vitamins K and B_{12} that are absorbed and used by its host. In turn it is provided an optimal environment and (normally) abundant food. Thus, under most conditions, it is a genuine symbiont. However, certain strains of *E. coli* may produce intestinal disease, especially in infants, and occasionally it produces infections of the urinary or genital tracts. Thus it is not totally without pathogenic capability. There are a number of other viruses, bacteria, and even parasites that are common in humans but produce effects of mild or insignificant nature. The pinworm is an example of a parasitic worm that is little more than a nuisance to humans.

Many of the organisms that fall in this category appear to be highly specialized for humans and generally do not occur in other vertebrates, even our close primate relatives. Thus many of our most virulent disease agents appear to be organisms that have only recently become associated with people and have yet to evolve a more nearly symbiotic status. Many of these virulent pathogens and parasites appear at the same time to be relatively harmless inhabitants of other vertebrates. More than 150 recognized diseases of humans are caused by organisms that possess "reservoir" populations in other vertebrates. The protozoan parasites causing yellow fever and African sleeping sickness in humans, along with the bacterium that causes plague but exists as a mild or harmless inhabitant of a number of species of rodents, are good examples.

Thus we may expect to find that part of the cause of many of our most serious diseases is the disturbance of environmental relationships under which various disease agents have attained a relatively stable, nonepidemic relationship with humans. Included in this disturbance is the acquisition of new disease agents by their transmission from other animals.

Studies of the incidence of various diseases among still-surviving groups of primitive peoples, such as the scattered Indian tribes of the Amazon Basin, support this generalization. Most of the major infectious diseases so prominent in recorded human history—smallpox, measles, cholera, tuberculosis, and many others—are apparently not sustained in these isolated, low-density populations. Should a disease of this type appear, it spreads rapidly through an individual population, often causing heavy mortality. Survivors gain resistance and the disease agent dies out. Apparently the only infectious diseases occurring in these tribes under primitive conditions were those that produced relatively mild effects, persisted in individuals for long periods, and were capable of periodically becoming reactivated in the population.

With the development of civilization and the growth of urbanized society, conditions favorable to the occurrence and spread of major epidemic diseases appeared. Smallpox may have appeared as an important human disease only in the first century A.D., measles in the sixth century, and cholera in the sixteenth. Syphilis spread through Europe in an epidemic wave in the late fifteenth and sixteenth centuries, its origin still uncertain. (The idea of its introduction by Columbus' sailors is a medical folk tale.) The appearance of such diseases in populations previously unexposed to them and lacking resistance due to previous exposure or genetic selection resulted in great mortality. The inadequacies of public health services in early civilized societies allowed many of these diseases to attack in infancy. Poliomyelitis, known originally as infantile paralysis, appeared as a disease of infants, apparently in the eighteenth or nineteenth century, and rose to prominence in the latter parts of the nineteenth century.

This brief historical account serves simply to demonstrate that disease has very strong environmental relationships and that human activities profoundly and continually modify these relations. We can also see that the disease relationship is a constantly evolving one, so each of our activities in public health, preventive medicine, and disease treatment represents a new selective force upon organisms admirably adapted to rapid evolutionary responses.

The environmental and evolutionary context that people create for infectious disease in the modern world is unique. It is characterized by greater human population densities than ever before and a greater interchange of materials, people, and therefore diseases between distant locations than ever before. In addition, it is characterized by the application of massive programs of prevention and control by means of powerful chemical agents including vaccines, antibiotics, and pesticides.

In this environment certain diseases, such as viral influenza, appear to be highly successful. Many of the new, minor strains of influenza apparently arise as a result of mutations of RNA structure which make the previously existing antibodies less effective and the virus strain more infectious. Occasionally, however, a radically different influenza virus capable of producing a serious pandemic arises. In 1917–18 an influenza pandemic killed perhaps 20 million persons throughout the world and led to the death of about 500,000 from influenza and secondary complications in the United States. In 1968–69 more than 51 million cases occurred in the United States, with between 20,000 and 80,000 deaths recorded. The strains responsible for these pandemics apparently possess protein antigens of strikingly different nature. It is probable that they originate by genetic reorganization of the RNA material in the tissues of certain domestic animals infected by several distinct viral strains. There appear to be, for example, two distinctive influenza strains in horses, two in swine, and several in poultry. Occasionally these strains pass to humans, and human strains pass to these animals. In their tissues, therefore, contact between different RNA molecules and occasional reorganization of RNA structure may occur. The passage of a distinctive new form back to humans may then initiate an influenza pandemic. The probability of such an event occurring is obviously greatest where man and domestic animals live in close physical association, as is the case in many parts of southeastern Asia, where some of these strains have apparently arisen.

Thus we can see several ways in which environmental conditions influence viral influenza. Other viral diseases, including forms of hepatitis, encephalitis, venerial herpes, and dengue and yellow fevers, may be capable of the same evolutionary response.

The increased interchange of people and materials throughout the world has also meant the introduction of disease agents and vectors to new areas. Rocky Mountain spotted fever, caused by a viruslike microorganism transmitted from host to host by a tick, was originally localized in parts of the western United States. Now, however, it has been introduced into the southern Appalachian region, where it has found a suitable vector in the form of a different species of tick, previously not a disease carrier. The same has occurred for malaria, yellow fever, and several other mosquito-borne diseases, since related members of the major genera of mosquito vectors are nearly worldwide in distribution.

Wide World Photos

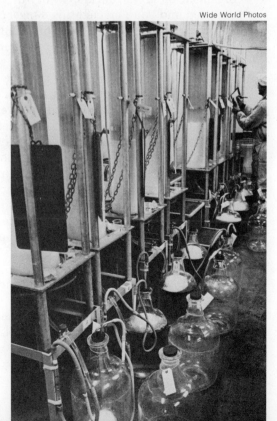

Glass vats used to filter swine-type flu virus cultures in beds of salt.

329

In addition, people have created distinctive conditions for the transmission of diseases by animal vectors in large urban areas. Free-roaming populations of dogs have become a serious problem in many cities. Over 40 infectious and parasitic diseases are transmittable to man by such animals, including rabies and several roundworm and tapeworm parasites. Urban rat populations also pose a serious disease threat, particularly since these rats are now acquiring a degree of genetic resistance to certain of the major rodenticides used against them. Should a high level of such resistance be developed, the threat from urban rats would become a very serious one.

Although we like to think that we are on the verge of eliminating many of the serious diseases of mankind, the rapid evolutionary response of many disease agents and their vectors, together with the extraordinary vulnerability of human populations due to their density and contact, mean that infectious disease will be with man for a long time to come. The fact that these new diseases must be dealt with by massive, expensive crash programs in increasing frequency has ominous implications. Consider the following policy questions, raised recently by William Reeves in his retiring address as president of the American Society of Tropical Medicine and Hygiene:

1. When an epidemic requires massive use of a yet unapproved and unlicensed chemical on a crash basis, how will the decision about this be made?
2. When an epidemic resulting from evolved resistance of a disease organism or vector occurs, who will be blamed for not having detected and counteracted this danger?
3. When the supply of a control agent against a pandemic is inadequate, who will be responsible for the allocation that is made?
4. As costs of developing more and more sophisticated controls against new pandemic agents rise, who will assume financial responsibility for their continuing development?
5. What will occur when aid in counteracting a serious epidemic is requested by nations whose economies, politics, or social attitudes clash radically with those of nations in a position to assist?
6. Who will be held responsible when cutbacks in research and control programs related to infectious disease result in our inability to prevent or control a major pandemic?
7. How long can society afford to pay the costs of massive prevention and control efforts, regardless of the ability of the individuals affected to pay the costs of such efforts?

Under these circumstances, and given the increasing financial difficulties of governments throughout the world, it seems inescapable that increasing responsibility will fall to the individual to be informed about disease threats to his own person and to protect himself against these threats.

Nutritional diseases, as well as infectious diseases, possess important relationships to the environment. Goiter and rickets are two environmentally related nutritional deficiency diseases that modern man has come largely to understand and control. Goiter is an iodine deficiency disease that results in inadequate production of thyroid hormone and the consequent sometimes drastic swelling of that gland in the neck. Although in developed countries such as the United States goiter is uncommon, on a worldwide basis 200 million or more people suffer from the disease.

Goiter is strongly localized geographically. Close to the seacoasts of the world it is rare, since iodine is relatively abundant in seawater and thus in seafoods. Soils of coastal areas are generally high in iodine, since it tends to be carried inland and deposited in precipitation. However, in many mountainous areas, such as the Alps, Himalayas, Pyrenees, and Andes, soils are highly deficient in iodine. Other inland regions tend also to be deficient. In the United States a "goiter belt" extends from the upper Great Plains eastward and southward across the Great Lakes region and the upper Appalachian area. (Incidentally, where iodine is somewhat low to begin with, soybeans and some cabbage-type vegetables may trigger goiter.) Today, of course, goiter has been eliminated in most areas by the addition of small amounts of iodine to salt and other basic food constituents.

Rickets, a bone disease involving inadequate calcium deposition in growing bones, is related to a deficiency of vitamin D, a steroid compound known as *calciferol*. Calciferol is not actually a vitamin but a hormone. Its action is one of regulating mineral metabolism by the body, in this case, that of calcium.

Calciferol may be acquired by the body in various ways, but in man it is unique among hormones in not being synthesized biochemically within living cells. A precursor substance (7-dehydrocholesterol) is, however, produced in the outer layers of the skin. Under the action of ultraviolet radiation, it becomes converted into calciferol, which is then absorbed into the bloodstream and carried to the appropriate action site. This "sunlight synthesis" serves as an adequate source of calciferol for many people.

In certain parts of the world such as northern Europe, this mechanism of calciferol production becomes inadequate during the winter months when days are short and the sun stays low in the sky. Dietary supplement is therefore necessary. Some foods such as cod-liver oil are rich in calciferol, a fact that gave rise to a common after-meal practice much hated by children of past generations.

Rickets was one of the first diseases to become magnified by man's creation of urban air pollution. The introduction of coal for heating purposes and industrial use in England in the 1600s brought with it the first form of urban air pollution. In the late 1800s, when medical attention became focused on rickets, the incidence of the disease proved to be greatest in urban-industrial parts of the country. The densely packed tenements lining dark, narrow streets and the smoky pall due to widespread coal burning reduced the rate of "sunlight synthesis" of calciferol below critical levels in some areas.

Nowadays calciferol deficiency is remedied by addition of a very similar compound, ergocalciferol, to certain foods, particularly milk. Ergocalciferol is derived from ergosterol, a plant steroid, by artificial irradiation with ultraviolet light and identified as vitamin D_2 in the materials to which it is added.

In the developed parts of the world many of these specific nutrient deficiencies can be dealt with by means of food additives. For the underdeveloped world, however, this is oftentimes impossible. Further, deficiency problems in many of these areas may involve not only specific items such as iodine but major dietary components such as protein or even caloric intake as a whole. Protein deficiency malnutrition, known also by the African name of *kwashiorkor*, is one of the most prevalent problems in the world of today. It is particularly serious in the case of growing children. Without adequate protein growth is retarded, various skin and intestinal disorders appear, and fatty materials are deposited in excess quantity in the liver, tending to produce a "swollen" abdomen. Serious retardation of mental development also occurs, an effect that does not seem to be mitigated by improved nutrition later in childhood.

On a world-wide basis, kwashiorkor is perhaps the most widespread nutritional disease. It has been estimated that more than two-thirds of the 800 million children existing in the developing countries will suffer disease or disability caused or brought on by protein-deficiency malnutrition. In the United States the problem is less severe, but it is still of significant proportions. Studies by the U.S. Public Health Service in 1969 showed that between 10 and 15 million Americans had

Child suffering from kwashiorkor.

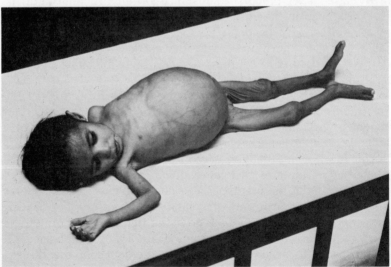

Fujihira/Monkmeyer

inadequate food supplies. These studies also revealed an appreciable incidence of kwashiorkor, goiter, and rickets among low-income populations in several parts of the country.

Unfortunately, the incidence of protein-deficiency malnutrition is favored in many areas by international patterns of trade in food products. In parts of the humid tropics major cash crop farming systems evolved during colonial periods. These systems, involving bananas, cacao, coffee, and other export crops, occupy the most fertile land areas and tie up much of the native population in seasonal labor activity. Consequently these people are unable to pursue patterns of well-balanced farming on good land. Many of them are forced to cultivate starchy foods on marginal land, thus favoring the incidence of nutritional problems such as kwashiorkor.

Serious problems have arisen in several areas as a consequence of programs of distribution of powdered milk. Certain human populations are physiologically intolerant of lactose, a sugar abundant in both cow's milk and human milk. This characteristic is apparently at least partly genetic, with intolerant individuals losing at an early age the ability to produce the enzyme required to split this double sugar into simple sugars that can be absorbed by the intestines. For such individuals lactose in food materials can produce severe intestinal disturbance. Intolerant individuals can gradually become conditioned to tolerate a certain amount of lactose in the diet. Black Americans come principally from agriculturalist African groups and possess about 70 percent intolerance of lactose. Generally, due to acquired tolerance, it causes few problems. However, it represents a situation of nutritional inefficiency in metabolic use of a particular carbohydrate that is one of the major foods promoted for general use in our society.

Many other examples could be given to illustrate health-related examples of the interplay of humans and our nutritional environment. For a final dramatic one, one of the dangers of the intensive promotion of "miracle" grain varieties is that these may replace acreage used for protein-containing plant foods (for example, beans and lentils) to the detriment of overall nutrition.

TAKING ACTION

1. Identify the infectious and parasitic diseases that exist in your area and for which reservoirs exist in other domestic or wild animal populations. What control or counteractive practices are used against these diseases? What is your particular vulnerability to them due to your residential area, job, or recreational preference?
2. List the infectious, nutritional, or hereditary diseases that have occurred in members of your family. How have these changed from the time of your grandparents and parents to the present? Discuss.
3. Discuss the evolutionary implications of the use of pesticides and antibiotics against various disease agents and vectors.

The intimate involvement of many features of the environment with important aspects of human health makes it essential for us, as informed citizens, to participate actively in programs for the improvement of this environment. This responsibility exists both at the local level, where the immediate self-interest of the individual lies, and at national and global levels, where our management of the environment ultimately relates to our survival as a species.

The Health of the Local Environment

The economies of the United States and Canada have grown up in a frontier atmosphere—a context in which vast, untapped resources await development and exploitation. We still think in these terms; every day we hear of "new frontiers" to be conquered in such areas as arctic Alaska and Canada, the continental shelves, and even the seabed itself. The economy that is geared to develop these new frontiers and exploit their resources is what Kenneth Boulding, a noted resource economist, has termed a "cowboy economy." It is an economy geared to getting the job done fast, obtaining the maximum return for a unit of investment, and cutting corners in the interest of expediency.

Most of our problems of environmental health, particularly those related to physical and chemical pollution of our living and working environments, result from the expediencies of "corner cutting." As long as populations were sparse, cities small, and industrial use of raw materials in its early stages of growth, use of the air and water environments as free dumping grounds for waste materials resulted in little detrimental feedback on human health. To some extent, as the growth of human populations and industry occurred, it was expedient for all concerned to ignore the developing problems of environmental health. The improved standards of living of workers, due to their growing incomes, offset to a degree the impacts of deteriorating environmental conditions upon their health.

In spite of the "unconquered frontiers" that we may hear about, largely in advertisements, our world can no longer afford to continue operating under the conditions of a frontier economy. Gains in material living standard resulting from production and consumption activities that create waste discharges are being offset more and more by the detrimental effects of pollutant wastes on human health. Clearly, we must speed the conversion from our present "cowboy economy" to a "spaceship economy," in which our population growth is regulated, our use of resources made more efficient, and our level of environmental health given much greater consideration.

How can we work toward this end at the local level? The strategy of environmental improvement is one of counting all of the costs, considering the whole system, and emphasizing efficiency. Many of the costs associated with the products and services we use are at present not included in the price of these items. They are in some cases paid by society at large or in other cases deferred until some future time. By permitting high exhaust pollutant levels from vehicles for many years, we allowed the costs of pollution to be paid by all those exposed to the resulting smog conditions rather than by the purchasers of automobiles. In effect, society was subsidizing the motorcar at the expense of its health. Similarly with regard to dumping industrial wastes into our waters. Our objective must thus be to identify these costs, internalize them so that they are paid by those who create them, and, of course pay for them in ways that prevent health damage from occurring. To do this we must consider the entire human ecosystem and not simply the small part that may seem at first glance to be involved.

Most forms of environmental pollution result, in one way or another, from the high rate of materials and energy use in our society, which are a function in turn of both affluence and large numbers of people. There are several basic ways that we may intervene into processes related to use of materials and energy to increase efficiency and improve environmental health conditions. These can be grouped into the following seven basic categories.

1. *Improving environmental waste inactivation capacity.* Natural and seminatural environments carry out a great deal of useful work in waste disposal. Ecological "engineering" may be applied to make these functions more effective, however. Tree plantings may serve as natural sound insulators in areas where noise reduction is desirable. Sewage treatment ponds, in which artificial aeration may be supplied to speed organic decomposition and to which other treatments may be applied to inactive particular toxins, may be designed. Techniques by which waste materials may be dispersed in other environments may be devised, such as the spraying of treated sewage water into designated areas of forest land.

2. *Exporting harmful wastes to points outside the biosphere.* For certain permanently toxic or highly dangerous materials such as radioactive wastes, systems of exportation to points from which reentry into active biospheric circulation is impossible may be devised. Storage in deep salt mines or injection into deep geological strata are examples of this approach.

3. *Reduction of harmful component per unit waste discharged.* Treatment of wastes prior to discharge may effect a reduction of amounts of the more serious components present. Emission control devices are examples of this approach, serving to reduce the quantities of incompletely burned hydrocarbons in automobile exhaust. Techniques that reduce the harmful action of a substance, following its release, by manipulating the time or location of discharges may also be considered to fall into this category. Controls over the time of rush-hour traffic in areas subject to photochemical smog may allow peak emissions to occur when there is less sunlight to produce dangerous chemicals.

4. *Reclamation of harmful materials from wastes.* This approach—in essence, recycling—leads to a reduction of usable materials in bulk wastes. Sulfur, lead, mercury, and other substances representing health

335

hazards constitute valuable raw materials upon their recovery. The "mining" of solid wastes for various metals has likewise been shown to be profitable. Recycling of organic wastes as fertilizers is still another obvious possibility.

5. *Improving the efficiency of production processes.* Changes in extraction and refinement of raw materials and in the processes of their manufacture into final products may be made so that the quantity of toxic waste generated per product is reduced. Obviously, internalization of costs related to current patterns of waste disposal will act as a strong force toward this end. One practical way to achieve this is through residual charges: a tax levied upon an operation in proportion to the quantity of toxic waste discharged. A related method is to tax the operation on the basis both of the quantity of toxic waste discharged and the size of the human population exposed to it.

6. *Changes in product specifications.* Design of manufactured items and particularly of their associated packaging may be modified so that a smaller quantity of harmful wastes are associated with their production, use, and disposal. For example, smaller cars and modifications of automobile engines to use lead-free gasoline and produce fewer nitrogen oxides because of a lower compression ratio would fall into this category.

7. *Reduction in consumption rates.* Increased product lifetime is one obvious way to reduce wastes generated per unit time. Greater emphasis upon repair, as opposed to replacement, is another. Changed societal emphasis from product consumption to increased spending for personal services constitutes another manner of reducing the patterns of materials and energy consumption that leads to pollution.

At the local level, various opportunities exist for individual action favoring reduction of forms of physical and chemical pollution. The individual must examine the patterns of materials and energy use that he or she is involved in, determine changes that may improve the health environment, and select an appropriate course of action. An initial response, of course, is personal example. Lewis Moncrief of Michigan State University has characterized one of the dominant features of the modern American lifestyle as being the absence of personal moral direction in environmental matters.

A second opportunity for action is through voting. Increasingly matters of environmental quality and community planning are gaining representation on ballots. Active participation in election activities and support of politicians sympathetic to environmental matters is essential to the democratic resolution of many problems.

Finally, active membership in environmental action groups can constitute a powerful force for environmental improvement. Responsible groups of this nature have demonstrated their ability to exert strong action through education, the news media, and the courts. The seriousness of human health challenges relating to environmental pollution give such action groups a strong legal basis from which to operate.

1. *Compile a list of environmental planning and action groups active in your area. Contact each of these groups and inquire about their current activities on problems relating to environmental health. Consider joining such a group.*
2. *Select several major sources of environmental pollutants with significant health impacts. Discuss changes representative of the foregoing seven basic types that could be implemented to reduce the impact of these pollutants.*
3. *Obtain a list of pending legislation at the local, state, or national level that relates to environmental health. Compile the views of your class on these items, and prepare a summary letter to be sent to the appropriate officials.*
4. *Keep a candid list of your normal activities involving consumptive use of energy and products. Estimate the portion of this activity that could be dispensed with or done in alternative fashion so that you might still enjoy the same material comfort or pleasure with a lesser amount of waste production.*

The Health of the Global Environment

At the global level environmental health is related to the capability of major environmental systems to provide renewable resources, including calories, protein, and other nutrients, and to absorb waste outputs. The capabilities of such systems are limited, and we may thus speak of the carrying capacity of the global environment for human populations. An idea of the determinants of this carrying capacity may be gained by examining the energy levels at which various natural and human-dominated systems operate.

Eugene Odum, director of the Institute of Ecology at the University of Georgia, has suggested that world ecosystems fall into four major classes, based on the energy level at which they operate. These are as follows:

1. *Natural, unsubsidized sun-powered ecosystems.* These systems, examples of which are upland forests, grasslands, and the open ocean, operate at an energy level basically determined by the level of solar radiation incident upon them. They cover by far the greatest fraction of the earth's surface and possess an annual level of energy conversion of the order of magnitude of 2000 kilocalories per square meter.

2. *Natural, subsidized sun-powered ecosystems.* Systems of this sort such as estuaries, deltas and floodplains, and ocean upwelling regions possess not only the regular inputs of solar energy but also subsidies provided by tidal action, stream flow, or ocean currents. These flows, which require energy, concentrate food materials, fertilize and irrigate land areas or bring nutrient-rich water to the ocean surface in localized areas. Due to these subsidies, natural rates of energy conversion reach the order of magnitude of 20,000 kilocalories per square meter per year, or about 10 times those of unsubsidized systems.

3. *Human-subsidized sun-powered ecosystems.* These agricultural systems highly manipulated by humans receive natural solar inputs

and a variety of other inputs, including fertilizers, pesticides, and mechanical cultivation, all of which require energy. These subsidies permit a higher rate of energy conversion but one that is roughly of the same order of magnitude as that of naturally subsidized systems, 20,000 kilocalories per square meter annually.

4. *Fuel-powered urban-industrial ecosystems.* Systems of this sort are highly subsidized energy-importing ecosystems. They are dependent upon energy and materials supplied from other systems and particularly upon accumulated geological supplies of energy in the form of fossil fuels and other materials. Their average level of energy conversion is about two orders of magnitude greater than other subsidized systems, or about 2 million kilocalories per square meter per year.

All of these systems are essential to the human ecosystem. The vast, unsubsidized ecosystems of the earth's surface provide limited yields of certain useful materials such as lumber and beef, but they are even more essential as "life support" systems that accept and counterbalance many of society's waste discharge activities. It is these systems that act as sinks for materials such as carbon monoxide, sulfur dioxide, photochemical-pollutants, heavy metals, persistent pesticide chemicals, and many other substances with particular health hazards. The extent of the useful work that these systems carry out is often not appreciated until their capacity is exceeded and man has to supplement their capacity by expensive technological approaches.

Subsidized systems, both with subsidies of natural and human origin, are the systems that humans depend on for food and other renewable resources; these are absolutely essential to our existence. Systems with natural subsidies are limited in extent, and since their subsidies are "free," it is clear that we should both protect and take maximum advantage of those that exist. As the human population grows, however, the areas and capacities of human-subsidized systems must increase. Each unit expansion of such systems is inevitably harder to accomplish. The easily subsidized environments—prime agricultural lands—are already in use. The costs of subsidizing new agricultural lands will be greater. For considerations of human health we should note that the quality of the foods produced on the marginal lands into which agricultural activity must push will become harder and more expensive to maintain. Thus environmentally related nutritional problems may be expected to become more prevalent in the future.

Fuel-powered ecosystems are the centers of.cultural productivity, where raw materials are converted into useful products and where human intellectual activity has become concentrated. The intensity of the energy use by these urban-industrial systems, compared to those of other systems, explains a great deal of their impact. Charles F. Cooper of San Diego State University has characterized this relationship as "the concentration of dispersed energy." In other words, energy stored over long periods of geological time and over broad regions of the earth's surface is increasingly being drawn to urban-industrial centers, where it is consumed. This consumption is the major cause of patterns of chemical and physical pollution of the environment. Fuel-powered systems are the systems of pollution production.

The dominant trends for the human population of the world are rapid growth and accelerating urbanization. Population growth, for the world as a whole, now equals about 2 percent per year, corresponding to the addition of nearly 80 million people each year. The percentage of this population living in cities is increasing, meaning that the growth of urban populations is occurring at a rate greater than 2 percent. Projections of current trends suggest that by 2000 or 2010 A.D. areas such as the New York City–northern New Jersey megalopolis may reach 30 million in size. At the same time cities of 36 to 66 million population may appear in India. Should the trends involved continue, it is clear that the special health problems associated with crowded urban life will intensify greatly. Zero population growth is clearly an urgent need; there is now evidence that significant progress is being made in this direction.

World economic and industrial growth is also growing. The average rate, as suggested by the rate of energy consumption, appears to approximate 5 percent per year. This rate of growth corresponds to a doubling of the processes involved each 14 years, and it is these processes that are responsible for many of the forms of environmental pollution having serious health implications.

It is agreed by all that unlimited growth in a limited environment is impossible. For the global human environment, however, estimation of the safe carrying capacity is difficult. Attempts to apply techniques of mathematical modeling of demographic, economic, and ecological processes at a global scale have recently been made by a group known as the Club of Rome. The most recent efforts of this group have involved developing a world model that includes submodels for 10 world regions and gives predictions of future trends in variables such as population, nonrenewable resource supply, food per capita, pollution, and industrial output per capita. These models are subject to a variety of criticisms, but they do demonstrate that, barring sophisticated responses of human society, the carrying capacity of the world ecosystem will soon be exceeded.

Of the various requisites for global equilibrium, perhaps the most important is stabilization of the human population, a stabilization that can only occur by reduction in birthrates or increase in death rates. For the first time there is now some evidence that significant progress is being made by world birth control efforts. Barring genuine stabilization due to voluntary and induced reduction of birthrates, the solution to continuing growth in a finite environment must be a death-rate solution. Death-rate solutions to temporary imbalances have occurred in the past; their mechanisms are war, pestilence, and famine.

TAKING ACTION

1. *Compile a list of incentives that might be employed to encourage couples to have smaller families without eliminating freedom of choice or imposing severe penalties upon the children who are born.*
2. *Discuss the manner in which economic changes could or should be initiated to convert from a product-oriented economy to a more service-oriented economy without creating massive unemployment problems.*
3. *Identify the problems of health and disease that are likely to increase in magnitude with further population and economic growth in the less-developed countries of the world. What dangers do these pose for the inhabitants of the developed countries, and how can these dangers be combatted?*
4. *Organize a discussion of a Club of Rome project with special reference to more recent predictions of things to come.*

DISCUSSION Environmental relationships are one of the major determinants of the state of human health and disease. The environment of primitive human beings exposed them to certain patterns of ill health but protected them from others. With their emergence as agriculturalists, humans assumed an even greater capacity for modifying their environment and achieved greater population densities. In this changed environment they became subject to new diseases and problems of health. With the growth of cities and the advent of industrial societies, a still different health environment has emerged. This environment is characterized by a variety of forms of physical and chemical pollution of both the living and working situations. It includes factors that reach people through the air, through the water, and even in our food. It also includes relationships of a psychosocial nature—factors that impinge upon our senses and produce strain or physiological stress. The complex of infectious diseases and parasites to which we are exposed and are most vulnerable is also related to the particular conditions of our environment. Even our basic nutrition may be affected by external, environmental relationships.

People have recognized and attacked certain important problems of environmental health, particularly those dealing with transmission of infectious disease and with certain dietary deficiencies. Other aspects of environmental health have been largely ignored, however. Many health problems associated with environmental pollution, for example, reflect basic tendencies inherent in the urban-industrial systems that form a dominant force in modern developed societies. These systems act, first, to externalize many of the cost factors associated with production and commerce, creating as a result various forms of physical and chemical pollution. Second, within the occupational environment they tend to regard the worker as an inanimate component of the production process. The conditions of the working environment are controlled on the basis of maximum levels of physical and chemical factors that can be tolerated rather than on the basis of levels optimal for worker health. Pollution conditions long common in the working place are only now reaching the public at large.

The costs associated with diseases caused by pollution in the community and occupational environments are much greater than generally recognized. However, strong vested interests within business, industry, and government often act to weaken and slow efforts to deal with these problems.

The organization of modern urban-industrial society is also reflected in patterns of psychosocial disease and in dietary and infectious diseases. Crowding and intense interpersonal contact in urban societies is being recognized more and more as a factor in the production of the inner-city syndrome. Nutritional diseases, such as protein deficiency, still occur in developed countries and are promoted in many underdeveloped areas by patterns of international food product commerce. Among infectious diseases a number of rapidly evolving, highly contagious viral diseases appear to have been favored by the environment of modern society. Elsewhere the incidence of various parasitic diseases has been augmented by inadequately planned developmental projects intended to bring about rapid modernization and increase in agricultural production.

The educated citizen has a responsibility to work for improvements in environmental health conditions at local, national, and global levels. Local action requires, first, the establishment of a personal, moral commitment in environmental action—a commitment evident through personal example and child-rearing practices. In addition, it requires active participation in the political process and in the activities of citizen planning and environmental action groups.

At the global level we all need to recognize the impossibility of continued population and economic growth with their associated destruction of the environment in a finite system. The intrinsic value to human beings of both the developed and undeveloped portions of the life-supporting earth cover must be recognized. Consumption of natural resources needs to correspond to what spaceship earth can support. Stabilization of the world population is an essential aspect of this adjustment. This stabilization must occur through reduction and regulation of birthrates. Alternatively, an adjustment by increased death rates will be forced upon man in the form of war, pestilence, and famine.

FOR FURTHER READING

Cox, George W., 1974. *Readings in Conservation Ecology.* 2d ed. New York: Appleton.

An anthology of 40 articles by environmental scientists, dealing with the origin, nature, and solution of problems of environmental quality and environmental health.

our health and
society

Farvar, M. T., and Milton, J. P., 1972. *The Careless Technology: Ecology and International Development.* Garden City, N.Y.: Natural History Press.

Fifty original papers dealing with unforeseen environmental problems resulting from hastily conceived international development projects.

Levine, Norman D., 1975. *Human Ecology.* Belmont, N.C.: Duxbury Press.

A wide-ranging text examining the environment, physical and cultural evolution, and future of humans from an ecological perspective.

Mesarovic, M., and Pestel, E., 1974. *Mankind at the Turning Point.* New York: Dutton.

The second report of the Club of Rome, analyzing, by computer methodology, the future of man in relation to economic and environmental interrelationships.

Miller, G. T., Jr., 1975. *Living in the Environment: Concepts, Problems, and Alternatives.* Belmont, Calif.: Wadsworth.

A comprehensive, detailed, and thought-provoking examination of all aspects of humans' environmental relationships.

National Institute for Occupational Safety and Health, 1973. *The Industrial Environment—Its Evaluation and Control.* Washington, D.C.: U.S. Government Printing Office.

A series of 50 short chapters by specialists on all aspects of the industrial environment.

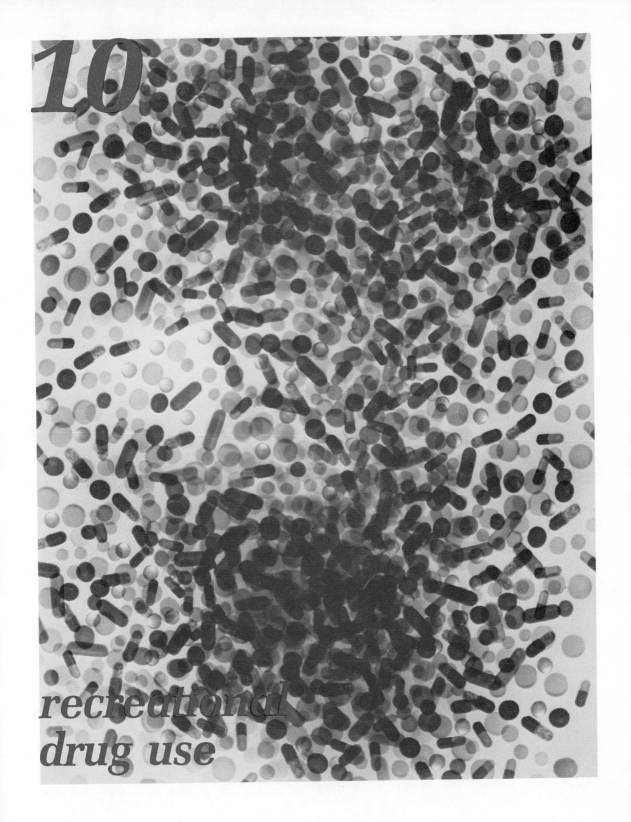

10

*recreational
drug use*

OVERVIEW

*There are many ways of classifying drugs and the ways they are
used, none of which is satisfactory for all purposes. Here we deal
with drugs that are used recreationally. We emphasize the
importance of pleasure to health and indeed survival. We then
describe the possible role of drugs in helping to provide pleasure
in life, and we identify a number of substances that often find
recreational use. However, due to such factors as the potential for
producing dependence or minimal "recreational payoff," most
drugs have such a precarious niche in the recreational drug
category that they are dismissed after brief consideration.
Others—namely, beverage alcohol, cannabis (grass, pot) and
nitrous oxide—evidently qualify as "recreational" drugs to a great
many people. Finally, the reader is challenged to try to clarify her
or his values with respect to possible relationships with
recreational drugs.*

INQUIRY

1. What is a drug? What is recreational drug use?
2. Is it possible for recreational drug use to be incorporated into a
   healthy lifestyle? If so, how?
3. What are the chances of effective prohibition of drugs with
   recreational potential?
4. How might people be harmed by alcoholic drinks if they don't get
   drunk?
5. Is the use of cannabis to obtain pleasure worthy of less respect than
   the use of opera performances, TV shows, or sports as a means of
   obtaining pleasure?
6. What drugs should be prohibited?

INTRODUCTION In its broadest sense the word "drug" has been used to refer to any
chemical that alters the structure or function of an organism. Because
this is such a broad definition, which includes plant and animal toxins,
air and water pollutants, pesticides, and even nutrients, many categories and subcategories of drugs have been established. No single way of
organizing drugs is adequate for all purposes. One person will find
"stimulants, depressants, and hallucinogens" an adequate troika (or
threesome) of subcategories for the broader category of "psychoactive
drugs." But another may argue, "But LSD doesn't produce true hallucinations, and alcohol sometimes does, so you can't properly consider
LSD an hallucinogen and alcohol a depressant. You need a different set
of categories." But which?

For purposes of this chapter, there's no need to resolve this particular dilemma. Rather than grapple with how to categorize *drugs*, let's
consider *drug usage*. To simplify things still further let's define only
the category of drug usage directly pertinent to this chapter—

recreational drug use. By "recreational drug use" we mean *the discretionary use of chemicals primarily in order to gain pleasurable feelings.* Such use may occur when the person is alone or with others. It is not essentially motivated by the desire for some result beyond immediate pleasure such as a desire to ward off unpleasantness or disease, to create a utopian society, or to become more productive.

THE IMPORTANCE OF PLEASURE

Let's assume that your health is your fitness for living a "good life." A healthy lifestyle for you, then, would be one which would maintain or increase your suitability for living a fine, full, fruitful, creative life. Although you, your classmates, and philosophers may debate what should be meant by a "good life," you probably will agree that any definition that would be acceptable would have to include the stipulation that the life must be perceived as being "good" by the person who is living that life.

Pleasurable feelings such as pride, eager anticipation, joy, comfort, hilarity, euphoria, tender affection, and erotic excitement seem to encompass more than just "feeling good." If we don't get enough pleasure, we won't thrive and develop properly. Good evidence of the need for basic pleasure has come from studies of infants. They are more limited in the ways they can obtain pleasure than are more fully developed humans. Perhaps this is why it is among infants that we have the most striking examples of "pleasure-deficiency disease." Infants whose need for food, clothing, shelter, and so forth have been met but who haven't received enough pleasurable stimulation via their skin, eyes, and ears manifest a syndrome called marasmus or "failure to thrive." Some literally "wither and die," and others fail to develop their genetic potential for healthy living. During our development as humans our repertoire of potential sources of pleasant feelings becomes much greater, largely because of our ability to manipulate symbols such as words. If we're fortunate, our world is a garden of potential sources of pleasures—pleasures we *need* to help us buffer the effects of the adversities and pains that are also parts of our lives. If we get too lean a ratio of pleasure to pain in our lives, we seem to become "brittle," and our health disintegrates.

We now know that to a very large degree our behavior is determined by its consequences. Those actions that are closely followed by pleasurable feelings tend to be repeated. Those that appear to result in pain or unpleasant feelings tend to be avoided. This appears to be a fundamental, psychobiological mechanism programmed into us and other creatures with the help of eons of evolution. Generally speaking, the mechanism works pretty well. It helps fish to locate themselves in water with better rather than poorer conditions (for example, salinity, oxygen, and temperature). Similarly, it helps us learn to keep our hands off hot stoves and to increase our dealings with people who "are good for us."

However, the mechanism can sometimes be fooled. It's especially

345

likely to malfunction when we're faced with situations that are relatively novel from an evolutionary point of view. For example, it is phylogenetically novel for rats to have electrodes implanted in "pleasure centers" of their brains. Rats wired up in this way appear to find the results of pressing the activating bar so pleasurable that they'll press it rather than drink water, eat food, and engage in the other pursuits necessary for basic survival and health. Similarly, people in the ecstasy of new love may neglect eating, sleeping, study, and play.

Essential Pleasure from Nonessential Sources

A useful analogy can be developed in which pleasure is to the sources of pleasure as a specific vitamin is to the sources of the vitamin. For example, butterfat and Swiss chard are generally excellent sources of vitamin A (or its precursor, carotene). But even if we never eat butterfat or chard, we can obtain sufficient vitamin A for robust health from other sources such as carrots and broccoli. The point is that probably no single source of pleasant feelings is essential in adulthood to "living a good life," just as no single food is essential to adequate vitamin A nourishment. Some sources of pleasure are particularly rich, and for most of us there are considerable advantages to ensuring that we get these. Sexual activity can be a reliable and good, though nonessential, source of essential pleasure. For most of us it is a good idea to cultivate the source. The sense of satisfaction from a job well done is another nonessential source of essential pleasure that most of us can wisely include in our lifestyle. Essential pleasure can also be obtained through the use of various chemical substances—recreational drug taking.

Sometimes a source of the vitamin A is not a "good" source. Although rhubarb leaves contain plenty of the vitamin precursor, carotene, they are just not a "good" source of vitamin A for people in general. The leaves contain so much oxalic acid that they are considered poisonous. And polar bear liver contains so much vitamin A that it's poisonous! Analogously, electrodes implanted in the "pleasure centers" of rats supply too much of a good thing. It might be said with justification that such a source of pleasure is so concentrated that it is poisonous.

Furthermore, some foods can be dependable sources of vitamin A for many or most people but not for others. It's not ordinarily wise for someone allergic to cow's milk to depend on ordinary cheddar cheese as a source of vitamin A. And if beef liver makes you feel like vomiting, in most cases you would be wise not to depend upon it to protect you from vitamin deficiency.

Personal Decisions

Since time immemorial people have used various chemical ways to obtain pleasure. And just as it's possible to wind up feeling that a particular way of obtaining sexual satisfaction or vocational gratification hasn't been worth it, so is it possible to find that a particular chemical mode of obtaining essential pleasure wasn't "profitable." Recreational drug use *can* cost us more than it gives us. Pleasure feels good and a certain minimal amount of it is necessary. To that extent it *is* good. But there appear to be no "free rides" in this universe. Although one cannot and should not try to run a cost/benefit analysis prior to taking each and every action, the recreational use of drugs may well be one area in which you would be wise to size things up. Different people come up with different balances.

Intelligent decisions concerning recreational drugs are complicated by the way we have been psychobiologically programmed to "approach and love" whatever gives us pleasant feelings and to "avoid and hate" whatever is associated with unpleasant feelings. As any beginning student of behavioral analysis can tell you: in order for behavior to be shaped effectively, the consequences of the behavior must become apparent shortly after the behavior occurs. It could be predicted that if we use a drug for recreational purposes and it produces pleasant feelings quickly enough for us to associate the drug with pleasure, we'll be likely to use that drug again. It could also be predicted that if some sort of recreational drug use resulted in pain, but that the pain didn't occur until so far into the future for it to be associated "at the gut level" with drug use, the unpleasant consequence wouldn't be effective in motivating us to avoid that particular type of drug use. It's important to keep this in mind. Generally speaking, "natural" human activities that tend to be good for us (that is, result in pleasant feelings) in the short run also tend to be good for us in the long run. Similarly, those things that are damaging to our short-term health (that is, things that are painful, unpleasant, or diminishing) tend to be bad medicine for us in the long term as well. Unfortunately, we're only human—and imperfect. Sometimes our naturally programmed tendency to avoid actions with painful consequences protects us only in the short run, but in the long run we come out losers. Avoiding the pain of a visit to the dentist may result in our having a happier, healthier day that day, but it may also result in enough pain for us in the future that our natural, understandable behavior resulted in our dealing ourselves a short hand. Withdrawal from drugs on which we have become dependent such as tobacco, alcohol, or opiates may actually make us sicker before it makes us healthier. To take actions that hurt now in order to be more suited for living a fine, full, fruitful life in the future often takes concerted application of our human powers of rationality—and perhaps a little help from our friends.

DRUGS WITH QUESTIONABLE RECREATIONAL POTENTIAL

Heroin

Heroin was first manufactured in the late 1800s by the heating of morphine together with acetic acid. It is not found naturally in opium, as are such other drugs as codeine and morphine. Ironically, this highly addicting drug was first touted as an effective cure for morphine addiction! Only about 2 or 3 percent of heroin addicts report that they obtained very pleasant sensations from initial trials. Another small minority of heroin *users* are those who have used it sparingly for years, perhaps once a week, without becoming addicted. Evidently, unless

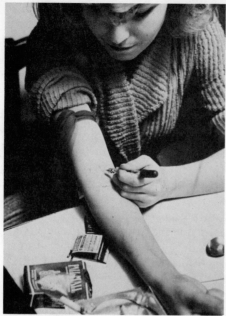

I. Howard Spivak—DPI

there's a good deal of suffering going on at the time, the user is unlikely to experience anything particularly pleasurable. But because of its ability to relieve the impact of one's physical and psychological pains, heroin and other opiates are highly likely to be resorted to more and more frequently. During the process the user builds up a physiological tolerance for the drug, and thus more of it is required to produce the same effect. Of course, addiction, an actual physical dependence upon the drug, is then in the process of becoming established.

Heroin use in the United States is primarily found in large urban centers, with an estimated one-third of the addicts located in New York City. The age at which addicts most commonly first experiment with heroin has dropped from the late teens to the early teens. Typically, most contemporary heroin addiction begins with quasi-recreational use. People don't usually have it pushed on them by someone else. Instead, the incipient addict seeks heroin for the purpose of being admitted into a circle of peers who are already using the drug. The way the famous blues man, Ray Charles, was hooked is classic. As a kid he begged older musicians with whom he worked to let him in on heroin use. They used to go off without him after work rather than use heroin in his presence. Of course, not wanting to be treated as a kid, Charles begged to be allowed to join in. The older musicians did their best to discourage him, but he finally prevailed upon them to be allowed to participate. (*Not typical* is the way Ray Charles decided on his own, largely for the sake of his son, to break his heroin addiction. He voluntarily admitted himself for treatment and insisted upon withdrawing "cold turkey," which he did successfully.) After a few weeks or months, depending on the frequency of the use, the quasi-recreational use tends to fade and addiction sets in. We call it "quasi-recreational" because the motivation seems to go well beyond trying and then repeating the heroin experience as a pleasurable end unto itself. It's heavily laden with using the drug as an entrance ticket to a peer group.

Amphetamines

This is a group of synthetic drugs that includes amphetamine (Benzedrine), the stronger dextroamphetamine (Dexedrine), and methamphetamine (Methedrine). The potential of these drugs for producing "highs" in many people seems to be the basis for playing with them. Although the drugs are generally taken orally, some people "speed" by injecting themselves, usually with Methedrine. Although drugs in this group produce euphoria in some people, in others a psychological agitation that they experience as distinctly unpleasant is brought on. Those who have found speeding to be to their liking appear to be in great jeopardy of moving from recreational drug use to a clearly unhealthy dependency, to say nothing of hepatitis. One emaciated speeder acknowledged that the way in which he was living would probably kill him in half a year. He then insisted with apparently great sincerity that when he injected Methedrine it made him feel so good that he would rather live for four months speeding than for 40 years feeling "the way straights feel." It's pretty hard to argue with something like that. Of course, just as we have no way of knowing what he felt like when he was speeding, he had no way of knowing what "straights" feel like. Rather, he knew what *he* felt like when *he* wasn't speeding. To feel like a nobody at one instant and then like superman the next is bound to be an impressive experience one is apt to seek to repeat. "Something that feels that good must be very good."

One of the troubles with seeking fun via amphetamines is that frequent use tends to cause an "uneven tolerance." The same amount of the drug that used to make you feel great becomes insufficient to give the same result. So you have to step up the dose if you want to keep on getting those highs as often as you've been doing. But your tolerance to some other effects of the drugs may not develop at the same pace, so you're apt to find your highs coming at the expense of unpleasant "jumpiness" and inability to sleep. This phenomenon has led quite a few to seek to bring themselves back down with sedative drugs, such as barbiturates. Trying to juggle uppers and downers is a game that soon becomes about as pleasant as any other sort of rat race.

Other Attempts at Chemical Recreation

To try to list and discuss even in a highly abstract way all the chemicals that a greater or lesser number of us have played with would be way outside the scope of this chapter. Fun seekers, as well as the seriously disturbed, have tried everything from methadone to morning glory seeds, gasoline to LSD, horse tranquilizer (Phencyclidine) to cocaine, Spanish fly (cantharides) to sleeping pills (barbiturates), and aspirins washed down with Coke to Valium (diazepam) in their pharmacopoeia.

Even when you know what you are using, the situation is complex. As Helen Nowlis (1969, p. 9) puts it, "The human organism is continually producing chemicals and modifying both the chemicals it produces and the chemicals incorporated into it. In studying the effects of drugs on this complex system we are trying to uncover the effect of a known chemical substance upon an unknown system."

There seems to be a trend toward multiple drug use. A decade ago there was much fanfare about the generation gap and the way youth were switching to cannabis and away from the alcohol (with all its inherent dangers) that the decadent older generation was wont to use. Of course, we know that now both drugs tend to be used not only by the same people but by the same people at the same time. Start mixing drugs and you multiply the uncertainty of the short- and long-term outcomes.

Often the drugs, obtained via extralegal routes, are of unverified purity. Those who don't even know what they're taking are trying to cope with the effects of unknown substances on an unknown system— their own! Russian roulette and rolling dice are both games of chance, but the implications of playing them are considerably different.

TAKING ACTION

If you are in contact with illicit drugs or sources thereof, find out how you can get "street samples" analyzed in your area. Then have one or more samples analyzed. How does the analysis report compare with the purported content of the drug?

A FEW DRUGS WITH GREATER RECREATIONAL POTENTIAL
Ethyl Alcohol

Ethyl alcohol is most likely the oldest and most widely used drug. It is convenient to classify alcoholic beverages according to the ways in which they're made. Although there are other ways to "cut the alcoholic pie," we'll consider wines, beers, and spirits.

Wines Wine is probably the oldest type of alcoholic beverage. It was most likely discovered independently at many points in time and space by prehistoric people as a result of ingesting wine produced by the accidental fermentation of sugars in berries, various plant juices, honey, and milk. Airborne yeasts that metabolize sugars and produce alcohol as a by-product easily find their way into such naturally occurring substances. The concentration of alcohol in terms of volume varies from approximately 2 percent in a certain Oriental wine made from mare's milk to 14 percent in fortified wines. Natural fruit wines tend to have 8 to 12 percent alcohol, but many American wines are "fortified" with additional distilled alcohol to bring the alcohol content up to 12 to 14 percent.

Beers Beer production was also developed ages ago. Beers are formed when the starch in grains is converted to sugar, which is then fermented. Various primitive peoples have learned to convert starchy foods into fermentable material by chewing them, thus allowing the amylase in their saliva to convert starch into sugar. Beers vary in strength from approximately 2 percent alcohol in some Scandinavian types to as high as 8 percent. Most American beers are in the 4 to 5 percent range.

Spirits Distilled beverages, or spirits, haven't been on the scene nearly as long. Distillation is said to have been accomplished first around A.D. 800 by an Arab known in the Occident as Geber. His name, associated with his syncopated writings on distillation, is thought to be the root of our word "gibberish." Although Geber concentrated the alcohol in naturally fermented wine, he evidently didn't get excited about the potential of the distillate for medicinal or beverage purposes.

It wasn't until the 1200s that distilled alcohol came to be widely recognized as a substance that could produce special effects when consumed. By the 1400s a leading German physician, Hieronymus Brunschwig, reported that *aqua vitae*, as it was called, had the power to do all sorts of good things for people. Among them were: combating cold-related diseases; comforting the heart; healing sores; causing hair to grow on one's head; bestowing a good color to the skin; killing external parasites; protecting against deafness; relieving toothache; sweetening breath; healing canker sores; improving one's facility in speaking; benefiting appetite and digestion; freeing one of belches and farts; easing dropsy, gout, and jaundice; reducing painful, swollen breasts; curing urinary tract diseases, including the dissolving of kidney stones; serving as an ingredient in an antidote for food poisoning; restoring shrunken, malfunctioning sinews; eliminating fevers; healing mad dog bites and foul wounds when they're washed with it; giving the courage of youth; improving memory; and purifying "the five wits of melancholy and of all uncleanliness." However, Brunschwig cautioned that this potent panacea was to be ingested only in the morning on an empty stomach, in a daily dose of five or six drops with a spoonful of wine.[1]

The alcohol in wines and beers is distilled in order to concentrate it, thus producing various forms of spirits. Vodka, gin, whiskies, rum, brandies, and liqueurs usually contain 40 percent alcohol (80 proof) to 50 percent alcohol (100 proof) by volume.

Alcohol in Ancient Times

By the dawn of recorded history alcohol had obviously been around long enough and used widely enough to have left its impact. The

---

[1]Berton Roueché, 1960, *Alcohol: Its History, Folklore, Effect on the Human Body.* New York: Grove, pp. 23–24.

Babylonian Code of Hammurabi, the oldest legal code known (circa 1770 B.C.) provided for the regulation of taverns, including who could sell what and at which price. About 15 percent of the written medical prescriptions of ancient Egyptian physicians (circa 1500 B.C.) included alcoholic beverages. Translations of ancient Egyptian and various Mesapotamian recordings have revealed that what today we call alcoholism existed then as well, causing many of the same sorts of problems it does today.

The ancient Jews incorporated wine into their culture in a fashion that has enabled their descendants through the centuries to enjoy many of its attractive features while minimizing its inherent liabilities. For starters, they usually diluted their wine with water, one or two parts water to one of wine. This produces a drink with 4 to 7 percent alcohol or less, rather than the 8 to 12 percent concentration naturally found in most wines (at this latter concentration the alcohol kills off the yeasts that are responsible for producing the alcohol). Then this diluted wine tended to be used quite frequently as a thirst quencher as well as an adjunct to their numerous ceremonies and celebrations. Drinking to the point of drunkenness was definitely discouraged.

Who hath woe? Who hath sorrow? Who hath contentions? Who hath babbling? Who hath wounds without cause? Who hath redness of eyes? They that tarry long at the wine.

(Proverbs 23:29)

To this day members of the Jewish community are less likely than the general population to become drunkards or alcoholics. But they are

Jewish family celebrating the seder with wine.

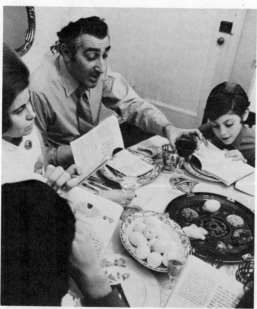

Len Merrim/Monkmeyer

also less likely to be total abstainers. Reflecting his Jewish background, even the Apostle Paul, certainly not a man who was inclined toward "pleasures of the flesh," urged his followers to "Drink no longer water, but use a little wine for thy stomach's sake and thine often infirmities (I Timothy 5:23)."

The early Greeks and Romans also usually drank their wine diluted. The drinking of undiluted wine was considered a sign of barbarism, as well as being likely to damage permanently one's mental abilities. Plato (Laws II) advised that boys should abstain from all use of wine until they were 18 on the basis that it's wrong to add fire to fire! Here is another point about ancient prescriptions concerning alcohol that may be of interest, even importance, to you personally. Biblical warnings against the evils of "strong drink" were not intended to be prohibitions against all beverage alcohol. Instead, they were aimed at undiluted, evidently nasty-tasting draughts known in the Roman world as "posca" (strong drink). People would drink posca not in the ordinary dietary and/or ceremonial ways but simply to obtain the intoxicating effect of the alcohol. Proverbs 31:6 advises "Give strong drink unto him that is ready to perish, and wine unto those that be of heavy hearts." Presumably, if you only had a "heavy heart" you should stick to the diluted wine. But if you were about to die, posca would be in order. It was posca that was offered to Jesus toward the end of his crucifixion.

The Islamic religion, formed in the seventh century, prohibited the use of wine by Muslems. Followers of Buddha and adherents to more recently developed religions such as the Mormons and Seventh-Day Adventists have also rather effectively shut the door on alcohol-induced suffering as well as alcohol-induced joys for the faithful. The "dropouts" from their ranks are less likely than those never protected by religious taboos to be able to drink healthfully.

Alcoholic Beverages as Food

According to Leake and Silverman (1966, p. 75), when alcoholic beverages are consumed "... *as foods, with foods* and at regular meal times, their nutritional, physiological, and psychological values are at a maximum and their potential dangers at a minimum .... Just as abstainers can live happily and healthfully without alcohol, moderate drinkers can also live happily and healthfully with alcohol."

When the caloric value of alcoholic draughts represents a "small percentage" of the total in the diet, the alcohol in the beverages, like fats and carbohydrates, can serve a useful role in sparing proteins. Alcoholic beverages should not be added to a diet that is already adequate in caloric value or you'll become fat. Of course, this applies to any other food in the diet.

Beverage Alcohol and Medicinal Care

Alcohol is a "drug" in at least two ordinary and nonrecreational senses of the term. That is, it has the potential of producing a life-diminishing dependency, and it can be used in the prevention or therapy of disease, thus enhancing the quality of life. Many contemporary Americans have been surprised to learn that some physicians here and many in other parts of the world generally recognize that beverage alcohol has a legitimate place in their practice. The history behind the tendency of American physicians in the past few decades to deny that beverage alcohol has a role in legitimate medical practice is rather interesting. In a nutshell, during the national attempt at prohibition Americans could legally obtain alcoholic beverages upon prescription by licensed physicians. A number of physicians found that they could make much more money by selling prescriptions for beverage alcohol than they could by conducting a medical practice. Also, this was the heyday of hucksters who sold bottled cure-alls at traveling shows. Of course, the main active ingredient in these panaceas was ethyl alcohol, and they did a booming business. Organized medicine in the United States launched a campaign against these nefarious practices. And the general public was convinced that only a quack would say that alcohol can be good medicine. However, increased numbers of American physicians appear to be getting in step with the worldwide medical community, which from thousands of years ago until the present time has continued to use various types of alcoholic beverages in health-care regimens.

As with any drug, self-medication with alcohol can be hazardous. Certainly alcohol can be taken as a tranquilizer, either under a physician's guidance or in a self-prescribed and regulated manner. Similarly you might treat an infection with an antibiotic (say, one that was intended for use on farm animals and was obtainable without a prescription) and be fortunate enough to produce entirely satisfactory results. However, it has its hazards. It has been said that a person who engages in self-medication has a fool for a patient and an idiot for a doctor.

Other Constituents of Alcoholic Beverages

Although we usually consider ethyl alcohol to be *the* active ingredient in wines, beers, and spirits, these beverages contain various amounts of other chemicals that influence the rate at which the ethyl alcohol is absorbed into the bloodstream, the taste, aroma, and color of the beverage, and the tendency for the beverage to produce a "hangover." These chemicals include butyl, methyl, and propyl alcohol, fusel oil (amyl alcohol), various acids, aldehydes, esters, ketones, minerals, phenols, tannins, and vitamins. Incidentally, in the days before modern brewing technology developed the clear, filtered types of beer with which most of us are familiar, the yeast in beers contributed more significantly to the overall nutrition of those who drank them than do today's commercially available products.

A scientist who was conducting research in an oceanographic institute, where he had access to a gas chromatograph, once analyzed samples of a few commercially available brands of spirits, including rum, whisky, and vodka. He was unprepared for what the instrument revealed. In addition to the large concentration of ethyl alcohol he had bargained for, he was surprised to discover that his beverages contained many of the aforementioned "impurities," which he knew to be highly poisonous. The vodka, which in essence is distilled ethyl alcohol diluted with water, was the "purest" by far, and he resolved that henceforth *if* he would ever bother to "go drinking" again, he would stick to "screwdrivers" or "Bloody Marys." His resolve lasted for a few weeks.

Prohibition of Ethyl Alcohol

Ever since the time of the ancient Babylonians, governments have tried to devise laws that would promote public order and moderation in the use of beverage alcohol. They have also generally hoped that the regulations would produce a tax income that would be used to effect a net gain for the public good. But throughout history these attempts repeatedly have been followed by efforts at prohibition—so often that it can be inferred that government leaders from time to time have concluded that the costs of alcoholic beverages to society were greater than the benefits. These governmental efforts at prohibition have never been very successful. As already alluded to, religiously motivated efforts at prohibition, such as in the Far East, have tended to be more successful, though not entirely.

The legacy of the American prohibition that was in effect from 1920 to 1933 includes an organized crime system that still plagues us almost half a century later. In less drastic efforts to mitigate the costs to drinkers and nondrinkers alike of unwise, unhealthy alcoholic use,

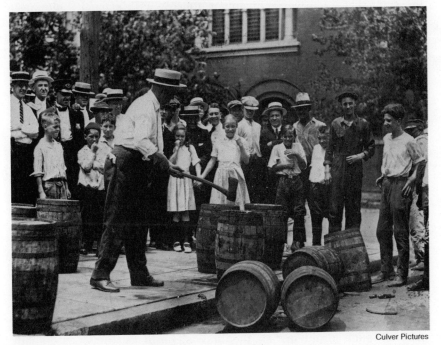

Federal agent smashing barrels of liquor during Prohibition.

Culver Pictures

various governments have passed laws regulating the nature of the places in which you may buy alcoholic beverages and the location of these places, the times you may buy alcoholic beverages, how old you must be in order to buy, the concentration of alcohol permitted in the beverages you may buy, and the way in which alcoholic products may be advertised, packaged, and priced. Sweden, Finland, and the state of Ohio have tried to prevent overdrinking by issuing ration books to those who wish to buy drinks. In Sweden the system was abandoned after 38 years. Evidently they concluded that those who wish, or are driven by reason of addiction, to overdrink will find ways to get their alcohol despite such a scheme.

The Chinese *Shu Ching* ("Canon of History"), written about 650 B.C., noted that to eliminate all drinking of alcoholic beverages, or even all drunkenness, was beyond the power of even the wisest people. Therefore, advice on moderation and warnings about the abuse of alcohol were provided.

The Prevention of Drunkenness

The ethyl alcohol in alcoholic beverages is absorbed directly into the bloodstream, no digestion being necessary. The rate at which it is absorbed depends on a number of factors over which you have some control. For example, if you "drink a quick beer" after undergoing considerable dehydration from sweating, it's apt to "go to your head" surprisingly quickly.

Furthermore, beverage alcohol taken on an empty stomach is absorbed more quickly and produces a higher blood alcohol level than if the same beverage were consumed after or with a meal. Enjoying a relatively nonconcentrated alcoholic beverage along with food providing starch and fat will retard the rate at which the alcohol is absorbed into the circulatory system. Thus for a given amount of alcohol drunk with a meal the concentration of alcohol in your blood would never reach as high a peak as compared to what would happen if an empty stomach were involved. Alcohol dehydrogenase, produced primarily in the liver, has a chance to help break down some of the ethyl alcohol before the rest has even begun to arrive on the scene.

The white-collar practice of having a predinner cocktail or two after "a busy day at the office" *need* not be but often is found in conjunction with a number of factors that increase its hazard. That is, too little physical activity tends to result in a battle with obesity. Ill-conceived plans for combating the fatness often lead to the skimping on or skipping of breakfast and/or lunch. By dinner time, the person has been undergoing a rather lengthy fast, in some cases since the heavy meal of the evening before. Blood-sugar levels are likely to be lower than optimal. Whereas our muscles can burn either fat or sugar for fuel, our central nervous system requires sugar. If the brain's energy supply is relatively short, it's apparently more vulnerable to intoxication.

To a large extent, the elimination of drunkenness would help to prevent such problems as the brawls, child beatings, automobile

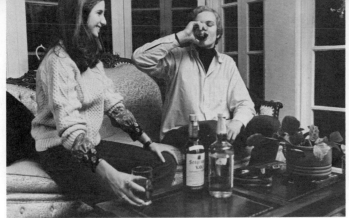

Teenage drinking and alcoholism appear to be on the rise again.

smashups, fires, and so on that frequently result from drunken behavior. It may also be true that many of the people who become alcoholics (and approximately one in ten "social drinkers" *do*) would not do so if they had consumed their alcohol in ways that didn't make them drunk. However, a strong case can be made for the point that we have placed undue emphasis on the *effects* of drinking rather than the *amounts* drunk. This emphasis may well have helped to develop the silly notion that as long as you can hold your booze you're more admirable if you drink a lot than if you drink a little. Many people subscribe to the idea that it's all right to drink as much as you want as long as you don't get drunk, drive your motorcycle or car while under the influence, or the like—and at first glance this argument has a good deal of appeal. It's easy to forget that it's the *amount* drunk that produces various undesirable effects.

It's not very widespread knowledge that some drinkers can and do intoxicate themselves in the literal sense of the word (that is, poison themselves) without ever appearing "drunk." In many respects the concept of drunkenness isn't very helpful. The word itself means so many different things to so many different people. Perhaps in an attempt to cope with the ambiguity of the concept of drunkenness, an old English drinking house song came into being:

> He is not drunk who from the floor
> Can rise again and drink once more;
> But he is drunk who prostrate lies
> And cannot drink and cannot rise.

Although we are physiologically equipped to cope with ethyl alcohol, too much of it, even at concentrations far lower than would qualify as drunkenness according to this song, can cause changes in us resulting in alcohol addiction and liver damage.

Some physiologists were once puzzled as to just why alcohol dehydrogenase is found in horses. Investigation into the problem revealed that a certain amount of ethyl alcohol was produced by natural fermentation in the gut, approximately the amount in a pint of

357

beer a day. This probably also explains why humans are naturally equipped to deal with alcohol. But our evolutionary history did not equip us to handle, healthfully, the amounts with which some of us load the system. And, as with all aspects of our humanity, we vary widely. Some people are inherently able to cope with more alcohol than are others without suffering ill effects. There is no sure way to determine how much we could handle without stressing ourselves to the point of eventual breakdown. Certainly it isn't whether or not we can drink our friends under the table!

Not many years ago it was generally believed that the liver, heart, and brain damage frequently produced in alcoholics was due to inadequate intake of nutrients such as vitamins and proteins. It's since been established that ethyl alcohol and acetaldehyde, a by-product in the metabolism of ethyl alcohol, are themselves directly poisonous. For example, in those who drink frequently, acetaldehyde concentrations in the liver rise enough to damage that organ, and thus it loses its ability to detoxify the acetaldehyde. This, of course, is a vicious cycle in which those who need to get rid of more of the toxic metabolite are precisely those who can handle less of it!

An Additional Note on Alcoholism

For decades most research into the roots of alcohol-induced problems have focused on the sociocultural realm. So it is not surprising that some of the most widely supported and interesting theories are to be found there. For example, one recipe goes something like this. Take people who're suffering, who have some "big, bad thing" they'd like to

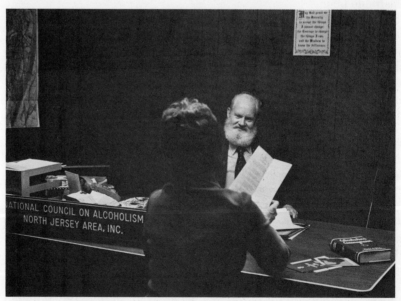

Counseling session for an alcoholic.

Sybil Shelton/Monkmeyer

go away. Then, juice them with alcohol in such a way that they get dramatic relief from that "big, bad thing." Learning theory predicts they'll be more likely to get juiced that same way the next time their big, bad thing appears. Soon a good percentage will move from psychological dependence to physiological addiction, trapped in a double bind: sick if their system runs out of alcohol and sick if they get it. To get an even bigger crop of alcoholics, add to the recipe the ingredient that alcohol had a prior "special significance" for the subjects. Usually this means they become frightened by the power of alcohol, either by seeing an alcoholic parent or by being raised in a teetotal environment where alcohol was viewed as an invention of the devil (even though, ironically, the central worship figure of many of these people is reputed to have changed water into wine for a wedding celebration).

Some relatively recent research sheds light upon apparent biological roots to alcoholism. For example, Peter Wolff[2] discovered differences in physiological responses to ethyl alcohol when he compared persons of Japanese, Taiwanese, and Korean ancestry with people of European ancestry. Such findings may help explain why there's a lower incidence of alcoholism among the former groups. People of Oriental ancestry were found to respond to alcohol with a greater amount of skin flushing. They also reported significantly more alcohol-induced symptoms, such as warmth in the stomach, palpitations, rapid heartbeat, muscle weakness, dizziness, and sleepiness than did the Caucasoid subjects studied. Differences were observed in infants as well as adults, therefore ruling out the possibility that individual differences in experience with alcohol could account for the differences between the groups. It may well be that the greater sensitivity of the Asian peoples to both the objective and subjective effects of alcohol may help to prevent many of them from drinking hazardous amounts of alcohol.

Donald Goodwin and colleagues[3] conducted a classic study of the "nature-nurture" issue relative to alcoholism. The study involved 55 men who, in infancy, had been taken from their biological parents, one of whom had been diagnosed as suffering from alcoholism. Because of the extreme difficulty in properly conducting such a study in the United States, the study was conducted in Denmark, where there is relatively little immigration and emigration, and access to national registries concerning adoptions, psychiatric hospitalizations, and criminal records could be obtained for purposes of the study. Control subjects were matched by age, sex, and time of adoption with the men who were raised apart from their biological family in which alcoholism existed. None of the subjects in the study was a total abstainer from

[2]Peter H. Wolff, January 28, 1972, *Science* 175:449–450.
[3]Donald Goodwin et al., February 1973, *Archives of General Psychiatry* 28:238–243.

alcohol. The groups didn't differ significantly with respect to the subjects' being classified as heavy drinkers or problem drinkers. However, those who had a biological parent who had been diagnosed as an alcoholic were significantly more likely to have experienced alcohol-related hallucinations, to have wanted to stop drinking on a particular drinking occasion but been unable to do so, to have engaged in repeated drinking in the morning, and to have received treatment for their drinking problems. Furthermore, those with alcoholism in their immediate biological background had nearly four times the alcoholism rate as did the controls. A more recent report of the ongoing Danish study[4] revealed that whereas 10 of 14 alcoholic adoptees had biological parents who were alcoholic, there was no known alcoholism among the biological parents of 119 nonalcoholic adoptees. The adoptive parents of the two groups did not differ in socioeconomic class, mental health indices, or drinking histories.

TAKING ACTION

1. *Get together with a group of five or six people of your choosing. Draw up a list of undesriable consequences that could possibly come from drinking alcoholic beverages. Then see how many of the untoward consequences could be prevented by altering the circumstances or the manner of the drinking rather than by completely eliminating the drinking.*
2. *Form a small committee to question physicians about their views on drinking. Standardize your questions. Ask such things as: Do they advise against drinking generally? Do they ever recommend it? Do they ever prescribe it? What do they consider to be criteria for "alcoholism"?*
3. *Talk with junior and senior high school students about their attitudes toward drinking. How do they feel about laws forbidding them to drink? How do these laws affect their behavior?*
4. *Have gas chromatograph analyses run on a number of alcoholic beverages about which you have decisions to make.*

Cannabis *Cannabis sativa* is the botanical name for a plant that has been widely cultivated both for the hemp fiber and for a variety of compounds it contains—compounds which are able to produce a variety of drug effects. Cannabis was thrown upon bonfires and the smoke inhaled as long as 2500 years ago on some of the Mediterranean islands and centuries ago on the African continent (Brecher, 1972, p. 311). It was used for its psychotropic effects more than a thousand years ago in India and, to a lesser extent, in China. During the next 500 years its use as a drug spread to the Middle and Near East. It was probably brought to Europe by soldiers returning to France from Napoleon's wars. But cannabinoid drugs didn't become well known there until the 1800s.

---

[4]Donald Goodwin et al., May 1975, *The Journal of Nervous and Mental Disease* 160:349–353.

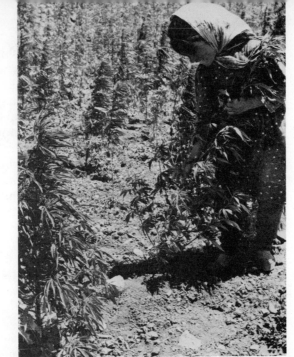

Lebanese girl picking cannabis plants.

Wide World Photos

Not until the 1900s did it become widely used in North America as a giver of pleasant feelings. Even then, until the 1960s its use was not common among middle-class "Anglos." It was used mainly by Mexicans and Afro-Americans and jazz musicians and their companions.

Relatively Mild Preparations   When the leaves, and sometimes the stems, flowering tops, and seeds, of the cannabis plant are dried and broken up, the result is marijuana. This sort of preparation is given different names in various parts of the world. For example, it's called "dagga" in South Africa, "kief" in North Africa, and "bhang" in India. It is currently believed that the principal psychoactive chemical in marijuana is delta-9-tetrahydrocannabinol (THC).

Although factors such as length of growing season, amount of sunlight, soil fertility, and water supply may influence the potency of marijuana produced by hemp plants, genetic variation seems to be the factor most responsible for the differences in potency. Contrary to a popular belief, female plants do not produce more potent marijuana than do male plants. The strength of street samples of marijuana has been found to vary anywhere from less than 0.01 percent to over 4 percent total cannabinoids by weight. Typical samples have a shade over 1 percent total cannabinoids.

The THC and other cannabinoids in marijuana can be taken into the system not only via the respiratory tract (the way most familiar to Americans) but also by the gastrointestinal system. In addition to eating the proverbial "hash brownies," one can obtain drug effects by drinking "tea" made from marijuana.

361

Higher-Potency Cannabis Preparations   Hashish, called "charas" in parts of India, contains a higher percentage by weight of the psychoactive cannibinoids. It is produced by gathering resin from the cannabis plants. Street samples of hashish have been analyzed and found to vary from slightly less than 3 percent to more than 25 percent total cannabinoids by weight, with somewhere around 10 percent being more or less typical.

Just as relatively weak wines, rather than stronger alcoholic drinks, were part of traditional religious rites, so was the weaker marijuana used instead of hashish. For example, the Indian bhang has long played an important role in Hindu practice, but not the more potent charas.

Health Implications   Cannabis, especially the less potent forms, appears to have "rather low" acute and chronic toxicity.[5] But smoking it is definitely not good for one's lungs. A drag of smoke from a marijuana cigarette contains about 50 percent more tar than a drag from a high-tar tobacco cigarette. Some argue that despite this fact the recreational smoking of marijuana is not as bad for the lungs as is the typical tobacco smoking pattern because you don't smoke marijuana as often. For some this assertion is true. However, it is not the case for the many marijuana smokers who are *also* tobacco smokers. That's adding insult to injury!

It also appears likely that inhaling marijuana smoke is considerably more stressful for one's heart than is breathing even tobacco smoke, let alone fresh air. Aronow and Cassidy[6] compared the effects of smoking marijuana to those of smoking high-nicotine tobacco on patients who had suffered angina pectoris (literally "pain in the chest," a condition brought about by insufficient blood flow to the heart muscle). One measure of the effect of smoking on the circulatory system was obtained by multiplying the systolic blood pressure times the heart rate. When this measure increases, it indicates a greater work load on the heart. Whereas smoking a high-nicotine cigarette increased this measure by 36 percent, smoking a marijuana cigarette increased it by 54 percent. The length of time these people were able to perform a standardized physical work task before chest pain appeared was decreased 23 percent by the smoking of a high-nicotine cigarette. The marijuana cigarette had an even greater impact, reducing the exercise time 50 percent.

The bulk of evidence indicates that it is hazardous to operate machinery, such as motor vehicles, when under the influence of marijuana. Research supports the street lore that experienced marijua-

---

[5]S. J. Yaffe et al., July 1975, *Pediatrics* 56:134–143. See also Brecher (1975).

[6]Wilbert S. Aronow and John Cassidy, May 1975, *Clinical Pharmacology and Therapeutics* 17:549–554.

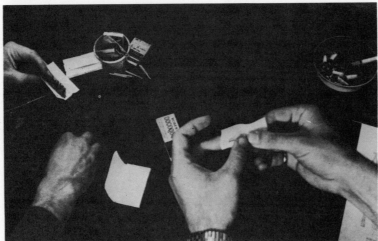

Rolling up some joints.

Wide World Photos

na smokers tend to be more sensitive to the sorts of marijuana effects that reduce psychomotor performance than are nonexperienced people who smoke for research purposes.[7]

At this point in history, and undoubtedly for some time to come, the topic of cannabis has myriads of controversial facets. One of them is its alleged potential for lowering testosterone levels in males, bringing on impotence and lowering sperm counts significantly. There has been research in which such effects were carefully looked for but not found.[8] But there has been some apparently excellent experimentation that is reported clearly to have demonstrated such effects.[9] However, no one seriously claims that "moderate" recreational use of cannabis produces these effects. Rather, it is "heavy" usage (for example, five "joints" daily over a period of weeks) that has been implicated. Also there is general agreement that if such effects are produced, they can be reversed by abstaining from cannabis. This same sort of reversible pattern has been seen in cases of males whose heavy cannabis use appears to have resulted in the development of enlarged breasts. Perhaps it is important to point out here that apparently no one has ever seen a case of a female whose breasts enlarged after heavy marijuana use and atrophied after she withdrew from the drug. Furthermore, for the sake of fairness, many males and females report finding sexual activity especially pleasurable when they are stoned.

[7]G. Salvendy et al., June 1975, *Human Factors* 17:229–235; and Stephen L. Milstein et al., July 1975, *Journal of Nervous and Mental Disease* 161:26–31.

[8]Brecher (1975); and *Science News* 108:374, December 13, 1975.

[9]*Time* 106: 45–46, September 29, 1975.

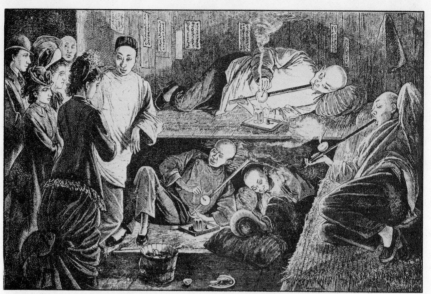

Americans visiting an opium den in China at the turn of the century.

Culver Pictures

Cannabis in Medicine   Before cannabis became such a controversial substance in North America, it enjoyed a degree of respectability here as well as in other parts of the world. At least some American Indians, among them the famous Sitting Bull, included marijuana in the mixtures they put in their peace pipes. They must have considered it good medicine. During the nineteenth century it was even recommended as a "therapeutic aphrodisiac" in a marriage guide.[10] It seems to have been a young Irishman, W. D. O'Shaugnessy, who introduced Western medicine to the use of cannabis. He practiced medicine for some time in India, where he became familiar with cannabis. Cannabis tended to be ingested rather than smoked during this time, and there were physicians in both Europe and North America who enthusiastically used it in treating people with such problems as menstrual cramps, insomnia, migraine headaches, and withdrawal from opiates, as well as for reducing tremors and suppressing coughs. Recent research indicates that oral preparations containing cannabinoids are indeed effective analgesics.[11] However, taken orally they are rather slow acting, sometimes not taking full effect until one or two hours after ingestion. Also, the doses of cannabinoids necessary to reduce pain in some patients are great enough to produce psychological effects that they find distinctly unpleasant, even terrifying. Of course, smoking cannabis would produce faster results, and it has the added advantage

---

[10]Commission on Inquiry into the Non-Medical Use of Drugs, 1972, *Cannabis.* Ottawa: Information Canada, p. 14.

[11]Stephen L. Milstein et al., 1975, *International Pharmacopsychiatry* 10:177–182; and Russell Noyes, Jr., et al., July 1975, *Clinical Pharmacology and Therapeutics* 18:84–89.

of allowing individuals to control more effectively the amount taken in. But smoking has its own very real drawbacks. In hospital settings there's often danger of fire (for example, smoking in bed, in the presence or concentrated oxygen or around explosive gases). At any rate, the cannabinoids are more effective in reducing pain than aspirin, but less so than the opiates.

Research done by the U.S. Army during the 1950s led those who wrote the reports to emphasize the low toxicity of cannabinoids and to recommend that their use be explored for treating fever, pain, epilepsy, migraine headaches, hypertension, and mental illness.[12] There is also reason to think that cannabis preparations ought to be studied further for beneficial effects on glaucoma patients.

TAKING ACTION

Conduct a review of current literature reporting on investigations into the effectiveness of cannabinoid drugs in the treatment of various ailments. Present the results of your library research to your classmates in a manner agreed upon with your instructor.

Prohibition of Cannabis   In 1937 the United States Marijuana Tax Act was passed. In essence, the act created a condition of prohibition against cannabis. It is ironic that it apparently wasn't until after the Volstead Act of 1919 prohibited the ordinary use of beverage alcohol that conditions were ripe for the widespread recreational use of cannabis. By the time the federal government passed its prohibitive Tax Act in 1937, the District of Columbia and 46 of the then 48 states had passed laws that tended to put cannabis in the same category with what are now generally believed to be much more dangerous drugs such as heroin and cocaine. Relatively recently the federal trial of Timothy Leary resulted in the Tax Act being ruled unconstitutional. Since then, a number of states have "decriminalized" the simple possession and use of cannabis.

There exists a fairly impressive list of reports of officially appointed and highly respected groups who have investigated cannabis. No member of any of these bodies has ever apparently approached his or her task with an essentially "procannabis" attitude and emerged converted to an "anticannabis" stance. But there have been conversions in the other direction. For example, one of the men working with the 1970–1972 National Commission on Marijuana and Drug Abuse was the director of the Illinois Bureau of Investigation and a "hard-line narcotics officer" who could boast of a 97 percent conviction rate as compared to the FBI's 85 percent conviction rate in cannabis cases. At

---

[12]Commission on Inquiry, p. 33. (See footnote 10.)

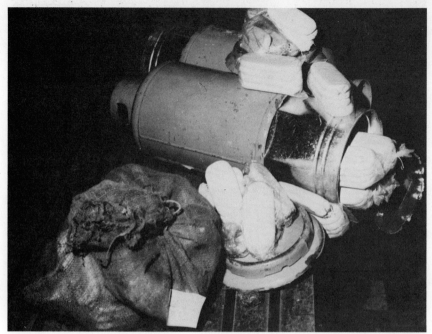

Hashish hidden in a butane gas tank to be smuggled into this country.

the end of one year of study, he called a press conference in Chicago at which he announced that he had been wrong in the past and that now he believed that there should not be criminal penalties associated with the use of cannabis (Grinspoon, 1973). Incidentally, this commission, which had been widely considered as weighted on the "conservative side," emerged from their two-year quest for truth with a report to the Congress and the President that the cannabis issue had been blown all out of proportion, especially in relation to America's really serious problem drugs—alcohol and tobacco.

As of this writing, the American Academy of Pediatrics' Committee on Drugs continues to adhere to its 1971 conclusion that the use and simple possession of marijuana should not be subject to criminal penalties, despite its adverse long-term effects on the respiratory tract when smoked.[13]

Now it might well be true that alcohol prohibition would, in the balance, be a good thing for personal and community health—except that it doesn't work! It's too easy to produce alcoholic beverages, and too many people insist on having them. Similar difficulties now exist with respect to cannabis. Perhaps 25 million Americans have tried the drug and as many as 10 million consider themselves current users. Obviously, the demand is there. And so is the supply. Because it's not legally available, all sorts of strategies have been employed to make it

---

[13]Yaffe et al. (See footnote 5.)

illegally available. For example, large bales of Mexican-grown marijuana have been dropped from low-flying airplanes. However, cannabis is so relatively easy to come by that it's not necessary to depend upon smugglers. Cannabis was cultivated here even before the American Revolution. It was grown for the hemp fiber that was so valuable in rope manufacture. But it escaped as a weed and is currently found growing wild over thousands of acres from Oklahoma to South Dakota and as far east as New Jersey. Highest population densities of wild cannabis plants seem to be in parts of Kansas, Nebraska, Iowa, and Missouri. And, of course, it is often planted these days especially to produce a crop of marijuana—cautiously in flowerpots, cleverly among other plants in the family's vegetable or flower gardens, and roguishly in the diggings of some unsuspecting neighbor or public park superintendent.

TAKING ACTION

Determine what is the current legal status of possession and use of cannabis in your state. Is there an amount you are permitted to possess without being liable to imprisonment? If so, what is it? If a fine is involved for possession or private use, how much is it? What are the current laws relative to selling cannabis? What is your opinion of these laws? Report findings for discussion.

Nitrous Oxide

Unlike beverage alcohol and cannabis, nitrous oxide is a drug with recreational potential that has been discovered relatively recently, in 1776, by Sir Joseph Priestley, the British scientist, clergyman, and author, who is more widely known for his discovery of oxygen. The British chemist Sir Humphrey Davy learned how to synthesize it later that year. Among those who enjoyed the effects of breathing the new "laughing gas" with Priestley and Davy were such well-known fellows as the poets Coleridge and Southey, the venerated potter Sir Josiah Wedgwood, and Peter Roget of *Roget's Thesaurus* fame. (As only a poet at heart could, Southey noted that the atmosphere of the highest of all possible heavens must consist of nitrous oxide.) Eighteenth-century Americans of repute who used the gas recreationally include the physician/author Oliver Wendell Holmes and the philosopher/psychologist William James.

A nineteenth-century member of the Hunterian Medical Society in Scotland, John Knox Stuart, advocated the establishment of "ethereal taverns," where patrons could enjoy highs from nitrous oxide. The gas was to be dispensed from "inhaling bags," a system very similar to that used recently at at least one folk festival where nitrous oxide was sold at the rate of 25 cents per balloonful. The tavern was to be well carpeted and cushioned in order to protect patrons from injury. He recommended charging about twopence per quart and making it available in the form of a "twopenny exhilarating breath," a "threepenny ecstatic breath," and a "fourpenny seraphic breath." He advised that those who

An artist's suggested use
for nitrous oxide in 1830.

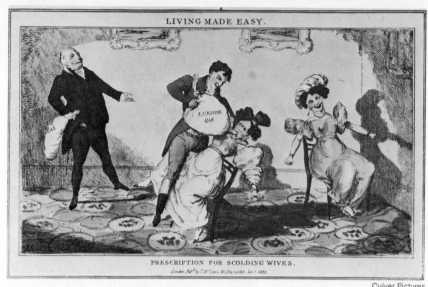

LIVING MADE EASY.

PRESCRIPTION FOR SCOLDING WIVES.
London. Pub.ᵈ by T. McLean, 26, Haymarket, Jan.ʸ 1, 1830.

purchased the one-quart size might be served at the bar, but those who wished to take advantage of the larger sizes would be required to go to the cushioned room, lest the motions accompanying the ecstatic and seraphic emotions result in injury. In describing the nitrous oxide experience, he referred to "irresistible mirth, exquisite pleasure, sensations of the most agreeable nature, toes, fingers, and the ears *thrilling* most agreeably, like cords [that is, chords] of musical instruments, a rapid flow of paradicial [that is, paradisiacal] ideas, . . . a propensity to laugh, dance, and lastly, a strong inclination to jump over chairs and tables, feeling so *light* as almost to be under the necessity to mount and fly."[14] Stuart went on to cite a number of advantages of nitrous oxide over the more ordinary tavern fare, summarizing with: "In short, it is a cleanly, time-saving, exhilirating, angelizing *ether*; whereas spiritous liquores are besotting, brutalizing, devil-inspiring draughts, which in the end clog the ideas, where the *ethereal oxide* sets them free."

Nitrous Oxide in Medicine Apparently the possibilities of nitrous oxide were first recognized about 70 years after the gas was first discovered. It happened this way. An American medical student named Gardner Colton was swayed from his medical studies by the desire to make a living selling recreational opportunities to others, with "laughing gas" as the medium. He staged a show in Hartford, Connecticut, at which the 25-cent admission charge entitled "gentlemen of the first respectability" (in order to ensure that the entertainment would be

---

[14]L. R. C. Agnew, April 1, 1968, *Journal of the American Medical Association* 204:159–160.

"in every respect a genteel affair") to a share of the 40 gallons of nitrous oxide that were available. One of the trippers tripped and cut his leg. He was amazed that the wound caused no pain. So was a young dentist, Horace Wells, who was in attendance and questioned the injured man. Wells arranged for Colton to pull out one of his teeth while he was under the influence of nitrous oxide. You can imagine his excitement when he learned that teeth could be extracted painlessly! Unfortunately, the enthusiastic Wells was laughed out of Massachusetts General Hospital a few weeks later when he demonstrated nitrous oxide anesthesia during surgery. The patient came out of anesthesia before the end of the operation, protesting vociferously.

Despite this inauspicious beginning, nitrous oxide has established a place in medicine as an analgesic (a 30 percent concentration can be used for analgesia) and as an anesthetic (typically it is mixed with other gases such as ether, halothane, and oxygen for this use).

Hazards in Nitrous Oxide Use   Compared with most other drugs that have been explored for recreational potential, nitrous oxide appears to be relatively safe. A physician who for years served as chairman of a medical school department of pharmacology believed that those who desire to use drugs recreationally should be encouraged to use this one. A major advantage it has over "street drugs" is that it can generally be obtained legally from reputable sources in a pure form. The doctor envisioned vending machines available in public places. Patrons could sit in a comfortable chair, and after placing appropriate coinage in the appropriate slot, breathe a measured amount of nitrous oxide for a measured period of time. The gas would come from a mask that would have to be held in the hand in order to be used. This would prevent the sort of accident that occurred when one individual breathed the gas through a tight-fitting face mask. An overdose of the gas rendered him unconscious; since he was unable to get air, he died. In another death from the foolish use of nitrous oxide, a young person sealed up a room, turned on the tank of gas, and asphyxiated himself.[15]

Because it is inhaled, the effects of nitrous oxide are rapid. The exhilarating effects are apparent within seconds of breathing it. One's powers of "straight thinking" are impaired for about five minutes after the last nitrous oxide whiff, and certainly one ought to wait that long before attempting to drive or write an exam.

Also, the fact that a drug has recreational potential seems automatically to go hand in hand with the fact that it has a potential for creating a dependence. That is, if someone is in a life situation where there is a great deal of stress, pain, and/or a minimum of pleasure, one can readily become conditioned to using something that dependably and readily provides relief from the pain or boredom. Thus the discretion-

---

[15]Lawrence Brilliant, December 31, 1970, *New England Journal of Medicine* 283:1522.

ary use of even such a relatively safe substance as nitrous oxide can, in some cases, slip out of the category of recreational drug use. Perhaps the case of Dr. P. W. S. Gray is a good example.[16] This British anesthetist was apparently a hard-working, conscientious member of his profession. He effected improvements in the operations of the hospital on which he was chairman of two committees. However, Dr. Gray's original recreational use of anesthetic gases had led to a dependency. Reportedly at a time when he was particularly depressed by professional responsibilities, some seven years after nitrous oxide and various mixtures of it with other gases had begun to be used in a relatively nondiscretionary way, Dr. Gray was involved in tragedy. A two-year-old child who was being operated on for hernia became anoxic and suffered cardiac arrest when Gray, alternately administering a mixture of oxygen, nitrous oxide, and halothane to the patient and to himself, became too stoned to perform his duties adequately. The child ultimately died.

An additional hazard that *might* be involved in nitrous oxide use is trouble with the law. In 1971 the state of Maryland initiated regulations intended to make the gas unavailable for recreational use.

TAKING ACTION

Determine what the current laws and regulations are in your state regarding the sale, possession, and use of nitrous oxide. Report your findings to your class.

RECREATIONAL DRUG USE, YOU, AND SOCIETY

We live in a generally confusing world, and so perhaps we shouldn't be surprised if we behave in an apparently confused way with respect to drugs. The media surround us with associations between all sorts of beautiful images and various drugs. They also worry us with admonitions against their use. There are a multitude of people with vested interest in getting us to do something about drugs. We hear generation gaps being widened with debates such as "Which is naturally worse for you, opium or alcohol?" We soon learn that the social, including legal, acceptability of a drug is not a dependable predictor of safety or desirability of using the drug.

But we seem not so quick at recognizing that there is no drug that invariably has pleasant effects for all people. Any chemical substance that can alter human emotions and perceptions has the potential of producing unpleasant and painful, as well as pleasurable, experiences in some people under some circumstances. Of course, the other side to

---

[16]*British Medical Journal* 1:308–309, January 31, 1959; *British Medical Journal* 1:376, February 7, 1959; and *British Medical Journal* 1:591, February 28, 1959.

the coin is that virtually any drug that has been touted as "a good trip" can be assumed to live up to its billing under some circumstances for some people.

In addition to having to make decisions about our own personal drug use (What? How? With whom? From where? When?), we are all involved in creating a community with a more or less rational attitude toward the gains and losses from drug usage. Isn't it your business when someone else is playing with drugs and this results in such unproductivity that the person needs to be supported by you and your more fortunate and/or wise comrades? Isn't it your business if irrational prejudices against some or all drugs, drug-induced good feelings, or recreational drug users hamper efforts to deal with drug-related issues in civilized ways?

Nearly all of us have prejudices that keep us from thinking clearly, feeling appropriately, and behaving wisely. These prejudices—for or against something—affect our thinking about many things, not just drugs. For example, most of us would be inclined to discourage a young woman we cared about from becoming a prostitute. We might point out to her that it is one of the few professions in which her earning power would decline as her years of experience in this field increased. We might also indicate that whores are apt to suffer from venereal disease and trauma to the reproductive organs. However, even though very comparable disadvantages could be pointed out to that same young woman's becoming a ballet dancer, we would not be likely to recognize them. It may be that the rational person would rank ballet dancing ahead of prostitution with respect to the general brightness of professional prospects. But wouldn't a rational evaluation have to recognize that ballet dancers as well as prostitutes tend to have to find other means of support as they age? Wouldn't such an evaluation have to recognize that problems such as premature osteoarthritis and deformed toes can be balanced against the medical risks encountered by prostitutes? Our prejudices keep us from seeing the advantages and disadvantages of both pursuits in reasonable perspective.

Which of the following scenes is easier to imagine?

1. Parents getting upset about their youngster's aspirations to join a rock band, arguing that persons who travel in such circles are more apt than the general population to fool around with and get hooked on dangerous drugs.
2. Parents getting upset about their youngster's aspirations to join the medical profession, arguing that persons who enter the profession are more apt than the general population to fool around with and get hooked on dangerous drugs.[17]

---

[17]The parental arguments in both of these hypothetical situations would in fact be true.

Broadening our experience, pursuing the novel, testing our limits are generally held in high regard when they are done in competitive athletics. People get patted on the back and can hold their heads high because of such undertakings. Coaches can make a respectable living encouraging youngsters to spend their time, energy, and other resources in all sorts of contests. We tend to focus on the bright aspects of athletics and to minimize the tarnished outcomes such as broken teeth, sprained knees, paralyzed bodies, damaged brains, and the learning of dishonest tactics. We minimize them by making serious efforts to reduce the incidence and severity of disadvantageous outcomes and to create circumstances that favor more desirable outcomes. We also minimize them by "playing them down" when they occur. But look how differently we are inclined toward "broadening our experience, pursuing the novel, and testing our limits" when playing with drugs is involved. People get cast out because of it and sneak about on account of it. Those who would try to coach youngsters in various sorts of drug-induced experiences, as did Timothy Leary,[18] are apt to be incarcerated or even killed. Those of us who tend to be accepted by society at large generally focus on the tarnished outcomes such as damage to psyches, paralyzed bodies, and serum hepatitis and to minimize the brighter aspects.

This atmosphere presents certain difficulties for those who would speak out for a reasonable approach to drug education. However, such voices are emerging. Edwin Brecher argues: "Just as we hope our children will drive an automobile more skillfully and responsibly, and a little less hazardlessly than we drive, so I believe our drug education goal should be to teach young people to use drugs just a bit more skillfully and responsibly, and a bit less hazardlessly than their parents do."[19]

The tendency to play has been programmed into humanity by evolutionary forces just as certainly as the tendency to sing has been encoded in certain birds.[20] If psychoactive chemicals are in our environment, and in a greater or lesser degree they are and will be, some people will play with them, just as others will play with other features in our environment. Perhaps we will be wise and try to be a bit saner about it than we have in the past.

TAKING ACTION

Here's a three-step exercise that can help you develop a better basis for decisions about the recreational use of drugs and a better insight into the

---

[18]To Leary drug use wasn't strictly recreational. He saw it more as a route to creating a better world.

[19]Quoted in Bernard Bard, December 1975, *Phil Delta Kappan* 57:254.

[20]For a thorough discussion of this concept, see M. J. Ellis, 1973, *Why People Play*. Englewood Cliffs; N.J.: Prentice-Hall.

actual thinking of your classmates about such use.

1. *Make a list of drugs which might provide pleasurable sensations. Do this and the next step outside of class.*
2. *Consider whether or not it's wise for you to pursue pleasure with these drugs. Reflect on your considerations in informal written fashion, analogous to the hypothetical examples presented here.*

Essential Which Is Being Sought

Vitamin A   Pleasant Feelings

General Type of Source Being Considered

Food   Drug
(as contrasted to injections,   (as contrasted to loving,
capsules, and so on)   reading, eating, playing, and so on)

Specific Source Being Evaluated and Hypothetical Evaluation

1) Carrots: not too expensive; easy to obtain; I like the taste; you don't get hassled by other folks for eating them; fairly rich source of Vitamin A, especially in relation to their caloric content.
2) Polar bear liver: not available in stores and would be extraordinarily difficult and expensive for me to obtain; also very poisonous (due to hypervitaminosis A); therefore scratch this one.
3) Other.

3. *All class members submit their lists anonymously to a designated person, who will "shuffle" and redistribute them. Make sure you don't take back your own paper. Then divide into groups of five to seven people to discuss the lists and your reactions to them.*

FOR FURTHER READING

Leake, Chauncey D., and Silverman, Milton, 1966. *Alcoholic Beverages in Clinical Medicine.* Chicago: Year Book Medical Publishers.

Includes much information on the chemical composition, pharmacology, and toxicology of various alcoholic beverages. Discusses the use of alcoholic drinks in the treatment of various medical conditions and health problems for which alcoholic drinks are contraindicated.

Brecher, Edward M., et al., 1972. *Licit and Illicit Drugs.* Boston: Little, Brown.

Cited by the American Library Association as one of the 43 books of outstanding merit published in 1972. Interesting and easy reading. Includes extensive sections on opiates, alcohol, barbiturates, tranquilizers, tobacco, cocaine, amphetamines, LSD and other psychedelics, cannabis, and a particularly revealing one on caffeine. If you were going to read just one book on drugs, this would be a good choice.

Brecher, Edward, et al., 1975. Marijuana: The Health Questions. *Consumer Reports* 40:143–149.

Evaluates in a readable fashion most of the key health-related arguments against marijuana use.

Grinspoon, Lester, Bozzetti, Louis P., Ungerleider, J. Thomas, and Fort, Joel, October 29, 1973. National Commission on Marijuana and Drug Abuse. *Audio-Digest Foundation, Psychiatry Series.* Vol. 2, no. 20.

Audio tape obtainable from medical libraries or your library's interlibrary loan service. Fascinating "inside information" on the workings of the "Shafer Commission," including vignettes of commissioners' experiences with drug authorities of other countries as well as here.

National Commission on Marijuana and Drug Abuse, 1972. *Marijuana: A Signal of Misunderstanding.* Washington, D.C.: U.S. Government Printing Office.

This is the "Shafer Report." The commission was initially widely criticized as being loaded with too much anticannabis sentiment, but the report was attacked as being too soft on marijuana.

Nowlis, Helen H., 1969. *Drugs on the College Campus.* Garden City, N.Y.: Anchor Books.

Outstanding for the wisdom concerning young people and drugs that the author brings forth. Such wisdom doesn't tend to grow less valuable with the passing of years.

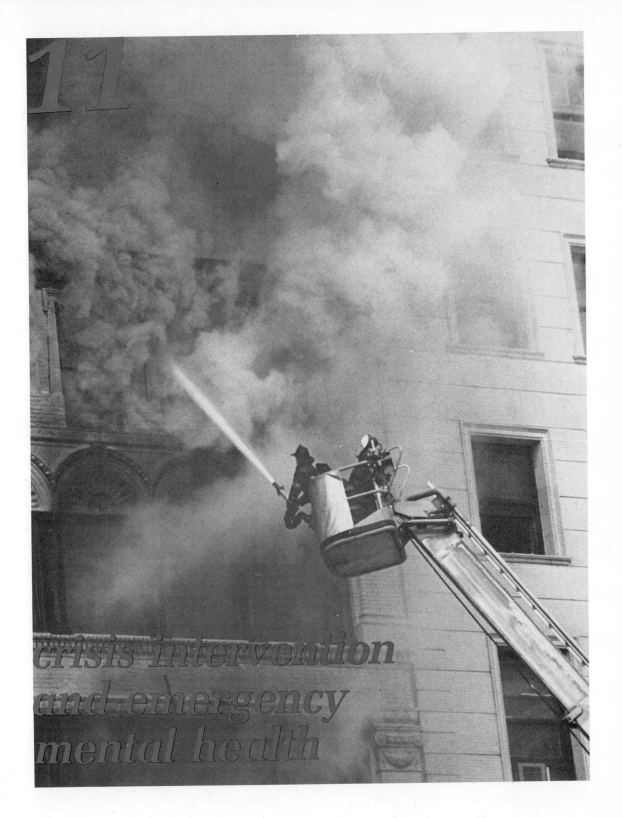

11

crisis intervention
and emergency
mental health

OVERVIEW

This chapter deals with the most prominent forms of mental health emergencies and emotional crises that occur in society today. Within the last decade most knowledgeable professionals have come to realize that difficulties in the mental health realm cannot be separated from social problems, which are of great concern among various cultural and subcultural groups. Social problems have a reciprocal influence upon emotional and mental health. Because crisis intervention procedures are closely related to social and economic problems, they have recently gained more recognition and emphasis nationally, both in the news media and in various levels of government. Poverty and health problems, especially among children, marital discord, frictions leading to child abuse, economic stress, difficulty in upward mobility, racial disturbances, housing problems, and inadequate preparation, emotionally and educationally, to take one's place in society are all interwoven into the mental health fabric of daily living.

In this chapter a special emphasis is placed upon the practical components of crisis intervention, including the role that volunteer work can play. The importance of training is underscored for professionals, paraprofessionals, and volunteer workers. The areas taken into account here include disaster relief, suicide prevention, rape, marital difficulties, and child abuse. Focus is upon psychological first aid for use in emergency mental health situations.

It is hoped that the information presented and the activities suggested will help readers function more effectively in the inevitable crisis situations of modern life.

INQUIRY

1. What are the available facilities for managing mental health emergencies in your community?
2. Are there any mechanisms in your community for handling crises associated with a major disaster?
3. What would you do if a member of your family attempted or committed suicide or was arrested for rape or drug addiction?
4. What effect will economic conditions and changing times have upon services in the future?
5. Will mental health service delivery procedures follow the same treatment disciplines 20 years from now as those that are employed today?
6. Will future health services be focused upon the individual or oriented toward larger groups of the population?

INTRODUCTION Mental health crises appear daily throughout the world. Peak periods and special incidents are often publicized in the news media because large numbers of persons are affected or because of the sheer drama of a particular situation. Present-day crisis procedures have stemmed primarily from three sources: war experiences, catastrophic and natural disasters, and suicide prevention. All represent dramatic situations constituting emergencies that require immediate attention. Despite the fact that mental health crises have existed for centuries, it has been only during the past two decades that a sizable body of knowledge has appeared for teaching purposes in graduate and professional schools. A demonstration project in crisis intervention and suicide prevention in Los Angeles in the late 1950s contributed materially to the growth of this field. In 1974 the Federal Disaster Relief Act added a new dimension of interest to crisis work nationwide by providing mental health services in time of disaster.

Historically the first organized crisis intervention or suicide prevention effort in the United States is believed to have originated with the National Save-a-Life League, founded in 1906 in New York City. National standards are currently being established through the efforts of the American Association of Suicidology, which covers management, service, and training activities for professionals and nonprofessionals in the various facets of crisis intervention and suicide prevention work. Although most of these centers operate independently from community mental health centers, the programs of the latter include emergency service sections that have crisis intervention capabilities. Many crisis intervention programs are affiliated with health departments, hospitals, and clinics, although they often function as separately identifiable units. By the mid-1970s there were approximately 180 professionally operated suicide prevention centers in the United States, but if "hot lines," high school and college crisis lines, as well as personal contact projects were included, it is probable that the number would be well over a thousand. Moreover, there are approximately 600 government-funded community mental health centers.

The term *crisis* indicates a crucial or critical period. For mental health purposes, a crisis means the existence of any situation that so affects the emotional or mental equilibrium of the individual that intervention should be provided so as to avoid possible damaging psychological or physical consequences to the person or persons involved. Crises can be of differing intensities and for varying lengths of time—from a few minutes to several months. A mental or emotional crisis may wax or wane; it may also evolve into an emergency, necessitating more immediate and dramatic attention. Essentially the word *crisis* refers to a time span or interval, a state in a given sequence of events, whereas *emergency* implies a compelling need for action, which may be related to a particular crisis.

Mental health emergency denotes a sudden, urgent, pressing need, just as any emergency situation does. The quick change inherent in the problem suggests a marked intensification of symptoms. *Mental health emergency* means existence of an emotional or mental disturbance that requires prompt attention in order to preclude the possible loss of life

377

or injurious psychological and/or physical effects. "Emergency" is often defined arbitrarily as covering a time span of less than 12 hours.

Crisis counseling refers to any short-term method in which appropriate techniques are used to reduce emotional and mental stresses and problems related to the crisis. It is designed to assist victims of any situation causing psychological trauma or marked emotional disequilibrium. The source of such a disturbance may be a personal loss, a natural or man-made disaster, financial difficulty, a problem with school, or physical health. Any crisis procedure is intended to aid in the management of these disturbances at the time of occurrence so as to establish emotional and mental equilibrium and thereby restore the affected person to the useful pursuits of daily living. Crisis counseling may be appropriate at different points in time during or following a psychological trauma. The primary emphasis is upon short-term treatment. Other forms of mental treatment, such as long-term psychotherapy, may follow crisis counseling.

Figure 11-1

Schematic illustration of common crisis situations, courses of responses, and outcomes.

Various stressful situations in crisis, followed by common crisis reactions, may be seen in Figure 11-1. Such reactions evoke an initial

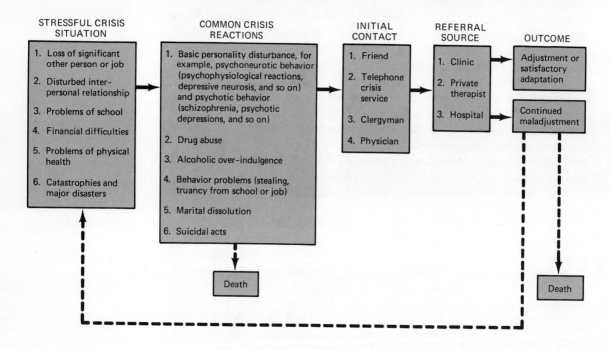

contact, which is followed by one of the common referral sources, namely, a clinic, private therapist, or hospital. After experience with one of these referral sources, the outcome leads either to a good personal adjustment or some other satisfactory adaptation to the problem or else to a continued maladjustment, depending upon the extent to which the individual has been able to utilize the services and the general effectiveness of the program offered. As you will note, crisis situations can lead to continued maladjustment, or even death. The most common areas where these phenomena are likely to occur have been connected by dotted lines in Figure 11-1.

A number of theories have been proposed to explain aberrant (abnormal or strange) reactions to crisis. One of the most time-honored explanations for a variety of abnormal behaviors, ranging from suicide to drug addiction, has been the concept of "anomie." In essence this theory states that when an individual has become adapted to a particular set of societal regulations and norms and that way of life becomes abruptly disturbed for any reason, the strain connected with the need for adjustment can become intolerable. Moreover, if there is a blocking of both legitimate and illegitimate avenues to successful behavior, such blocking acts as an additional causal factor in producing aberrant behavior. Sudden shifting in the life situation of the individual, whether it be in an upward or downward direction in terms of socioeconomic mobility, may produce essentially the same result. The chief difficulty with this concept is that it fails to explain why many individuals who experience these changes do not resort to such aberrant forms of behavior.

THEORIES OF ABERRANT CRISIS BEHAVIOR

The mental illness theory holds that when individuals engage in behavior that is different from what we expect, such behavior is rooted in psychopathology and should be regarded as some form of emotional or mental illness or moral weakness. One of the reasons for this view is the threat that unusual behavior poses to our own egos. The unconscious thought that "there but for the grace of God go I" becomes overwhelming, and we wish to put as much psychological distance between ourselves and such an individual as we can as a protective reaction. Some behaviors make people so uncomfortable that we declare them crimes, as in the case of drug addiction and suicide attempts. However, this theory does not stand the test of objective research. People who engage in most forms of crisis behavior have not been found to be mentally ill, even those who commit or attempt suicide or become alcoholic.

Inheritance or genetic theories have always been tempting means to account for that which is unknown. It is easy to ascribe phrases like "organ diatheses" and "weak nervous systems" to those individuals who display aberrant behavior. Still, solid evidence to support a genetic explanation of unusual behavior during crisis is even more tenuous than the mental illness theory. Despite any known inheritable weaknesses, including those where mental retardation existed, it is still virtually impossible to assign specific behavior to inheritance.

Learning theory and conditioning seem to provide the most plausible explanation for particular behaviors. Under stress our behavior is likely to be affected by what we have previously experienced. Other things being equal, past behavior is always the best indicator of future behavior. This holds for crisis behavior as well. Even though there may be other influences in crisis behavior, it is difficult to imagine any explanation of behavior without a strong learning component. The following model represents the learning sequence found in crisis: stress—→tension—→aberrant act—→relief—→shame and guilt—→tension —→aberrant act. The cycle then repeats itself. This model explains how the use of various drugs, such as energizers on the one hand or tranquilizing agents on the other, serve to establish or condition behavior rather than eliminate it. Both bring relief from tension and thereby effect a strengthening of the behavior as a rewarded act. To illustrate, drugs may be taken to relieve tensions. Once relief has occurred, the individual will be likely to repeat the same act that brought relief before. The more intense the emotional aspects are that have accompanied past events the more likely the resultant behavior will be to recur.

GENERAL PROCEDURES IN EMERGENCY MENTAL HEALTH

Psychological first aid can be of vital importance, just as physical first aid has been in the past. In the future it is hoped that psychological first-aid training will routinely go along with training in physical first aid. It can be a crucial component in the delivery of effective service in any crisis or emergency situation. Some of the general procedures for use by crisis workers are listed here:

1. *Be calm.* The crisis worker's own personal demeanor and bearing are crucial. The patient or victim in crisis may interpret from the worker what his own situation is likely to be. If he is seriously injured, disclosure of a negative or disquieting reaction can create often unjustified anxiety and panic on the patient's part.

2. *Provide honest reassurance.* Give supportive information that is truthful. To illustrate, if a person appears to be seriously injured upon cursory examination, and asks about his condition, the worker might respond by saying, "I don't know," or "I am not sure, but you have an injury, and we are going to see that it's taken care of." In this way the victim's trust and hope will be nurtured. Heightening the victim's anxiety should always be avoided.

3. *Attempt to engage the person in conversation if he is able to talk.* Conversation allows for a verbal catharsis, which can be tension-reducing and help to delineate some of the person's emotional difficulties. Such information may be extremely valuable for a professional therapist who may be working with the individual later. Moreover, it may help relieve the victim's mind or focus his attention away from some physical injury.

4. *Take a definite plan of action.* An action plan is important even though it has not always been made firm. As an example, one might say, "We are trying to arrange for you to be taken to a clinic or to Dr. "X," or some other comment that appears probable and appropriate. This gives the feeling that something tangible is being done to help. Nothing can be more anxiety-provoking than feeling that little or nothing is being done to assist the person under stress.

5. *Attempt to contact relatives or friends.* Input from other persons of significance can be valuable. Not only may friends and relatives exert a positive influence, but they may serve as adjunctive treatment resources. In the event that negative feelings toward such persons appear on the part of the victim, it is especially important to have this knowledge in order to plan appropriate follow-up procedures. For example, if an individual has attempted suicide in an effort to hurt a significant person in his life, that very fact may constitute the nucleus of an effective treatment approach.

6. *Mobilize the individual's own resources.* Although there are cases where dependency feelings can be accepted and nurtured temporarily, it is helpful to highlight the inner personal strengths of the individual as early as possible. Children and others may be depending upon him or her, and it may be very useful to build upon such relationships as an aid in restoring the person's psychological equilibrium.

7. *Provide reassurance.* The use of reassurances supplies immediate support of a very direct and critical nature to persons in crisis. It offers a vital first step in helping to mobilize the person's psychic reorganizational processes.

8. *Give appropriate advice and guidance.* Persons in crisis need direction. In formal psychotherapy advice is not regarded as particularly helpful, inasmuch as the individual is simply following the suggestions of another person rather than solving his own problems. However, during periods of psychological frustration and impotency, thoughtful advice can be a valuable tool in getting an individual to take tangible steps toward solutions to his problems. Thus both advice and guidance are supplied where needed.

9. *Scotch rumors.* It is important to discourage rumors, since the information from which they come may be inaccurate or may generate harmful emotional reactions that can become contagious and create group chaos. The person in crisis should not be flooded with information he is not prepared to handle. It is best to answer only what is necessary in order to alleviate uncertainty. In crisis definitive statements may be made in order to manage rumors effectively. A lack of direct response or parrying of a question can simply add to uncertainty.

10. *Promote activity.* Motor responses are extremely beneficial in alleviating anxiety, reducing panic, and motivating an individual to move away from depressed feelings. Simply using the muscles to accomplish a task may be extremely valuable. This can be done by encouraging the person to help someone else accomplish a task. Assuming that he or she is physically capable, an individual under stress might be encouraged to attend a community meeting, while giving another in need of a car a ride to the same meeting. If the experience turns out to be a positive one, personal confidence has been enhanced. If it should not prove especially rewarding, another activity can be suggested.

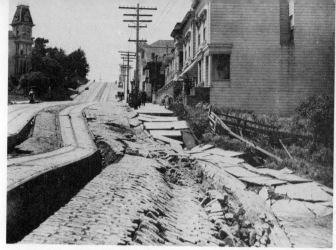

A San Francisco street, split open after the earthquake of 1906.

THE CRISIS OF MAJOR DISASTERS

In the 1971 earthquake in San Fernando, California, 74 people were killed and thousands suffered emotional disturbances. A large percentage of the children in the immediate area became psychological casualties. In June 1972 persistent rains caused rivers and streams to overflow in Rapid City, South Dakota, resulting in a loss of 237 lives, with hundreds left homeless and in need of psychological intervention. In February 1972 a torrent of rain in West Virginia caused a dam to break at Buffalo Creek. Over 100 people were killed, 1000 were injured, and 4000 were homeless. The psychological impact of that disaster has continued to manifest itself for years. And so it goes: tornadoes, hurricanes, fires. Most recently in 1976, Guatemalan earthquakes killed over 15,000, injured countless others, and destroyed entire neighborhoods. Dramatic as these examples are in numbers, they do not reflect the psychological consequences involved in surviving such incidents.

Until recently the personal loss and special stresses accompanying disasters have been overlooked as significant factors in the mental health sphere. A number of misconceptions still exist concerning personal responses during and after these events. Serious emotional and psychological problems follow, but not of the type customarily imagined. Rarely do persons become overtly panicky or run amok. On the other hand, disasters do not always unite or unify people. Such situations frequently bring about psychological disintegration along with physical injury and property damage. Although some people may assist their neighbors and other community members in times of disaster, many others do not respond in such a cooperative and helpful way. Surprisingly, some victims will often harbor feelings of resentment toward those who have been spared serious loss. Contrary to what one might expect, standard psychotherapy techniques are inappropriate during the acute phase of disasters. In terms of readily assessable damage, many of the physical results are often grotesquely apparent. Psychological damage, particularly of a long-term nature, is more subtle and often requires professional expertise to assess.

One of the reasons people are likely to believe that cohesiveness occurs after disasters stems from past national efforts during wartime.

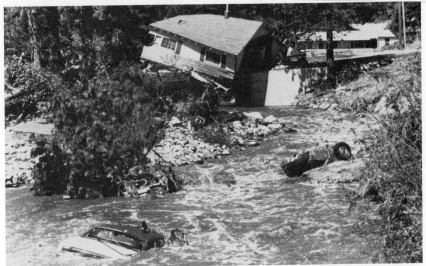

However, unlike during war, people affected by disaster frequently do not mobilize community resources and become a cohesive unit, working in concert toward a common cause. Some of the differences that appear are the following:

1. War is a continuous, ongoing process, which disasters are not. Jobs are made available specifically targeted toward the war effort, accompanied by various activities centering around both work and play, all focused upon effective production and winning the war. Disasters occur quickly and are over, leaving people with a feeling of frustration and impotency.

2. There is a gearing-up period in war efforts that does not occur in disasters. The nation's resources, both in the private and government sector, all assist in this period of preparation and mobilization of effort. Disasters, being of a shorter time frame, permit no such gearing up. There are no pep talks by leaders and no literature and entertainment geared toward the ongoing functions of persons involved in the alleviation of the trouble.

3. During war a nation's spirit has been insulted or challenged, which does not obtain in disaster situations. There is no "rallying around the flag" movement during disasters. There is only a temporary call for cooperation, which does not persist in people's minds since they know that the disaster has already occurred and that the focus is chiefly upon mopping-up operations. Rebuilding is cast in an individual light rather than as a group responsibility.

4. There is a firm personal and societal resolve during a war to right a wrong, which does not obtain in time of disaster. In war another nation has stepped on our toes, so to speak, and created a great misdeed or injustice that must be undone. Disasters are seen as fateful events over which we have little control.

383

5. As a rule, wars do not occur quickly and precipitously, whereas disasters do. There is no time for preparation or fighting back. In effect, disasters occur on a hit-and-run basis. Generally if an opponent strikes us and remains on the scene, we can often muster the courage to fight back; when there is nothing present to fight, our self-concepts are of little use in the process of reorganization or reconstruction.

An important variable in the psychological reaction to disaster appears to be the time factor. Disasters that occur over a period of several days, such as hurricanes and floods, appear to take a greater toll psychologically than those occurring rapidly since in the latter case recovery measures can begin immediately. Some of the most specific reactions commonly seen in disasters are noted in the following discussion.

Problems Affecting Children

A variety of emotional and mental health problems in children have been reported following disasters in the past few years. The most prominent of these seem to be phobias (irrational fears) concerning the elements and future disasters, sleep disturbances, and lack of responsibility. To illustrate, the tornado that struck Xenia, Ohio, the earthquake in San Fernando, California, and the Buffalo Creek flood disaster in West Virginia all left these problems in their wake. An unexpected result is the fact that these disturbances have been observed consistently in children even a year or two later. Moreover, such problems have been reported in a large segment of the children in the affected community. For example, in Xenia, Ohio, the area Inter-Faith Council reported that following the tornado 86 percent were less happy, 70 percent showed a loss of interest in school, and 70 percent experienced nightmares and severe problems. After the earthquake in San Fernando, California, the local Child Guidance Clinic noted that scores of children literally clung to their mothers, hid under beds, and refused to go to school for protracted periods of time.

Problems Affecting Adults

Frequent symptoms among adults are those of initial anxiety, followed by anger, resentment, and hostility. This in turn leads to depression and loss of ambition. The commonly expected reactions of panic, followed by community cohesiveness, love, understanding, and mutual assistance, do not always manifest themselves. Hostilities often develop that are directed toward others nearby. For example, anger is transferred from disastrous events themselves to neighbors, family members, children, helping personnel, and others in the individual's life space. This is followed by feelings of self-blame, often resulting in depression and hopelessness. In some instances suicidal or even homicidal acts occur.

It is frequently helpful to avoid references to mental health assistance in standard terms. The notion that anyone would need psychological or psychiatric help may constitute a threat in itself. The view has been perpetuated in many parts of the country that it is a sign of

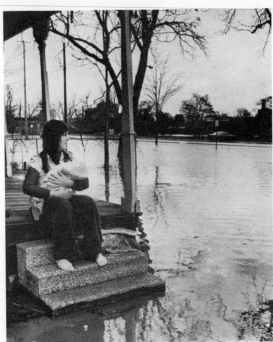

Mother cradling her baby in Lansing, Michigan, as the Grand River creeps up to her doorstep.

Wide World Photos

disgrace and moral weakness to need psychological counseling. The idea of being able to stand on one's own two feet, straighten up, and get a hold on oneself are all ingredients of the rugged individualist so admired by North Americans. Although such a feeling of independence has merit for some occasions, it is totally inappropriate in many forms of emotional and mental disturbance. It prevents the receipt of needed services. Self-treatment for serious emotional disturbance is likely to be ineffective and self-defeating.

The traditional physical model for evaluating disasters does not suffice in the mental health realm. This model arbitrarily categorizes disasters into the following phases: warning, threat, impact, inventory, rescue, remedy, and recovery. A more suitable mental health model would simply list a generic sequence: (1) *the event*, (2) *the perception of the event*, (3) *attempt at adaptation*, (4) *residual aftereffects*, and (5) *reorganization*. An event is established initially by definition. This is followed by a particular perception of it, which may bring about fear and a number of other reactions varying with the individual and severity of the disaster. Attempts to adapt may include flight or freezing behavior in a primitive manner, such as many lower animals do. Immobilization is a traditional response. Anxiety is an immediate reaction, whereas other responses and feelings such as depression, anger, hostility, persecutory thoughts, psychophysiological symptoms, and sleep disturbances often follow. Some of these may occur rather quickly, but in general they are not part of the immediate disaster reaction.

385

What to Do during a Disaster   Disasters, characteristically, are relatively short-lived, depending upon the type. Earthquakes may last only
a matter of seconds, whereas flood and hurricane activity may last for
much longer periods. In such a situation:

1. Think and act in a deliberate manner. This will also affect other
persons.
2. Watch for falling objects and broken wires.
3. Stay away from chimneys and mirrors.
4. Get under a strong desk or table, or stand in a doorway.
5. Do not run outdoors, since the danger of falling objects is
enhanced.
6. Stay away from elevators and stairwells because they may be
broken or jammed with people. Elevators may fail and be hazardous.
7. Move slowly to a suitable exit after surveying the situation.

What to Do after a Disaster   Following a disaster there are a number of
sensible steps you should take. The following list is typical.

1. Make sure that you are not injured; then you may proceed to
assist others.
2. Check for fire hazards and fires.
3. Check all utility lines and appliances, such as observing gas
leaks and electrical connections.
4. Make sure that you wear a good pair of shoes to protect your feet
from sharp objects and broken glass.
5. Do not eat or drink anything from open containers that have
been near shattered glass. Liquids may be strained through a
clean handkerchief or cloth if danger of glass contamination is
thought to be present. Check refrigerators and electric outlets to
make sure that electricity is working properly. Outdoor charcoal
broilers can be used for emergency cooking.
6. Do not use your telephone, except in an emergency. Turn on the
radio.
7. Do not spread rumors. They can create great harm.
8. Do not explore the surrounding area. You may create more
problems than you solve.
9. Apply both psychological and physical first aid where appropriate. In brief, helpful first aid measures are: reassure and relax the
injured person; obtain information through direct questioning;
determine the patient's level of consciousness orientation, alert-
ness, and emotional state; and check breathing and circulation.
If the individual is unconscious, you can simply observe whether or not the chest is moving and place fingertips on the carotid
artery just under the jaw at the side of the neck for a pulse check.
It should be somewhere in the neighborhood of 70 beats per
minute. Check to make sure there is no blockage of the airway
and breathing apparatus.

10. Take note of the victim's complaint, since he may pinpoint his own problem.
11. Visually scan the person's entire body from head to foot.
12. Look for injuries to any part of the body, and observe unusual bleeding, odors, or temperature. Watch for convulsions and pain sensitivity. Check arms and legs in terms of skin color, temperature, texture, position, sensation, and tenderness to touch and movement. Report all your findings to the medical technician or another individual capable of handling the problem later. *Do not move or manipulate the victim! Observe only!*

TAKING ACTION

Preparedness training of persons to manage difficulties ahead of time is of vital importance if people are to respond sensibly. How would you manage in a crisis? Some definite steps in the action process are listed below. Follow through with as many as you can during a period of one week.
1. *Set up emergency situations in class. Role-play the handling of them. Evaluate.*
2. *Obtain and distribute printed matter, cassettes, or films for discussion so as to acquaint your community with problems of disaster.*
3. *Find out if there are local safe building codes with efficient inspection and firm enforcement. Modern engineering can provide structures that will resist many kinds of disasters, especially earthquakes. If there are no codes or regulations in your community, explore ways to enact such procedures with community officials.*
4. *Teachers and parents should instruct schoolchildren in what to do in terms of disaster. Contact local principals and PTA groups to determine how your community is prepared. Fire drills have long been a standard procedure in schools. Other kinds of disaster and first-aid procedures, including psychological first aid, ought to be established as an integral part of such a program.*
5. *Check your own home, whether you own it or are a tenant. Water mains, gas mains, fire extinguishers, and so on should all be made available and should be secured and fastened.*
6. *Rehearse with those with whom you live action to be taken in event of various disasters. Each family member can be assigned tasks to be done at regular intervals, such as checking for gas, electricity, and so on. First-aid kits can be examined. Water can be made available in bottles. Flashlights can be checked to make sure the batteries are working. Radios of a transistor or portable type can be checked to make certain that they are in working order.*
7. *Discuss emergency actions to be taken in different locations: at work, while driving, in a theater, and at home.*

THE CRISIS OF SUICIDE

The incidence of suicide has increased steadily in recent years. For practical purposes, *suicide may be defined as any willful act designed to bring an end to one's own life.* Any person who ingests a handful of aspirin with the belief that such an act will end his or her life possesses

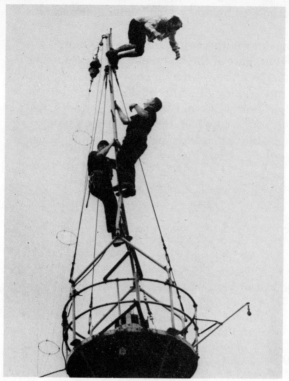

A man jumping to his death from the mast of a ship docked in New York.

Wide World Photos

the necessary frame of mind to justify the classification of suicidal behavior. On the other hand, if a housewife ingests a dose of lethal medication a few minutes prior to the time she expects her husband home from work, the act may not be so clearly suicidal but may be in part an attention-getting device to make her husband save and feel sorry for her. All suicidal acts, even those that do not have an apparent cause, should be taken seriously because many suicidal threats turn out to produce tragic results. Generally it is a mistake to dismiss any kind of suicidal behavior as a mere gesture or attempt to obtain attention. There is everything to lose by taking the threat lightly, and everything to gain by taking it seriously.

Let us examine some brief case illustrations.

1. Josephine is a 16-year-old girl who has had a number of quarrels with her mother and has received little support from a rather weak and ineffectual father. Her mother is quite self-centered and makes strong demands upon her daughter, which the latter feels are unreasonable. The girl turns to a boyfriend for psychological and financial support, which he is unable to supply. At that point she believes that her boyfriend is rejecting her. Is she a suicidal possibility?

2. John is a 20-year-old college student who has done reasonably well in his studies, is quite bright, and is capable of doing even better. His father, who was rather well-to-do, died from a heart attack when

John was in his early teens. The father, an attorney, was absorbed with the pursuit of his career and the achievement of financial success. During the period of his secondary education, the boy was sent to a private boarding school. Although John was given most of the material things he requested, he has always believed that the mother in particular and the father to a lesser extent favored a younger brother. Is John a likely suicidal risk?

3. Joanne is the wife of a successful, middle-class businessman. She has two attractive and well-liked teenage daughters and appears to have experienced a happy marriage. She is approaching her forty-seventh birthday but has recently suffered pangs of anxiety, coupled with feelings of depression and loss of motivation. A favorite aunt, with whom she lived as a child, took her life while in a mental hospital when Joanne was 13 years of age. Her physician has prescribed an antidepressant medication and decided to hospitalize her for a few weeks to permit her to get away from the stresses of daily living. Is Joanne apt to take her life?

Josephine will probably not commit suicide, but she may attempt it. John and Joanne are high-risk cases, with a marked probability of suicide, if skillful intervention does not occur. Teenage girls, as a rule, are attempters rather than committers, although there has recently been some increase in suicides among younger females. Young males who have never had a satisfactory relationship with their fathers, who tend to become isolated and lacking in focus, with feelings of rejection, are serious cases for concern. Among persons at highest risk one finds the middle-aged female who experiences menopausal problems and feelings of depression. For both John and Joanne, there have been losses of important figures in their lives, a fact that correlates highly as a prognostic indicator of suicidal behavior. Suicide is the third leading cause of death among persons of both sexes in the age group from 15 to 25 years, and it is the fourth leading cause of death among persons of both sexes between the ages of 25 and 45. Interestingly, the other significant causes of death among the younger age group are (in order): accidents, homicide, malignant neoplasms, and diseases of the heart.

Psychological Equivalents of Suicide

Crisis workers often cast deaths into this grouping according to intent: intentional, unintentional, and subintentional. The definition of an intentional death is reasonably clear. It means that an individual is seriously intent upon taking his or her life. An unintentional death is one in which it is obvious that the individual had no idea that he was going to die, as in an unavoidable accident. A subintentional death is the psychological equivalent of suicide. Examples of this type may be seen in the way an individual maltreats himself when drinking to excess or overeating. This category probably accounts for the largest number of suicidal deaths, even though they are not reported as self-induced. All kinds of deaths wherein the degree of intent is uncertain are taken into account, like various accidental deaths or neglecting one's personal health in the face of a known infirmity.

Self-induced deaths may be clarified when placed on the continuum in Figure 11-2. Self-assaultive behavior is characterized by personal

Figure 11-2

Scale of behavior showing psychic intent to end one's own life.

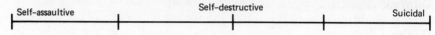

Self-assaultive   Self-destructive   Suicidal

abuse of oneself without total awareness of its life-threatening components. Self-destructive behavior suggests more awareness. An example could be an individual who possesses a known physical problem and yet neglects taking proper steps to care for himself. Specific illustrations would be smoking after developing emphysema or improper eating and the neglect of medication in the presence of severe diabetes mellitus. Suicidal behavior per se involves any overt act with a relatively clear plan and intent. Behavior that is self-assaultive and self-destructive can become suicidal, even though it would not be characterized as such initially.

Many psychological equivalents of suicide occur every day without being recognized. In addition to the neglect of the medical problems just noted, reckless driving constitutes an equivalent form of suicidal behavior, particularly of the individual who drives regularly under the influence of alcohol.

Causes of Suicide

Self-destruction is a complex phenomenon; several variables contribute to the actual act.

1. *Feelings of loneliness.* Invariably individuals who have made suicidal attempts, as well as those who have written about it in suicide notes, have commented upon feelings of persistent and pervasive loneliness. This feeling is one that tends to be rooted in rejection, perceived or actual, feeling of lack of confidence, loss of self-esteem, feelings of unworthiness and shame, and loss of love. Frequently a significant individual in the victim's life has been lost or has turned away.

2. *A quality of haplessness.* The cards seem to have been stacked against individuals who take their lives. A series of events has often taken place in which bad breaks seem to have been inevitable. These events may have been self-induced, in large measure, but they give the appearance of a hapless quality to the individual's demeanor. The person may have experienced continuing difficulty with an automobile, enduring numerous accidents, or he may have suffered some physical injury or medical difficulty, lost money, failed examinations in school, lost a job, and experienced a variety of other difficulties that suggest a series of bad breaks.

3. *Feelings of helplessness.* When an individual is feeling lonely and has experienced personal difficulty, he tends to feel helpless. The idea of being unable to manage one's own life becomes a pervasive and deleterious concept. The thought that an individual is unable to do anything to help himself tends to undermine feelings of self-worth,

self-esteem, and confidence necessary to function effectively. The ability to ask for help from another person, in time of need, can have a salutary effect, but many people feel as if they ought to be able to manage their lives without seeking help from others. Helplessness is debilitating in itself and is a likely accompaniment to depression.

4. *Feelings of hopelessness.* The loss of hope is likely to be the straw that breaks the camel's back. When an individual has experienced a hapless series of events, becomes consumed with helplessness, and then sees little hope, it is as if the entire world has collapsed before his very eyes. The loss of hope brings down the final curtain on the person's perception of his life situation and carries with it a finality, which can be seen as irreversible. Although many people experience one or two of these feelings occasionally, most of us do not feel or experience all of them simultaneously.

When individuals feel hapless, helpless, and hopeless, it suggests an imminent suicidal act. This can be called the "syndrome of the three Hs," namely, *haplessness, helplessness,* and *hopelessness,* as indicative of self-destructive behavior.

Identification of Suicidal Behavior

Self-destructive acts contain the "three Ps" as courses of action for the crisis worker who is to intervene, whether professional or nonprofessional. The three Ps will serve to remind the worker that suicide is *perceptible, predictable,* and *preventable.*

Perceptibility If we can learn to observe the way an individual behaves, we can increase our sensitivity to suicidal acts. Through talking with those who know the individual, crisis workers will realize that certain signs were recognizable all along. Clues to suicidal behavior are both overt and covert and appear as verbal and behavioral indicators. Frequently the youngsters in lower socioeconomic groups are products of an unwanted pregnancy, become problems even as preschoolers, are one of many other youngsters, have been given an inadequate amount of responsibility, and have had unattainable goals and expectations pushed upon them. If a personal loss is part of the picture, the probability of suicide is always increased.

Verbal indicators are those whereby an individual states openly or covertly that he or she has entertained the notion of suicide. This may be done by saying flatly that he intends to take his life or that he is fed up with living. More subtle forms include inquiring about insurance policies, discussing the hereafter, or asking about procedures for leaving one's body to a medical school after death.

Behavioral indicators that may assist in identifying suicidal behavior include such actions as the purchase of lethal instruments, such as a gun, ropes, pills, or knives. More hidden and less obvious behavioral clues involve those of depression. These are characteristically loss of appetite, loss of weight, loss of libido, loss of sleep, loss of energy,

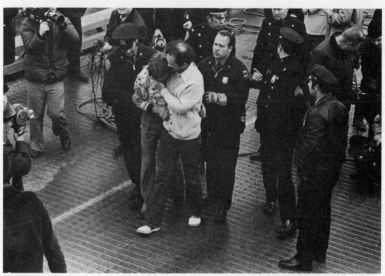

Attempted suicide victim being comforted by a police rescue squad.

fatigue, mood changes, isolation, withdrawal, and heightened irritability. Sudden changes of behavior on one's job or in school, in the home, or throughout the neighborhood, may signal an incipient suicidal act. In recent times heavy ingestion of drugs, as well as alcohol, have been contributing factors.

Depressive symptoms may not always be clearly apparent, especially among young people. Some depressive signs may appear in youngsters, but all of the classical symptoms noted above are not usually apparent. It is an error to believe that an individual will not take his life unless he is depressed. Many persons kill themselves who are not depressed, while some who are depressed do not make suicidal attempts. Nevertheless, it is always cause for concern when depression persists and goes untreated.

The following behavioral patterns or circumstances are typically evident in self-destructive youth.

1. There is poor communication with relatives. Part of the difficulty stems from the fact that there is often a communication gap between young people and older ones, like parents, who might help them. A potentially suicidal individual is more likely to communicate with another interested individual or peer than with his own parents. If it seems that a young person cannot talk to his parents, the listener should be alert to any subtleties that may signal a serious problem.

2. The victim often gives away items of personal value. A personally treasured possession may be given away with the comment that it is no longer needed. This act may signal a feeling of finality and hopelessness in the person's life.

3. Isolation may become apparent. The tendency to withdraw and isolate oneself from others is an ominous sign. Even if the person is

naturally retiring, a change from customary behavior will still be evident. Moroseness of mood is a corollary to this sign. Less frequently, a forced jolliness will appear as an effort to cover up the feelings underneath the mask. The *I Pagliacci*, or heartbroken clown, syndrome can manifest itself in this way.

4. Insomnia and worry may appear. Sleeplessness, worry, and loss of appetite are some of the clues to depression in adults, but they may not always show themselves in adolescents.

5. Frequently young males have lost their fathers. Through death or divorce many young males have not experienced a good and enduring relationship with their fathers. This loss usually occurs before the age of 16 years. The fathers are likely to have been quite successful in business or in a profession when this phenomenon appears in the middle classes.

6. Young women are apt to have self-centered mothers. Among females who attempt suicide, there is likely to be a rather domineering, demanding, and narcissistic mother and a weak father figure. The girl may frequently think she is pregnant, whether she is or not.

7. Heavy smoking is usually very apparent, a fact that suggests the presence of severe tension and anxiety.

8. Job or academic performance often drops. Performance in school and general efficiency are likely to decline rather sharply from previous levels.

9. Substance abuse may be in evidence. Heavy ingestion of drugs or alcohol is likely to accompany anxiety, depression, and self-destructive thoughts.

10. Prior acts of suicidal behavior often exist. A history of previous attempts or threats is apt to be apparent and may have gone unnoticed or been disregarded. Instances of prior self-poisoning can be indicators, even though they may appear to have been accidental.

11. Child abuse may contribute. If a pattern of child abuse has been observed, this is cause for serious concern. Clinical evidence continues to show that future violence, including suicidal acts, may be related to child abuse. Feelings of psychological abuse, which are more difficult to assess, are also to be considered in the same category.

In addition to the foregoing behavioral indicators, verbal attitudes also provide useful clues. Verbalizations about martyrdom or expressions of hostility or resentment toward another person should be noted. The wish to take one's life and be martyred and the desire to even a score by punishing those survivors left behind are frequent components in suicidal behavior. Verbalization may be indirect, with another person the focus of the conversation, but the content will reveal suicidal ideation.

Predictability Having perceived the important clues that may add up to suicide, it is quite possible to predict the likelihood of its occurrence. Although one can never be certain, since suicidal thought may be present and not acted upon, the likelihood of preventing a tragedy increases tremendously when predictability is based upon the perception of solid clinical evidence. The rating scale shown in Table 11-1 can

Table 11-1	SUICIDAL BEHAVIOR CHECKLIST AND RATING SCALE*			
	Factor	Low	Medium	High
	Sex			
	Sexual orientation (female, male, homosexual): female heterosexuals are generally low; male heterosexuals are high; homosexuals are medium to high)	1	3	5
	Marital status			
	In general married persons are lowest, single persons next, divorced next, and widowed among the highest	1 2	3 4	5
	Plan			
	Lethality of method: Ingesting a few pills of a benign type would likely be low, whereas ingesting pills of a more lethal variety or self-inflicted gunshot wound would be high	1 3	5 7	10
	Availability of method: Benign pills—low; lethal pills or firearms at hand—high	1 2	3 4	5
	Specificity: No evidence of plan—low; carefully laid plan—high	1 3	5 7	10
	Cause of death			
	Natural—low; homicidal—medium; accidental—medium to high; suspected suicidal—high; homicide may be victim-precipitated	1 2	3 4	5

Ratings for suspicious accidental deaths:
1 Falls, clearly fortuitous
4 Falls, not clearly fortuitous
2 Fires and flames
3 Electric current
3 Gas and vapors
3 Drowning
4 Solids and liquids
4 Personal medical neglect, such as diabetic coma
3 Firearms and explosives, self-inflicted
5 Cutting and piercing

Stress
    Recent death of significant other person, 1 3   5 7   10
        upsetting divorce, loss of job, time in
        jail, and so on; personal reaction
        determines level

Behavior symptoms
    Disturbances in sleep, eating, sex habits, 1 3   5 7   10
        mood, fatigability; feelings of
        haplessness, helplessness, and
        hopelessness; presence of known
        alcoholism or drug abuse

Agitated mood
    Agitation alone, 1 to 3; agitation plus 1 2   3 4   5
        depression, 4 or 5

Self-blame
    Suspected but not clear, 1 to 3; clear, 4 1 2   3 4   5
        or 5

Personal resources
    Adequacy of available friends, family, 1 3   5 7   10
        employer, clergy

Rejection by "significant other" person
    Suspected, 1 to 5; clearly in evidence, 7 1 3   5 7   10
        to 10

Medical status
    Medical health reasonably good, 1 to 3; 1 2   3 4   5
        serious medical problem, 4 or 5

Personal interaction
    Ability to interact and communicate with 1 2   3 4   5
        others, 1, 2, or 3, if depression not
        apparent; if difficulty in
        communication, and withdrawal or
        despondency are evident, rating is 4
        or 5

Total score _____
(sum of all scores in each row)

Probability of suicide: <50 = low,   >50 = high

Low	*Relatively Low*	*Relatively High*	*High*	*Extremely High*
40	40–50	50–60	60–70	>70

---

*The author is indebted to N. L. Farberow, R. E. Litman, and the staff of the Los Angeles Suicide Prevention Center for part of the information contained herein.

provide a helpful index for the prediction of suicidal behavior. The
factors listed are generally regarded as the most significant ones in the
assessment of suicidal behavior. Until quite recently age was considered to be of significance in the prediction of suicidal acts, but with the
increase in suicide among the young, it no longer seems to be. For that
reason age has been left out of the checklist. As you may note, the
checklist includes comments about each factor in making a determination with respect to the rating scale. For example, although females
attempt suicide, they do not commit the act with the frequency that
males do. One reason for this is the method employed, since ingestion
of pills occurs more frequently with females, whereas guns and
explosives are used by men. To be sure, the lethality of method is an
important component, regardless of which sex employs it. Among the
causes of death one may establish ratings for suspicious accidental
deaths by utilizing the number suggested by each event. To illustrate, if
a fall is clearly accidental, it would receive a rating of only 1, whereas if
there was much doubt about whether it was accidental, perhaps with
some indication that the individual may have jumped, then it would
receive a rating of 4, even though the evidence was not conclusive.
Those aspects of predictability that receive a possible score of 10 as the
high point are clearly the most significant. An individual who is going
to be an effective suicide prevention worker would need to be especially adept in determining those aspects of the prediction scale. The total
score is obtained by simply adding all of the columns and then
summing the rows, or in other words, adding the total points scored for
each factor. The probability would be determined with 50 as a
midpoint, which would separate the probability of suicide into high
and low categories.

Preventability The following preventive procedures may be employed by both the professional and nonprofessional in rendering
psychological first aid and dealing with the crisis of suicide.

1. *Listen.* The first thing that anyone in a mental crisis needs is to
have someone available who will actually listen to what is being said.
So often do we have preconceived notions that we wish to superimpose
upon the potential victim that we shut off effective communication.
Every effort should be made to understand the feelings behind the
words expressed.

2. *Evaluate the seriousness of the person's thoughts and feelings.*
All suicidal talk should be taken very seriously. If the person has made
carefully laid plans, then clearly the problem is a more acute one than if
his thinking is less definite.

3. *Evaluate the intensity of the emotional problem.* A person need
not be openly upset to be suicidal. It is quite possible, on the contrary,
that a patient may be extremely upset but not actually suicidal. On the
other hand, sometimes patients who have made a decision to take their
lives can appear calmer than we expect. If the individual has been

depressed and suddenly becomes agitated, moving about in a restless manner, it is cause for alarm.

4. *Accept each complaint and feeling that the patient expresses.* Do not make the mistake of undervaluing and dismissing what may seem to be a minor complaint. To the patient it may be very serious and indicative of a critical problem. In some cases the person may express his difficulty in a low key, but beneath a seeming calm, deeply disturbed feelings are apparent.

5. *Do not be afraid to ask the person directly if he has entertained thoughts of suicide.* Suicide may be suspected, but not really mentioned, during an emotional crisis. Experience has shown that little harm is done by inquiring into such thought at an appropriate time. This should be done after the interview is well along in time. Frequently the person in crisis will welcome any direct inquiry and will be willing to discuss the subject openly.

6. *Beware of apparent quick recoveries.* Frequently the person will experience initial relief after talking about his problem and will mistakenly state that he is past the crisis. Subsequently, however, the problem may recur, and follow-up is crucial in ensuring an effective intervention program.

7. *Be supportive, yet affirmative.* Stable guideposts are an absolute necessity in the life of a disturbed person. In essence, provide the individual with your strength by giving the impression that you are in command of the situation and intend to do everything possible to prevent him from taking his life.

8. *Evaluate available resources.* The person may have both inner resources (psychologically) and outer resources (in his environment). His psychological resources are those of intellectualization and rationalization, with the hope of strengthening himself in the future. If these are all absent, the problem is a serious one, and additional support and observation will be necessary.

9. *Act specifically.* It is very important that something tangible be done for the patient, such as arranging for him to see a professional person or a clergyman later. It is frustrating for a person to feel that he has received nothing from the interview.

10. *Be ready to ask for assistance and consultation.* One should feel free to call upon whoever is needed, depending upon the severity of the problem. It is unwise to try to manage everything alone. An attitude should be conveyed of composure, so that the potential victim will feel that something appropriate and realistic is being done to help him.

11. *Never treat the individual with horror or attempt to persuade him to deny his suicidal thoughts.* Sometimes it is particularly damaging to comment that the person cannot actually mean it when he talks of suicide. This implicitly condemns the person's feelings, which are very real to him.

12. *Never challenge the potential victim or attempt to shock him out of a suicidal act.* For example, telling the person to go ahead and

take his life, with the belief that such a comment will shock him into clearer thinking, is fallacious and may precipitate a tragedy.

13. *Mention that if the choice is to die, the decision is irreversible.* As long as life exists, there is always a chance for problem resolution; death ends every possibility for improvement.

14. *Point out that depressed feelings will pass.* Depressions are self-limiting and tend to run their course. If the person will continue on, he can be reassured that matters will get better.

15. *Never leave the person alone during an acute crisis.* Isolation and lack of personal contact greatly increases the probability of suicide.

Professional persons, including psychologists and psychiatrists, are not the first individuals usually contacted in a suicidal crisis. It is more probable that clergy, teachers, parents, close friends, beauty operators, bartenders, or co-workers would be the first contact in time of stress. With this thought in mind, courses for bartenders have been set up in Wisconsin and California to help spot potential suicidal persons and establish a liaison with the local suicide prevention center. In particular, policemen need to learn how to handle suicidal crises because they are often called upon to deal with such problems. Unfortunately, in most instances, law enforcement officers have little training in psychological first aid and frequently make tragic errors. Everyone, however, is potentially a gatekeeper, and the principles for assisting in time of suicidal crisis are broadly the same. By keeping in mind many of the points mentioned here, it is possible that many lives that are unnecessarily lost by suicide could be saved each year.

TAKING ACTION

1. *Using the rating scale and checklist information found in Table 11-1, evaluate the death or attempted death of a person described in a newspaper or magazine.*
2. *If you know of a friend or family member who has experienced mental depression or suicidal thoughts, evaluate them with the scale, and discuss the results openly so that they may be encouraged to seek professional help, if that is indicated.*
3. *Role-play a crisis intervention session between crisis worker and potential suicide victim. See whether you can pick up clues to potential suicidal behavior.*
4. *Go to a crisis center, and interview a crisis worker about interactions with potential suicide victims.*
5. *Evaluate and discuss your community's activities involving crisis intervention services.*

**THE CRISIS
OF RAPE**   Forcible rape is the "carnal knowledge" of a woman through the use of force or threat of force. "Statutory" rape, or sexual intercourse with a girl defined a minor (under 14 or 21, depending on the state), will not be covered in this category because the "victim" is willing or even,

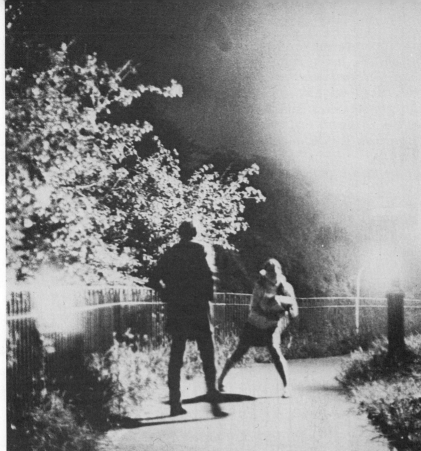

Lida Moser—DPI

perhaps, the initiator. The offenses classified are broken down by actual forcible rapes and attempted forcible rapes. There has been a suggestion by some professionals that any sexual activity against one's will constitutes rape. Although this may be so psychologically, such a view has not found support in the legal arena, particularly in a marital relationship in which the husband is supposedly justified in forcing the wife. Numerous other sexual assaults can justifiably be termed rape, such as those occurring among male prisoners. However, the emphasis in this chapter is on rape crisis involving an assault of a male upon a female. This phenomenon has led to the creation of numerous rape crisis centers throughout the country recently, as well as an increased focus of attention upon the problem.

A marked increase in forcible rape has occurred during the past several years. In the time span between 1968 and 1973 the percent change in the number of offenses increased 62 percent, while the rate per 100,000 inhabitants went up 55 percent, according to *Uniform Crime Reports* from the U.S. Department of Justice. Rape has continued to climb by several percentage points each year since 1968.

The age group most involved appears to be males between 16 and 24 years old. As an illustration, about 61 percent of the arrests for forcible

399

rape are for persons under the age of 25 years. Some 47 percent of the persons arrested for forcible rape are black and 51 percent are Caucasians; "all other races" comprise the remaining 2 percent. The term "all other races" traditionally used in keeping statistics by the number of city, county, state, and federal agencies is actually a misnomer. It should be noted that racial groups are often confused with color differences. This is apt to contribute to misleading statistical information.

Although a problem of reporting has existed, this appears to be lessening. Recently, a rate of 47 per 100,000 females reported the incident. The number of unreported rapes is still believed to be several times higher than those reported, however. For the core cities, with populations in excess of 250,000, the victim risk rate is about 100 per 100,000 females. In the suburban areas the risk rate is 35 per 100,000 whereas the risk rate is 23 per 100,000 in rural areas; thus, the urban rate has provided a clear contrast with those in suburban and rural areas. Statistics indicate that nearly three-fourths of all forcible rape offenses were actual rapes by force, with the remaining one-fourth being assaults or attempts to commit rape.

It is interesting to note that three out of every four adults arrested for forcible rape in a single year were prosecuted for this offense. Prosecution does not imply sentencing; it merely means bringing to trial on charges of rape. Various problems of prosecution account for acquittals or dismissals in nearly half of the cases.

Dos and Don'ts

What to do and what to avoid doing constitute practical components of interest to every female citizen. A number of procedures have been suggested, both anecdotally and in the literature, concerning the most advisable behavior in a rape crisis. It seems that the essence of a successful reaction in most situations is to do the unexpected. An unexpected response tends to disarm the would-be rapist so that the original thought or plan does not continue on its expected course. There is always a preconceived notion in the rapist's mind about how to carry out the act and how the event will go. He often begins by making a survey of apartment house nameplates, as well as of isolated laundromats, parks, or other places habitually used by women. He wants to make sure that the victim is alone. Statistics have shown that some three-fourths of the women are single. Thus in the rapist's mind the act has been designed to proceed in a definite and relatively trouble-free fashion. In a general way he may expect some resistance, but by and large he hopes for and even expects at least partial compliance. He dreams of himself as a strong, attractive, and irresistible lover. He is likely to fantasy the woman yielding to him, even passionately, after initial, mild resistance. In some investigations of this matter women who did not resist or did so halfheartedly were usually those who were raped. Contrary to highly publicized and popular opinion, most rapes do not end in murder. Hence the prevailing belief that women who strongly resist will be violently beaten and murdered is usually not borne out in fact. When a rapist's threats work, his preconceived image of the event is proceeding according to plan and the rape will be accomplished. Often the plan is not one of direct sexual intercourse but of variations of it. Anal and oral types of intercourse are more common than traditional vaginal penetration. Rapists assess their victims, where possible, in terms of the kind of response they are going to get. If the response is not an acceptable one, the rapist will usually not proceed. Unsatisfactory responses are not in line with the rapist's expectancies and plans.

There have been instances where the delivery of unusual responses turned the man off, so to speak. These have included such things as urinating, belching, vomiting, flatulence (farting), nose picking, or bursting into a patriotic song. These all fit the unexpected category and may serve to disarm the rapist—that is, disrupt his plan and defuse his ardor.

Procedures for Behavior in the Rape Crisis

A handy memory device, when confronted with a potential rape situation, is to recall the first letter of the word "rape" as a key to action: R—resist, A—attack, P—protest, E—escape. Resistance, like other aspects of successful action, can take several forms. Women can and should resist physically and attitudinally. Persons who are overly friendly, compliant, and soft are easy victims. Even though rapists may hate women consciously or unconsciously and possess many conflicting negative thoughts about them, they do not want or expect serious trouble.

When attacking the rapist, it is best to employ the most effective means at one's disposal. Useful procedures include kicking and elbowing. Scratching, biting, and hair pulling are less effective. The intended victim should kick sharply against the knee or shinbone with the heel or stomp on the foot. All such action should be violent and rapid. The chief reason for attack is to disable the attacker long enough to become free. Blows of these types will do the trick if practiced for effectiveness. Many women feel that carrying a sharp instrument, such as a long hatpin, a pair of cuticle scissors, a nail file, or a beer can opener, is of value. Although there is no doubt that, when properly used, each of these instruments can do some damage, there is frequently little likelihood that these instruments can be sufficiently applied when needed. Moreover, although most rapists are not homicidal, a mild painful injury could serve to anger them enough to harm the woman in question. One procedure that can be helpful, in some instances, must be deftly applied. A set of keys, inserted between the fingers in a closed fist, can do great damage to the eyes of a rapist. This procedure, like the others, must be applied quickly and with great precision. If the woman misses, it will merely scratch or cut the rapist's face and may not accomplish its purpose.

Of course, if the situation can be handled verbally and with noise,

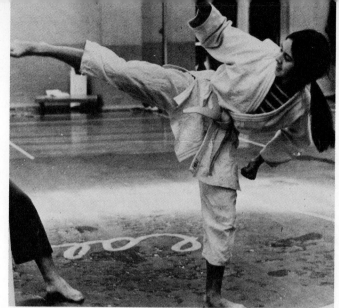

Young woman learning karate for self-defense.

Wide World Photos

that's safest. In protesting, the victim should do so loudly and repeatedly, so as to attract attention to the incident and frighten the attacker away. No rapist wants to be caught in the act by another man, who might inflict severe injury upon him. Any form of continuous loud noise will serve as an alarm; screaming, yelling, or using a whistle are examples. If a woman carries a whistle, she should keep it in her hand, ready for use. It is of little value buried in the bottom of a purse during time of need. Rapists sometimes anticipate a quick scream and may be prepared to clamp a hand over the mouth of the victim. They do not anticipate continuous noise, however. Making noise for help implies that there are or might be people around. Stay out of isolated areas!

When escaping, the intended victim should run to the nearest lighted and populated area. Rapists will rarely pursue a victim who is moving toward light and people. Except for teenage group assaults, rapes are not committed in front of other persons or in lighted areas. Darkness provides the necessary cover that makes the rapist feel most comfortable. Even when sexual assaults have been carried out in the victim's apartment, the lights are usually dimmed or extinguished by the rapist.

An Ounce of Prevention

Anticipating trouble is the best way to avoid it. Remembering these simple precautions will spare the potential victim much trouble.

1. Avoid lonely, darkened areas.
2. Avoid traveling alone.
3. Light entryways to your abode, and lock doors and windows.
4. Avoid displaying a telephone listing or mailbox nameplate that makes it obvious that the inhabitant is a female, especially one living alone or solely with other women.

402

TAKING ACTION

1. *Contact the various crisis centers in your community to find out where rape centers are located. Make arrangements to interview the staff or obtain information about procedures followed by the rape center, and jot down important points.*
2. *Make an appointment, through the clerk of a municipal or district court, to attend a hearing that is being held regarding any aspect of crisis behavior and mental health, including rape. A day in court can be very revealing.*
3. *Tape-record a conversation with a woman who has been raped. Play the recording to the class and encourage classroom discussion.*
4. *Check into the laws of your state concerning rape, including statutory rape.*
5. *Does your college have any kind of program designed to help rape victims or teach rape prevention techniques. Investigate and discuss.*

When marital crises continue to recur and are not resolved, they usually end in divorce. Divorce is a crisis itself and can carry with it emotional scars that should be handled in a therapeutic manner. Marital relationships that are basically sound can be salvaged through professional counseling; however, unions that lack such stability are likely to terminate in divorce, assault, suicide, or homicide.

CRISES IN MARITAL RELATIONSHIPS AND CHILD ABUSE

Most homicides occur primarily within families and frequently involve marital partners. Indeed, only one homicide in 10 involves a stranger. Violent behavior ending in homicide is associated with close personal ties and is largely a domestic crime involving wives, husbands, lovers, and children. Moreover, slayings usually involve offenders and victims of the same ethnic and racial group. Statistics reveal that only 6 percent of the homicides committed indicate that the offender crossed a racial line. When a man kills a woman, he is likely to take her life in the bedroom. Women kill their mates more often than men do, and they ordinarily do it in the kitchen. When a man takes the life of another man, he is just as likely to do it at home as away from home.

One of the most regrettable aspects of a bad marriage is the deleterious effect it has upon offspring. For example, 87 percent of the cases of male schizophrenia in one study were shown to come from families with marital incompatibility and discord, as compared to 13 percent in a control group. In an investigation of convicted female felons, roughly two-thirds had been married but became separated or divorced. In numerous instances of sexual deviance, such as in child molestation, rape, masochism, and sadism, bad marital relationships are in evidence on the part of the offender, as well as in his family background.

Parents who abuse their children come from a wide variety of educational, racial, and ethnic and socioeconomic backgrounds, but the majority come from the lower classes. Lower-class fathers, in particular, are more likely to threaten and abuse children than are

403

middle-class fathers. Some 90 percent of the families involved have been shown to have serious social problems, unhappy marriages, and financial difficulties. An ongoing state of anger and hostility is pervasive among abusive parents. Ordinary difficulties in child rearing will suffice to trigger a violent expression of anger against the child. Many parents reject the child and blame the youngster for the problem. Such parents have a history of emotional instability. Their own childhoods were usually marked by overly strict rearing and a deprivation of parental guidance and emotional warmth. A parent of either sex may assault or abuse children both physically and psychologically. There may be a tendency for mothers to kill female children more often than male children. Fathers are equally likely to kill a child of either sex. An additional tragic outcome is the fact that children who are treated cruelly by their parents are likely to develop hostile attitudes toward their own families, become deeply disturbed adults, and in turn abuse their own children. Thus the cycle is perpetuated into future generations.

Parental neglect and abuse of children do not necessarily occur together. When a child's basic needs are not met, the parent is neglecting his or her responsibilities. In our society there is a growing tendency to insist that children are entitled not only to food, clothing, and shelter but to the assurance that they are wanted and loved. Some forms of neglect are quite obvious, but many others are more subtle. Both neglect and abuse can be psychological or emotional as well as physical, although the former type is rarely reported or acted upon because it is more elusive and difficult to substantiate. Essentially parents abuse children for these reasons: (1) an immature parent sees the child's actions as annoying and does not know any other way to manage the situation; (2) the abusive parent was beaten by his or her own parents; (3) the offending parent is mentally or emotionally severely disturbed.

It will be useful for you to understand some of the psychodynamics underlying these reasons. None of the things listed can excuse child abuse, but they may serve to explain it. Hitting a defenseless child is inexcusable by any account. We must place squarely at our own doorstep part of the reason for child abuse, since it is inherent in the North American culture that punishment of children for wrongdoing is the order of the day. The mistaken assumption that punishment is character-building, plus the old principle of "an eye for an eye," comprise two notions underlying such a position. "What that youngster needs is a good whipping" is the prescription readily offered for unwanted behavior. Over 90 percent of American and British parents evidently follow this prescription. The prisons are full of inhabitants who got regularly "good whippings" as children. The Boston strangler recalled the nightly strappings he received from his father's belt—"whether I needed it or not," as he put it.

The parent who beats a child actually hates the child, hates other people, and hates herself or himself. The late A. S. Neill, who developed Summerhill, the famous experimental school for children in Britain, stated that it was incomprehensible to him how adults could consider themselves good Christians (or other religious believers) and still beat children. The thrust of his thesis was that children become what adults make them. Neill also held that any mother who has a loving, satisfying sexual relationship with her husband would not be likely to strike a child. There is little doubt that frustration takes its toll. Many of us have heard a mother, for example, scream at a youngster: "I'll beat you to within an inch of your life if you don't mind me." Such intense hostility and obvious hatred is being displaced from within the parent to the child. A person who hates wants to hit and strike out. The hostility is foisted upon a helpless youngster because the parent cannot often bring herself or himself to strike another adult. Any person who strikes another deserves, perhaps, to be hit in return, including parents who hit children; yet if a child strikes back at an adult, the latter's weak ego is threatened, and the youngster is further endangered.

Early on we should learn that we cannot get our way by going through life hitting people. Parents will sometimes delude themselves that they are punishing a child for his own good. This constitutes a foolish self-deception, where the parent plays the role of a dictator or god.

How often have we heard parents say, "Nothing seems to help. I spank him and he still doesn't seem to learn!" They have no conception of the rudiments of learning. What punishment does is to evoke fear and hatred in the child. The youngster associates the punishment with the punisher rather than the undesirable act that caused the parent to administer it in the first place. At best, it only suppresses the act for a short period. It will return because nothing has been taught to take its place, and resentment toward the punisher still remains, even if at an unconscious level. Youngsters will sometimes conform superficially for a time, out of fear, but the hatred of the parent has already been established. Punishment is always an expression of hatred. The child will read it as such. The resentment and hatred evoked in the child stimulates fear of further punishment and an unconscious feeling of shame for wishing the parent harm as a retribution. This may cause the child to cover it by an expression of regret or a display of affection, but it is a pseudo love that the child shows. The bitterness and hatred of the parent remain beneath the surface. Depending upon its intensity, at best the youngster will likely grow up to become an unhappy, punishing parent, or, at worst, one of the many criminals who fill our prisons each year.

Another factor contributing to the problem is the fact that we not only tolerate but glorify violence. The media and motion pictures continue to promote acts of this kind and give it a heroic quality. It is small wonder then that we have begun to produce more tyrannical leaders and have moved in the frightening direction of dictatorial control of society in recent times. Punishment is not the only way to learn or even the most effective way. Reinforcing desirable behavior and instilling personal responsibility through self-development are the cornerstones of maturity and self-reliance. Even though it is not easy to spare the rod, it will be the courageous and farsighted parents of the future whose children will be responsible, happy leaders. Those who are willing to painstakingly teach children to learn by accentuating the positive rather than attempting to eliminate what they perceive as annoying negatives through the use of physical and psychological punishment will contribute most to the world of tomorrow.

A basic view of motivation lies at the core of our attitudes toward children. Is a child born basically positive, negative, or neither? The terms "good" and "bad" are too halo-laden or negative and have been avoided here for that reason. Some believe that humankind is basically social ("good") because we must depend upon others for our survival, more than any other species. The human infant is the most helpless organism on earth. Survival is completely contingent upon others for appreciably longer periods of time than for infrahumans. This interrelationship of parent and child sets the stage for cooperation, mutual interaction, positive attitudes, and love in later life, so as to procreate the species. Humans require a particular kind of cooperation and affection in order to sustain life, both the life in themselves and in their offspring; otherwise, humankind would destroy itself. People's finest motives become sidetracked in the maelstrom of a negatively oriented society. When we drive our cars under a certain speed limit, do we do so because we fear getting a traffic ticket or for some better motive? All too often, it may be the former rather than the latter. We ought to drive at reasonable speeds because we wish to see and enjoy our surroundings more easily, we will place less strain on our nerves and our cars, and there is far less likelihood of inflicting injury upon someone else, and so on. It is just as easy, and critically important to society's welfare, to employ learning principles in a positive sense as in a negative one. In fact the future progress of the human race will hinge upon it as the world becomes more populated and living becomes more complex. Suicide can be traced in part to immaturity stemming from either overindulgence or severe punishment, while homicide is traceable to harsh rearing, characterized by severe punishment and violence.

A number of characteristics seem to set abusive parents apart from nonabusive ones. Some of the most significant are as follows: (1) the abusive parent subscribes strongly to the idea of physical punishment; (2) regardless of social class, most parents assert that the youngster should know "right" from "wrong" by the age of 12 months or sooner; (3) most of these parents prefer their children to be good—that is, obedient, nonrebellious, grateful, and respectful—rather than adventuresome or creative; (4) emphasis is placed upon cleanliness and materialistic values; (5) abusive mothers describe an ideal father in terms of one who is a disciplinarian and capable of providing financial support; (6) these mothers are far more authoritarian than nonabusive ones; (7) such persons tend to be compulsively oriented, as manifested by the tendency to be very good housekeepers (that is, well-ordered and neat); (8) mothers have poor self-control and are attracted to men with similar problems, often wishing to place the father in a bad light so they may appear sympathetic by comparison; (9) much marital discord is evident, with the occurrence of frequent separations and reconciliations; (10) the most common method of discipline is whipping and spanking, with scolding, shaming, and physical shaking following close behind; (11) reasoning or avoidance of conflict are procedures seldom employed, even with children old enough to comprehend; (12) abusive parents view small infants as deliberately misbehaving and in need of discipline; (13) they possess negative feelings toward the abused child; (14) emotional problems such as depression are common; (15) abusive mothers have usually shown uncontrollable actions in the past, including aggression against other women, some sexual promiscuity, and secret, compulsive spending, and they tend to be afraid of some man in their lives, either their own fathers or their husbands; (16) these mothers are lonely and have had poor relationships with one or both parents.

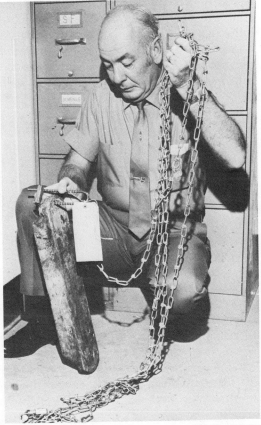

Policeman holding a 50-pound weight and chain found shackled to a 12-year-old girl by her father.

In order to spare a child from abuse, it is necessary to spot these problems early and secure help for both the parent and the youngster, as needed. Professionals should be alert to the fact that many children are born very close together. The pressures of child rearing, along with marital strain, financial difficulties, and isolation, tend to overwhelm young mothers. Premature births may provide an additional stress. Young mothers need to be taught basic concepts about health, growth, and development in children. This ought to include an understanding of the child's emotional as well as physical needs. Much of this material should be incorporated into the educational curricula of both elementary and secondary school systems. Young girls and boys can learn to appreciate the emotional needs of babies and other children, and they can act responsibly only in terms of their age levels. A common problem is the overexpectation and the unreasonable demands that abusive parents make upon their children. For example, when a young mother says she expects a child to be "good" and "act respectful," she is really expecting the youngster to act like an adult rather than a child. It will suffice to say that this is totally unrealistic and will lead to serious difficulty if not understood by the parent.

Appropriate birth control methods should be made easily available, since unwanted children are a high risk for child abuse. The intercorrelation between isolation, lack of education, unplanned children, and financial and marital strain produces the seeds that lead to marital discord and subsequent child abuse. Being alert to these difficulties can save marriages and children's lives as well.

Some Typical Signs of Child Abuse

The following are some typical signs of child abuse:

1. Bruises and abrasions on the back of the body or on the sides of the head and face.
2. Fractured bones, particularly on very young children and infants.
3. Evidence of burns, especially from cigarettes or cigars.
4. Tendency to offer excuses or other explanations for the incident by both parents.
5. Apprehension, fear, or avoidance of any discussion on the part of the child.

Most children who injure themselves from falls or other accidents will damage only the front part of the knees, legs, hands, elbows, and face; almost never the sides of the face or back of the body. Because of threats made toward youngsters, they are reluctant to discuss the issue and may be afraid they will be placed in an unknown environment, which is even more disturbing to them than their own homes. Curiously, some youngsters may appear to love abusive parents despite the injuries they suffer. Children will often seem to forgive parents much cruelty in return for an occasional display of attention, as evidenced by the purchase of a toy or some desired object, but deep hurt and resentment remain.

TAKING ACTION

1. *Consult your local county attorney's office and welfare office to seek answers to these questions:*
   a. *What constitutes child abuse?*
   b. *Are parents who spank their children committing child abuse?*
   c. *Is child neglect equal to child abuse?*
   d. *What are the procedures that should be followed in reporting suspected child neglect or abuse?*
   e *Can any citizen report suspected child abuse without running the risk of being sued for falsely accusing an innocent parent?*
   f. *Are professional persons and public officials liable to prosecution if they do not report suspected child neglect or abuse?*
2. *Make a chart of children's rights and parents' rights, based upon laws in your community.*
3. *Discuss the topic of "Children's Lib."*
4. *Discuss with your parents (or parents you know) their views on effective discipline. Discuss in class alternative forms of punishment to the age-old "spanking." When does spanking become child abuse?*

DISCUSSION

In addition to being only of relatively recent concern to mental health specialists, problems surrounding emergencies and crisis events have begun to reshape themselves in recent years. Traditionally mental health emergencies were viewed in the light of someone who was "crazy" or "dangerous," requiring incarceration. Little thought was given to the stresses of personal life and everyday living that affect most of the population—those who would not be included in these categories. The plain fact is that most persons encounter mental disorders or emotional crises at certain points in their lives, and at such times they are sorely in need of assistance. If handled in a timely and appropriate manner, most of these problems are short-lived and need not continue to plague the individual for protracted periods of time. Emotional crises are triggered or enhanced by numerous situations, such as biological stress accompanying menopause, pressures of school, economic and financial stress, loss of a loved one, or the consequences of an overwhelming natural disaster.

Besides the community mental health center movement, which has been government financed, numerous independent and private clinics and centers that focus upon mental health crises have mushroomed during the past several years. The spirit of the times is partly responsible for this burgeoning of interest. It encompasses such phenomena as the unpopular Vietnamese War, socioeconomic conditions and unemployment, problems accompanying drug abuse, and the disintegration of the family unit of the past. The younger generation has been particularly victimized by these phenomena. The need to emancipate oneself from parental authority and "do one's own thing" serves as a two-edged sword. The newfound freedoms, without stable guideposts, constitute difficulties that are often in themselves frustrating and

409

insurmountable. The various programs of the type mentioned have not really attempted to address themselves to these problems. The structural and organizational components of such operations have varied widely. Some of the differences that appear in these programs are worthy of note. Central among them is the fact that community mental health centers place emphasis upon program continuity, incorporating five essential ingredients in order to receive funding: outpatient treatment, inpatient treatment, partial hospitalization, consultation and education, and emergency mental health services. In contrast with so-called "hot-line" operations, essential criteria for suicide prevention and crisis intervention services include the utilization of such minimal standards as: 24-hour-a-day service, seven days a week; a basic training program for crisis workers; a walk-in service offering face-to-face contact; a referral system to appropriate community and professional resources; and access to professional consultation, when needed.

The staffing patterns of these centers may vary, depending upon the needs of the population to be served. Community mental health center programs customarily include personnel from all of the three major professional services: psychologists, psychiatrists, and social workers. Nurses and volunteer workers can also be active participants. The director may come from any of the professional disciplines, with appropriate training and experience. The staffing pattern of crisis intervention and suicide prevention centers frequently comprises a director, who is a professional person, professionally trained assistants, and volunteers of both a professional and nonprofessional type. The effective utilization of volunteers has been a crucial component in the crisis intervention and suicide prevention movement to a larger extent than any other single treatment effort in recent times. One of the primary strengths of these programs has been the widespread use of adaptable, trained, and dedicated members of society, who have been willing to serve with little or no monetary compensation. College students have often served well; you may wish to volunteer.

FOR FURTHER READING

Frederick, C. J., 1972. *Dealing with the Crisis of Suicide.* Public Affairs Pamphlet 406A. New York: Public Affairs Committee, Inc.

A comprehensive pamphlet dealing with the basics of psychological first aid.

McGee, R. K., 1974. *Crisis Intervention in the Community.* Baltimore: University Park Press.

Written for professional, paraprofessional, and volunteer workers in community mental health centers, the book emphasizes the value of a team approach in the development of crisis intervention programs.

Neill, A. S., 1960. *Summerhill.* New York: Hart.

A description of the philosophy behind a world-renowned British school for child rearing. It recognizes the innate worth of the child and places responsibility upon the youngster for his own behavior.

Wittenberg, C., 1971. *Studies of Child Abuse and Infant Accidents in the Mental Health of the Child*, J. S. Segal, ed. Public Health Service Publication 2168. Washington, D.C.: U.S. Government Printing Office.

The study disclosed that abused children are in serious jeopardy and may even die or become severely retarded as a result of parental neglect and abuse. The subjects constituted 50 former patients and their families from the Children's Hospital in Pittsburgh.

Wolfgang, M. E., 1969. Who Kills Whom? *Behavior Today* 3:55–75.

The author draws on his own and other investigators' studies. The concept of victim-precipitated homicide is discussed at some length.

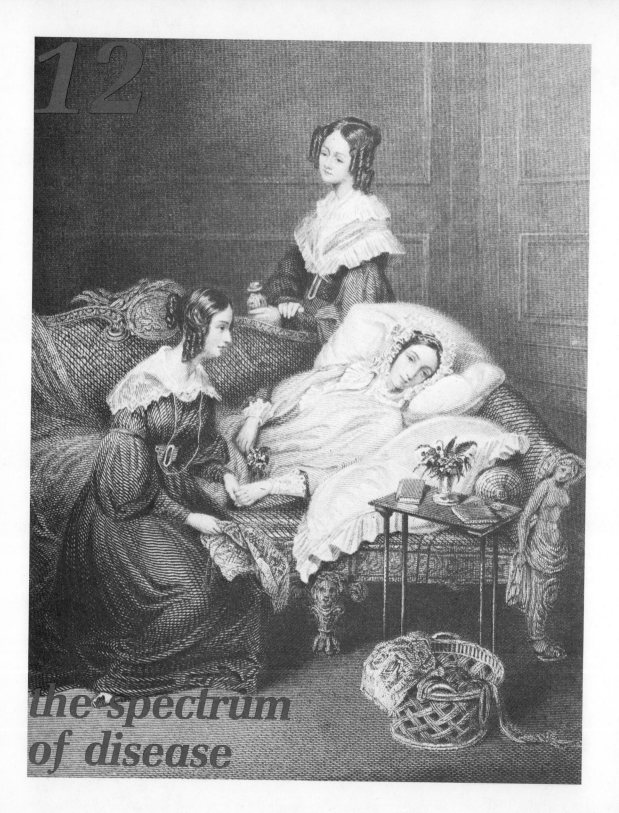

12

the spectrum
of disease

*We begin this chapter by reviewing the evolution of our concepts
of disease and our efforts to cope with them. This is followed by
an overview of the spectrum of disease in the United States and
around the world, with special reference to health problems of
young adults. The infectious diseases are described and
contrasted with the chronic diseases in terms of their frequency,
overall impact, and changing patterns over time. Recent medical
advances in cancer and other diseases are summarized. The costs
of medical care and research are then discussed in the context of
gross national product, the national budget, and private
expenditures for various necessities and luxuries. Selected
problems of particular relevance to young adults living in the last
quarter of the twentieth century include venereal disease, the
contraceptive pill, and smoking.*

INQUIRY

1. Can cancer be cured?
2. How does the contraceptive pill work?
3. What type of disease is increasing more rapidly among teenagers
   and young adults than any other today?
4. What disease causes more death and disability than any other in the
   United States?
5. What common disease continues to flourish because people won't
   talk about it openly?
6. How much money do we spend each year on medical research
   compared with that spent on alcoholic beverages, cigarettes, candy,
   hair sprays, and defense?

INTRODUCTION

Health is a word that cannot be readily defined. For want of a better
definition, it is often held to mean the absence of disease. This
somewhat negative definition of health poses a number of problems for
us. First of all, it is not precise in the sense that it depends entirely
upon one's definition of disease. The more conditions we consider to
be diseases the less likely is anyone to have good health. What is
disease? Whereas most of us would concede that cancer, kidney failure,
and pancreatitis are diseases, how about the common cold, an uncom-
plicated case of an upset stomach (gastroenteritis), or a simple skiing
fracture of the shin? These conditions imply that it is quite possible to
be healthy and yet to suffer from specific diseases.

To further complicate matters, there is the problem of our own
perception of disease and how this affects whether or not a diagnosis is
made. If we feel well, that is, if we do not perceive the existence of
disease and consequently do not seek the attention of a physician, we
are for practical purposes "healthy," despite the fact that some undiag-

413

nosed disease state (such as an early undetected tumor, an unsymptomatic leakage through a heart valve, or the like) may exist.

You may now understand why it is sometimes as difficult to define "disease" as it is "health." In ancient times diseases were believed to originate from supernatural causes, such as divine punishment for sinful behavior. Other ancient theories of pathogenesis (the development of disease) were based more on the scientific thinking of the day, however faulty, than on faith. For example, some diseases were thought to stem from an imbalance of the four body humors: phlegm, yellow bile, black bile, and red blood. However, metaphysical notions of disease causation have strongly influenced medical practice and community attitudes toward health throughout history. During the Middle Ages, in particular, advances in knowledge on human anatomy and physiology were frustrated because of religious opposition to autopsies as well as to the scientific methods necessary for clinical investigations in man. Even in modern times the belief that diseases can be cured by religious conviction persists among various peoples around the world.

Over the centuries health-related activities have been conducted at two levels: individual and community. Individuals have always sought to have their illnesses treated and, when possible, prevented from occurring. Physicians of one sort or another have been treating patients since the earliest days of recorded history. At the same time communities as a whole often took action to isolate the sick, to sanitize the environment, and otherwise to prevent or reduce the chances for the transmission of disease.

In the succeeding sections of this chapter our principal attention will be focused upon those diseases that are considered to be the most serious as measured by the degree of death and disability that they cause. For college students from South America, Africa, and Asia, quite a different spectrum of diseases would exist. Rather than such chronic conditions as heart disease, cancer, and arthritis, students from the "Third World" would be primarily concerned with many acute, communicable, and epidemic diseases (such as schistosomiasis, malaria, cholera, and so on) as well as with such chronic conditions as malnutrition and dietary protein deficiency. As we shall see, the reasons for the different disease spectra are biological, geographical, and economic, as well as sociocultural.

We will take note of some new developments in medicine, including a number of rather remarkable advances in the prevention or treatment of disease. This will lead us to a consideration of the costs of medical research and of medical care. We will examine these costs both in absolute terms and in relative ones—that is, by comparing them with other expenditures in the national budget.

THE MAJOR CHRONIC AND ACUTE DISEASES

Some diseases kill or permanently disable their victims. Others cause temporary illness or disability from which the patient recovers fully or partially, sometimes spontaneously and sometimes after specific treatment. Let's take a brief look at those diseases which are the principal causes of death and disability in our country today.

Principal Causes of Death in the United States Today

By far, more people die of some form of heart disease than of any other condition. In fact if we combine into one category all diseases of the heart and circulatory system, we can account for slightly more than half of all deaths occurring each year. These deaths may be classified for convenience as follows:

1. One-third are due to *acute myocardial infarction*—that is, a sudden heart attack.
2. One-third are due to *chronic ischemic heart disease*—that is, repeated attacks that affect the circulation of oxygenated blood to the heart.
3. One-third are due to a variety of diseases characterized by *arteriosclerosis* of major blood vessels—that is, stroke, hypertension, certain kidney diseases, and so on.

The second most common cause of death is cancer in one or more of its forms, which we shall be describing in more detail later. Taken by themselves, strokes or cerebrovascular diseases are the third most common cause of death in the United States.

By examining the statistics in Table 12-1, you should be able to confirm that the overall death rate in our population is now slightly below 1 percent. Keep this figure in mind as you read on.

The spectrum of fatal diseases in young adults is quite different from that of persons younger and older. In Table 12-2 you will find rankings of the 10 leading causes of death among males and females of different ages. What is the leading cause of death among persons of college age today? Compare the data in Tables 12-1 and 12-2. In the population as a whole, what percentage of annual deaths are due to accidents? What are the major causes of death in persons aged 15 to 34?

Declining Death Rates of Particular Diseases

Medical knowledge, both basic and applied, has been accumulating at an ever-increasing pace. For example, somewhat less than 100 years ago, with the exception of smallpox there was essentially no disease for which a specific preventive measure or effective treatment was known. Bacteria had not yet been classified, to say nothing of viruses that could not even be visualized under the microscopes of those days. Although surgical operations are known to have been undertaken in ancient Egypt and China, the benefits of what we would now call "modern surgery" did not become widely available until about the time of World War II. Ether anesthesia was developed about 100 years ago, sterile operative techniques some years later, and antibiotics during the World War II. These and other developments have made possible the relatively painless, clean, and safe surgery of today. Contrast this with the situation 75 or 100 years ago when operative mortality was close to 100

Table 12-1

MORTALITY FROM LEADING CAUSES OF DEATH
IN THE UNITED STATES, 1968

Rank	Cause of Death	Number of Deaths	Death Rate per 100,000 Population	Percent of Total Deaths
1	Diseases of heart	744,658	372.6	38.6
2	Cancer	318,547	159.4	16.5
3	Stroke (cerebrovascular diseases)	211,390	105.8	11.0
4	Accidents	114,864	57.5	6.0
	Motor vehicle accidents	54,862	27.5	2.8
	All other accidents	60,002	30.0	3.2
5	Influenza and pneumonia	73,492	36.8	3.8
6	Certain diseases of early infancy	43,840	21.9	2.3
7	Diabetes mellitus	38,352	19.2	2.0
8	Arteriosclerosis	33,568	16.8	1.7
9	Cirrhosis of liver	29,183	14.6	1.5
10	Emphysema	24,185	12.1	1.3
11	Suicide	21,372	10.7	1.1
12	Congenital anomalies	16,793	8.4	0.9
13	Homicide	14,686	7.3	0.8
14	Peptic ulcer	9,460	4.7	0.5
15	Infections of kidney	9,395	4.7	0.5
	Other and ill-defined	226,297	113.3	11.5
	All causes	1,930,082	965.8	100.0

Source: E. Silverberg and A. I. Holleb, 1972, *Ca—A Cancer Journal for Clinicians* 22:2–20. With permission of the American Cancer Society.

percent in most hospitals. Nowadays deaths due to an operation rather than to the underlying disease are a rarity.

Figure 12-1 compares the leading causes of death in the United States in 1900 and in 1968. Have you ever known anyone who had tuberculosis? Are you surprised that this infection of the lungs accounted for more deaths than any other disease as recently as 75 years ago? How many of the other causes of death might have been due to bacteria and other infectious organisms? Pneumonia, diarrhea, enteritis, and diphtheria would all fall into this category, as would certain cases of bronchitis. How does this situation compare with that in 1968?

Examine the disease mortality curves in Figure 12-2. They reflect the entries in death certificates filled out by physicians for all Americans

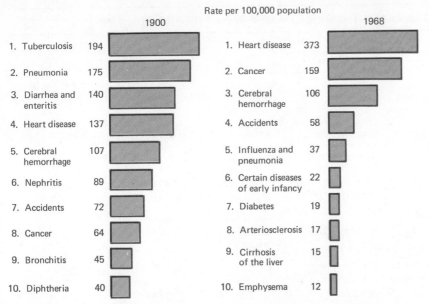

Rate per 100,000 population

1900		1968	
1. Tuberculosis	194	1. Heart disease	373
2. Pneumonia	175	2. Cancer	159
3. Diarrhea and enteritis	140	3. Cerebral hemorrhage	106
4. Heart disease	137	4. Accidents	58
5. Cerebral hemorrhage	107	5. Influenza and pneumonia	37
6. Nephritis	89	6. Certain diseases of early infancy	22
7. Accidents	72	7. Diabetes	19
8. Cancer	64	8. Arteriosclerosis	17
9. Bronchitis	45	9. Cirrhosis of the liver	15
10. Diphtheria	40	10. Emphysema	12

Figure 12-1

Leading causes of death in the United States, 1900 and 1968. (From E. Silverberg and A. I. Holleb, 1972, *Ca—A Cancer Journal for Clinicians* 22:2–20. With permission of the American Cancer Society.)

who died in the years given. When a person suffered from two or more diseases, the physician would certify the death to the more serious cause. Therefore these mortality statistics reflect not only the changing incidence of each disease but also trends in survival, efficacy of treatment, and to some extent the diagnostic judgments of individual physicians.

Note that only selected diseases are graphed. The figure shows that heart disease increased markedly as a cause of death between 1920 and

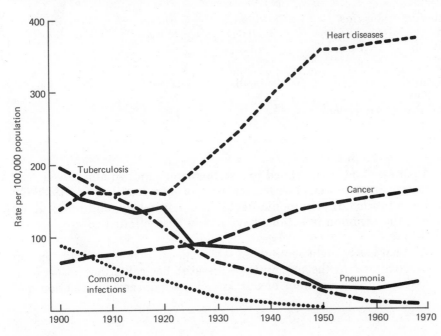

Figure 12-2

Death rates of selected diseases in the United States, 1900–1968. (From E. Silverberg and A. I. Holleb, 1972, *Ca—A Cancer Journal for Clinicians* 22:2–20. With permission of the American Cancer Society.)

Table 12-2   THE TEN LEADING CAUSES OF DEATH BY AGE AND SEX, 1968

	ALL AGES		AGE 1–14		AGES 15–34	
Rank	Male	Female	Male	Female	Male	Female
1	Heart diseases 425,610	Heart diseases 318,685	Accidents 8574	Accidents 4538	Accidents 28,563	Accidents 6893
2	Cancer 173,694	Cancer 144,853	Cancer 2095	Cancer 1665	Homicide 5624	Cancer 3181
3	Stroke 96,701	Stroke 114,689	Congenital malformations 1301	Congenital malformations 1141	Suicide 3780	Suicide 1432
4	Accidents 79,424	Accidents 35,440	Pneumonia, influenza 1144	Pneumonia, influenza 1048	Cancer 3646	Heart 1376
5	Pneumonia, influenza 40,562	Pneumonia, influenza 32,930	Heart diseases 319	Heart diseases 289	Heart diseases 2347	Homicide 1357
6	Diseases of infancy 25,879	Diabetes 22,571	Homicide 287	Homicide 227	Pneumonia, influenza 1109	Stroke 885
7	Emphysema 20,434	Arterio-sclerosis 18,923	Meningitis 227	Cystic fibrosis 201	Stroke 848	Pneumonia, influenza 880
8	Cirrhosis 18,821	Diseases of infancy 17,961	Stroke 210	Stroke 193	Congenital malformations 641	Complications of pregnancy 621
9	Suicide 15,379	Cirrhosis of liver 10,362	Gastritis, colitis, enteritis 200	Gastritis colitis, enteritis 155	Cirrhosis of liver 641	Cirrhosis of liver 486
10	Arterio-sclerosis 14,645	Congenital malformation 7,718	Meningo-coccal infections 198	Meningitis 153	Diabetes 444	Congenital malformation 471

1950 and that it continued to rise thereafter, though at a slower rate. Cancer has been on the increase more or less steadily since 1900. On the other hand, pneumonia declined precipitously, and tuberculosis and the common infections have nearly been eliminated as causes of death.

What has brought about these rather spectacular changes in medical practice and in the prognosis of disease? Basically, they result from explosive augmentation of our knowledge concerning infection and

Table 12-2 (Continued)

Rank	AGE 35–54		AGE 55–74		AGE 75 AND OVER	
	Male	Female	Male	Female	Male	Female
1	Heart diseases 55,943	Cancer 29,707	Heart diseases 209,917	Heart diseases 113,056	Heart diseases 156,723	Heart diseases 185,818
2	Cancer 26,282	Heart diseases 17,875	Cancer 96,317	Cancer 69,715	Stroke 50,066	Stroke 73,027
3	Accidents 17,648	Stroke 6880	Stroke 38,305	Stroke 33,585	Cancer 45,245	Cancer 40,478
4	Cirrhosis of liver 7934	Accidents 5785	Accidents 15,241	Diabetes 10,774	Pneumonia, influenza 16,477	Pneumonia, influenza 17,678
5	Stroke 7146	Cirrhosis of liver 4700	Pneumonia, influenza 13,169	Accidents 7423	Arterio-sclerosis 10,962	Arterio-sclerosis 16,079
6	Suicide 5531	Suicide 2755	Emphysema 12,589	Pneumonia, influenza 7316	Accidents 7954	Accidents 9649
7	Pneumonia, influenza 4161	Pneumonia, influenza 2564	Cirrhosis 8978	Cirrhosis 4270	Emphysema 6329	Diabetes 9271
8	Homicide 4051	Diabetes 2022	Diabetes 7960	Arterio-sclerosis 2710	Diabetes 5118	Infections of kidney 2340
9	Diabetes 2201	Homicide 1043	Suicide 4689	Emphysema 1979	Hyper-plasia of prostate 2152	Hypertension without mention of heart 2250
10	Emphysema 1452	Nephritis 840	Arterio-sclerosis 3489	Infections of kidney 1908	Infections of kidney 2112	Hernia, intestinal obstruction 2047

Source: E. Silverberg and A. I. Holleb, 1972, *Ca—A Cancer Journal for Clinicians* 22:2–20. With permission of the American Cancer Society.

infectious diseases. As you have seen, bacterial infections were among the deadliest of killers during the first decades of the twentieth century. Millions of people in the United States and in other developed countries died of acute infectious disease. Untold millions more in the less-developed countries succumbed to a variety of tropical infectious diseases.

In the 1930s came the discovery of the sulfa drugs and their

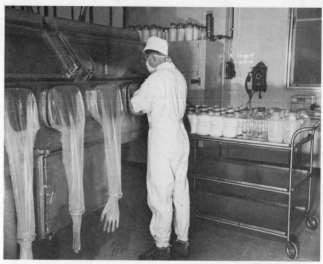

life-saving ability to inhibit the growth of deadly bacteria. Penicillin was developed during World War II, and shortly thereafter streptomycin and related substances, which are now called antibiotics. If you had developed tuberculosis of the lung in 1930, you would most likely have been sent to a sanitorium in the hope that the combination of good nutrition, sunshine, rest, and occasional surgery might enable your body to mobilize its defenses against the deadly tubercle bacillus. Nowadays most tuberculosis patients require very little hospitalization and are in fact treated mainly at home with streptomycin and other effective drugs developed over the past 30 years.

Thirty years ago death from poliomyelitis or infantile paralysis was a frightful possibility to parents of children everywhere. Shortly after the introduction of the Salk and Sabin vaccines some two decades ago, the attack rate fell markedly. Since 1963 only a handful of cases are detected each year in the United States as compared with the thousands expected in previous years.

The examples just cited offer a partial explanation for the decline in infectious diseases as a major cause of death. However, it would be incorrect to attribute the dramatic changes in our spectrum of disease to such specific health measures alone. The London cholera epidemic of 1848 was controlled by preventing contact with contaminated water. Many other infectious diseases are also waterborne. By separating water and sewer lines and by purifying the water that we drink, far more cases of typhoid fever, dysentery, cholera, and other potentially fatal infectious diseases are prevented than could be cured by specific antibiotics or eliminated by vaccination programs. Modern methods for the sanitary control of milk and milk products have markedly reduced the incidence of tuberculosis, brucellosis, streptococcal infections, and similar diseases.

Other diseases have declined markedly as causes of death, not because of any single scientific discovery but because of a multiplicity of improvements in our standard of living that have tilted the balance against serious infection and in favor of survival and recovery. A good example of this is the rather spectacular decline in both infant mortality and maternal mortality in the United States. Since the 1940s the death rate of infants has fallen in half and that of women giving birth has fallen to almost negligible proportions. These trends cannot be attributed to any specific factor. Rather, it is believed that a combination of factors is responsible, including improved nutritional status, wider availability of prenatal services to pregnant women, near elimination of home deliveries, improvements in obstetrical techniques, and steps taken by hospitals to reduce infections in nurseries for newborn babies.

It has been demonstrated that people in different socioeconomic classes suffer from different types of mental disease. In quite analogous fashion, the spectrum of many other diseases varies according to social class. Tuberculosis, bronchitis, stomach ulcers, liver cirrhosis, and cancer of the uterine cervix all seem to be more common among individuals in the more disadvantaged social classes. This is undoubtedly due to the environment in which they live, the foods they eat or do not eat, their knowledge and expectations about disease and medical care, and their ability to bring their health problems to medical attention.

In the United States the gap between the haves and have-nots is narrower than in most other countries. Federally and locally subsidized programs to provide medical care (such as Medicaid and Medicare), to improve nutrition (such as school milk and lunch programs), and to make people more health-conscious (health education programs) are narrowing this gap even further. The result is that, as compared with many other countries, our social class differences in disease frequency are rather modest insofar as most of the major diseases are concerned.

In a discussion of medical advances we cannot ignore the impact of the discovery of insulin. In 1920 a young person who developed sugar diabetes could generally expect to die within six months to a year. In 1922 insulin was discovered and crystallized; soon it was made widely available around the world. Within a decade the medical prognosis for the survival of diabetics changed from death to life.

The net impact of these specific and general developments has literally been to add years to our lives. In 1900, for example, the average American could expect to attain 48 years of age. At present life expectancy has risen to 70 years or so. We are not only living longer but more healthy—and therefore more potentially productive—lives.

Many of the diseases that kill also cause varying degrees of disability among the survivors. In addition, there are a number of diseases not usually fatal that disable large numbers of persons. The major causes of such chronic or long-term disability in the United States are listed in

Major Causes of Disability in the United States Today

Table 12-3

MAJOR CAUSES OF CHRONIC DISABILITY IN THE UNITED STATES	
Cause	Estimated Number Disabled
Heart and circulatory disorders	
Heart diseases and hypertension	
Hypertensive heart disease	12,670,000
Coronary heart disease	3,650,000
Rheumatic heart disease	1,510,000
Hypertension without heart disease	8,370,000
	26,200,000
Cerebrovascular disease (strokes)	2,000,000
Mental and emotional disorders	20,000,000
Arthritis and rheumatic diseases	16,000,000
Hearing impairments	8,549,000
Mental retardation	6,000,000
Visual impairment	5,390,000
Neurological disorders	
Epilepsy	1,500,000
Parkinsonism	1,000,000
Cerebral palsy	600,000
Multiple sclerosis and related diseases	500,000
Muscular dystrophy	200,000
	3,800,000
Diabetes mellitus	4,000,000
Cancer	940,000

Source: Facts on the Major Killing and Crippling Diseases in the United States Today, 1971. New York: National Health Education Committee.

Table 12-3. As you can see, heart and circulatory disorders are not only responsible for the majority of deaths but for most cases of chronic disability as well.

The extent of disability in cases of heart disease is highly variable. Some patients are bedridden, unable to work, and often even unable to carry on their normal activities of living. Other patients may be only minimally disabled, their disease well controlled by medication, and their disability scarcely evident to the casual observer. The same is true for most of the other causes of chronic disability.

For example, the large majority of elderly persons who suffer a stroke survive with a wide range of disabilities over varying intervals of time. Accordingly, the prevalence of stroke in the United States (that is, the number of cases existing at any given time) is approximately 10 times greater than the mortality from stroke in a given year. Try to confirm this from the actual statistics given in Tables 12-1 and 12-3.

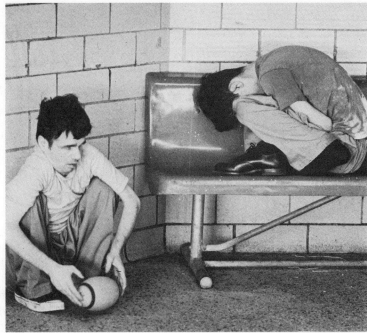

Two young men in a training school for the mentally retarded.

Does it surprise you that the second largest category of diseases responsible for chronic disability is that of the mental and emotional disorders? What does this amount to, in percentage terms? Bear in mind, however, that behavioral disorders, alcoholism, and a number of transient conditions are included here as well as schizophrenia, arteriosclerosis of the brain, and other more permanent or untreatable psychiatric diseases.

The various types of arthritis and the rheumatic diseases such as rheumatism do not usually kill, although they may severely disable. Therefore although they do not appear among the major causes of death in Table 12-1, they rank third in national frequency as a cause of chronic disability. Once again, however, we must remember the wide range of clinical manifestations and extent of disability that they produce. Although technically most elderly persons would be considered arthritic to one extent or another, relatively few are severely disabled by arthritic conditions.

Mental retardation is the fifth most common cause of chronic disability but is an insignificant cause of death. However, the functional disabilities it produces interfere with an individual's capacity to work, take care of his daily needs, and otherwise get along in our competitive society.

Do not be misled by the number of people with visual impairments listed in Table 12-3. Fewer than 10 percent of these (approximately 421,000) are legally blind. The remainder are individuals who have other forms of visual disability that are not correctable by eyeglasses.

423

The neurological disorders (those affecting the body's nervous system), as you can see, are a very important cause of chronic disability in the United States. Since the brain is part of the central nervous system, brain malfunctions caused by strokes are, in a sense, neurological disorders. Therefore the total number of individuals disabled by such disorders at any given time in the United States is actually about 6 million.

The other listed conditions are, on the whole, quite variable in the degree of disability produced. For example, the large majority of epileptic persons would be able to live essentially normal daily lives, provided that they maintained proper drug therapy. Unfortunately, public ignorance about epilepsy often results in much cruel and unfair ostracism. The same is true for children or adults with cerebral palsy, many of whom suffer much less from their physical disabilities than from the embarrassment that their condition seems to induce in classmates or associates. Except for Parkinsonism, the other listed neurological disorders all tend to affect young and relatively young individuals more than old.

Although, as we have seen, diabetes mellitus (sugar diabetes) is no longer a major killer, it remains one of the more common disabling conditions of young people. When diabetes begins in childhood it tends to be much more severe in its clinical manifestations. Relatively little functional disability is produced in older people who become diabetic in adulthood.

Cancer is also one of the most important causes of long-term disability. We have already seen that it is the second most frequent cause of death. Compare the numbers of Americans dying from cancer and suffering from cancer each year. What does this imply about survival rates from cancer? We shall return to this subject again. For the moment, however, these statistics should encourage us all.

TAKING ACTION

1. *Consider the following three individuals:*
   a. *A 5-year-old boy who suddenly went into a coma and was discovered to be suffering from diabetes.*
   b. *A 45-year-old father of three children who woke up choking for breath, experienced severe chest pains, and was rushed to the hospital, where a diagnosis of acute myocardial infarction was made.*
   c. *A 69-year-old grandmother, living alone on social security benefits, who noticed the development of increasingly disabling tremors and rigidity, which were attributed to chronic Parkinson's disease.*
   Discuss the impact of their diseases upon (a) the individuals concerned, (b) their immediate families, (c) their neighbors and associates, (d) their communities, (e) the state and federal governments, and (f) future generations.
2. *Rank the three diseases in terms of their impact upon (a) through (f). Explain your reasoning.*

3. *Discuss how you think such considerations might influence how individuals, communities, and the nation as a whole vote for new taxes to pay for medical care and health research programs.*

**Diseases That
Have Been
Declining in
Frequency and Why**

About a century ago, thousands of Americans suffered from leprosy all over the continental United States as well as in Hawaii. At present not a single leprosarium is open in our country because this dread disease has essentially disappeared here. Medical research has led to the discovery of a number of drugs that are extremely effective in treating leprosy. Unfortunately, in other parts of the world such as Southeast Asia, leprosy remains a serious public health problem because of the extremely crowded living conditions that are conducive to transmission of the disease and because of the poverty and inadequate standards of medical care. Cholera, a disease as old as history, is practically unknown in the United States. As is the case with tuberculosis and typhoid fever, the spread of cholera is encouraged by poor sanitation, poverty, malnutrition, and high population density—that is, conditions still existing in many parts of the world.

Most Americans have not heard of yaws or trachoma, but hundreds of millions of people suffer from these diseases each year. Yaws is a nonvenereal disease borne by an organism similar to the one that causes syphilis in the United States. It can be rather effectively treated with penicillin. Trachoma is a painful eye infection that may lead to permanent blindness or to partial loss of vision. It is shocking to consider that some 400 million people today suffer from one form of trachoma or another. As with yaws, antibiotics are very effective in the treatment of trachoma provided that the disease has not yet progressed to its irreversible stages. Unlike yaws, however, specific vaccines have not yet been perfected for the prevention of trachoma. Poor hygiene, poverty, and crowded living conditions are important precipitating factors for both trachoma and yaws.

Smallpox is a dreadful disease that has practically disappeared from our country since the introduction of smallpox vaccination programs many years ago. Unfortunately, thousands of cases still occur in less-developed countries, killing many and needlessly scarring the lives of countless others, especially young children. There is good reason to hope that this disease may be completely eradicated soon.

Malaria is an acute infectious disease which was once a serious health menace in the southern United States and has now been essentially eliminated. However, millions of persons in Africa, Asia, and Central America continue to suffer the ravages of this disease in spite of vigorous, even heroic, malaria control programs.

As we have already seen, tuberculosis is another serious disease that has markedly declined in frequency in the United States. Yet there are probably between 15 and 20 million persons in other countries with active infections. Conquest of this disease seems to require vaccination in order to prevent the development of the disease in persons who

425

come in contact with active cases; vigorously treating patients who already have the disease in order that the period of their infectiousness to others be minimized; and eliminating slums, improving nutrition, and pasteurizing milk. Finally, poliomyelitis (infantile paralysis), measles, and rubella (German measles), once responsible for considerable mortality and chronic disability, no longer pose significant threats to public health in this country or other "advanced" countries.

Trends in Chronic Disease

Thus far we have concerned ourselves with the disappearance or decline in frequency of a number of acute infectious diseases. How would you classify most of the diseases that are numbered among the leading causes of death in the United States today? With the exception of influenza and pneumonia, none is an acute infectious disease. Rather, these are usually termed "chronic diseases," for lack of a better description. As we shall see, heart disease, cancer, stroke, and the other chronic diseases are not, to the best of our knowledge, caused by the direct action of microorganisms or other agents upon the human host. Although such factors may well play important roles in the development of chronic diseases, the process almost certainly extends over many years and involves interaction between the causative agents, the defense mechanisms of humans, and the environment in which both of these interact. Mechanisms underlying the development of chronic disease are obviously far more complex than those responsible for acute infectious disease. It should not be surprising, then, that our understanding of the biological bases of the chronic diseases—and therefore the chances of our developing means to prevent or cure them—is still far from complete.

Nevertheless, considerable progress has already been recorded in reducing the human impact of a number of serious chronic diseases. Consider, for example, that the mental and emotional disorders we have seen are second only to heart disease as a cause of disability in our country. In 1955 there were about 558,000 patients confined to state mental hospitals. By 1969 the number was 367,000, a decline of 34 percent. By far the most important reason has been the development of new drugs that effectively control two of the most critical problems of mental hospital patients: the agitation and depression that often necessitate their incarceration for long periods of time. Tranquilizers and antidepressants now make it possible for the large majority of patients with mental illnesses to be treated at home or require only brief periods of hospitalization.

Not very many years ago cancer could be treated either by surgical removal of the diseased organ or by radiation. These methods were and still are of benefit to many patients, especially if undertaken when the tumor is localized in one organ and has not yet spread (metastasized) to other parts of the body. Unfortunately, by the time many patients are diagnosed, their malignancies are no longer localized. In such cases new types of treatment are urgently needed if the growth is to be controlled. In recent years cancer chemotherapy (the treatment of cancer with drugs) has become a reality for thousands of patients. Several highly malignant, though relatively rare, cancers have proved remarkably susceptible to chemotherapy. These include two childhood tumors—retinoblastoma of the eye and Wilm's tumor of the kidney—as well as two tumors of adults—choriocarcinoma and certain skin cancers. Many patients suffering from these neoplasms have essentially been cured of their disease by chemotherapy.

Patients with a number of other cancers, while not cured, have had their survival considerably prolonged through chemotherapy. Breast cancer in women and prostate gland cancer in men are malignancies that have been effectively controlled through the use of steroid hormones such as estrogen or testosterone. Temporary remissions have also been induced in a variety of other human cancers by means of these and other chemotherapeutic drugs.

Besides specific anticancer drugs and hormones, another category of agents has recently shown promise in cancer control. These are agents that act upon or stimulate a person's own immune defense mechanisms against foreign material such as cancer. Some of these agents act by inducing an immune or allergic reaction in the skin of patients who have undergone cancerous change. The result is destruction of the tumor without much effect on the surrounding normal tissue. Another approach, which appears very promising at present, involves the use of modified tuberculosis bacilli (BCG) in patients with skin and other tumors. BCG is a powerful stimulant of the human immune system and appears to be somewhat effective in destroying certain human tumors.

Of all cancers in man, leukemia and Hodgkin's disease have proved to be the most susceptible to chemotherapy. Whereas 30 years ago, for example, the average survival time for patients with acute leukemia

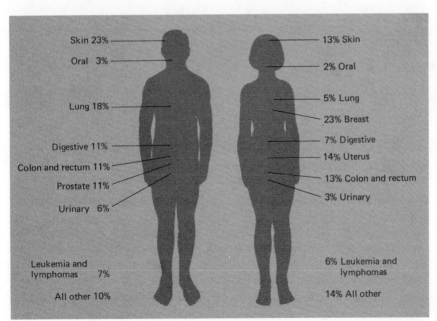

Figure 12-3

Cancer incidence by site and sex. (From E. Silverberg and A. I. Holleb, 1972, *Ca—A Cancer Journal for Clinicians* 22:2–20. With permission of the American Cancer Society.)

Skin 23%

Oral 3%

Lung 18%

Digestive 11%

Colon and rectum 11%

Prostate 11%

Urinary 6%

Leukemia and lymphomas 7%

All other 10%

13% Skin

2% Oral

5% Lung

23% Breast

7% Digestive

14% Uterus

13% Colon and rectum

3% Urinary

6% Leukemia and lymphomas

14% All other

was perhaps three months, it is now approximately a year or longer. Equally important, a number of leukemic children have survived up to 20 years or more following the onset of their disease.

One of the more common "metabolic" diseases is diabetes mellitus or sugar diabetes. Fifty years ago thousands of persons, both young and old, died prematurely of the complications of this chronic disease. Then insulin became available, and within a few short years the survival of diabetics improved dramatically all over the world. In more recent years oral drugs have been developed to reduce the need for insulin injections, but their effectiveness has not yet been confirmed.

Next to a stroke, Parkinson's disease is the most common serious neurological disorder of man. It is a chronic and progressive condition that gradually incapacitates its victims in walking, speaking, swallowing, and manipulating. Medical research has recently led to a spectacular breakthrough in both knowledge about and treatment of Parkinson's disease. It is now known that Parkinsonism is related to a deficiency of L-dopa in the brain. When patients are treated with this drug, the clinical symptoms of most are either reduced or eliminated without surgery.

Arthritis and the rheumatic diseases often extend over most of a life span and tend to be associated with pain and inflammatory reactions. Aspirin and other antiinflammatory drugs often provide relief, although side effects are a hazard. A related disease, gout, which has afflicted some of the most famous people, is now controllable in terms of both reducing or preventing its very painful attacks and dealing with

Gout victim in 1902.

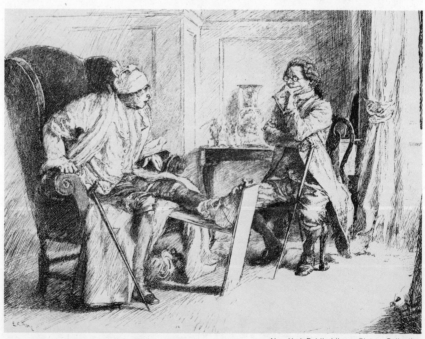

the inflammation and abnormal uric acid metabolism.

A number of recent advances have begun to improve the prognosis of coronary disease patients suffering from heart attacks. Anticoagulant drugs, which reduce the tendency for clots to form in the heart and blood vessels, have been shown to reduce mortality from acute myocardial infarction. Another promising development has been the establishment of "coronary care units" at hospitals all around the country. These are manned by teams of physicians, nurses, and technicians specially trained for the treatment of patients as soon as possible after their heart attack.

Much in the news these days are the federally sponsored programs to prevent coronary disease by identifying and treating those with the highest risk. Hypertension (high blood pressure), smoking, and cholesterol are three of the most highly suspect risk factors. Accordingly, attempts are being made to find those individuals in selected communities who are smokers, hypertensive, and have increased blood cholesterol levels. The objective is to reduce their smoking, treat their hypertension, attempt to lower their blood cholesterol levels by diet and drugs, and then determine whether their subsequent risk of heart attacks falls. The results of these clinical trials are being awaited with interest by the medical community.

HEALTH PROBLEMS OF YOUNG ADULTS

Let us now consider four health problems which are of vital importance to young adults: accidents, venereal disease, the contraceptive pill, and smoking.

Accidents

Motor vehicle accidents are responsible for the deaths of more young adults by far than any other cause. In 1972, for example, 25,700 individuals between 15 and 24 years of age died in accidents; of this total, 18,000 were killed in accidents involving motor vehicles, primarily private automobiles. The second most frequent type of fatal accident was drowning, with nearly 2200 such deaths occurring that year. Fatal firearm injuries, excluding military operations, killed about 800 young people, and poisons of various kinds killed another 700. The majority of the deaths from poisoning were due to drugs, medicines, mushrooms, shellfish and carbon monoxide poisoning; they exclude deaths involving fires, moving vehicles, or food poisoning.

The fatal accident rate among males aged 15 to 24 years is four times higher than that among females. Why is this the case? To some extent, of course, it is due to the perpetual love affair between young men and their automobiles, which, as we have seen, ends tragically for so many of them. Their rate of fatal accidents from all other causes is also considerably higher than that among their female contemporaries.

What are the trends in accidental death rates over time? The picture is very clear-cut. Over the past 10 years or so, accident death rates in general have been falling. This includes accidents at work, at home, and in the public domain; accidents due to falls, to fires, and to

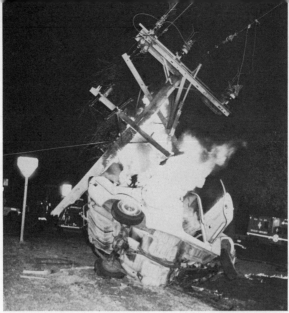

Speeding teenagers crashed into a utility pole and narrowly escaped death.

drowning. One type of accidental death rate, however, is continuing to climb and especially among young adults: motor vehicle accidents. There is a death from a motor vehicle accident every nine minutes of every hour of every day, on the average. There is a motor vehicle injury every 15 seconds every hour every day. As you might expect, the rates are highest during the summer months, when young people are most likely to be driving their cars frequently, and are lowest during the winter. Furthermore, fatal car accidents are much more likely to occur in rural areas and at night.

Four factors appear to be crucial in causing accidents or, at least, in increasing the chances of a fatal accident: alcohol, drugs, failure to use safety belts, and speed. In a recent study it was shown that 44 percent of fatally injured drivers under 20 years of age in Vermont had blood alcohol concentrations of 20 percent and more. Among those drivers aged 20 to 24, 69 percent had increased alcohol levels. Other studies have shown that the drivers who tend to show the highest blood alcohol concentrations are clustered among males aged 21 to 25 years.

In a study conducted by the United States Department of Transportation two years ago, 24 percent of the fatally injured drivers tested revealed evidence of recent drug ingestion. Barbiturates and amphetamines were those most frequently identified. It has been estimated that if all passenger car occupants used safety belts, more than 14,000 lives would be saved annually by preventing ejection from the vehicle and by reducing contact with the vehicle interior on impact. Excessive speed is the fourth major cause of fatal automobile accidents, especially among young adults. In 1972 three out of ten fatal accidents involved vehicles that were being driven too fast (or too fast for existing road conditions). These accounted for 16,000 excessive fatal motor vehicle accidents in that year.

When 10 million persons in the United States are without remunerative employment it is a major economic calamity. When 10 million are infected with a disease which, if it is not properly treated, brings dire and dreadful symptoms and in some cases death, it is a public health problem of major importance.

In the first named situation the whole country is stirred into frenzied action. The resources of the government, national and state, are levied upon to meet the emergency. Cost is given scant consideration as billions of dollars are spent to relieve distress and to save the people.

In the second named condition a vast blanket of silence covers the land. People conceal their alarms (those who have any) by refusing to discuss the peril. Only an intelligent few, who have overcome their puritanical instincts concerning an ailment that more often than not is associated with the subject of sex, are courageous enough to discuss the problem.[1]

The five most important venereal diseases are syphilis, gonorrhea, chancroid, granuloma inguinale, and lymphogranuloma venereum. Though they differ markedly in causative organisms and in pathology, these diseases are grouped together because their usual method of transmission is venereal—that is, by sexual intercourse. Of the five, syphilis and gonorrhea are the most important because of their relatively high frequency. Syphilis itself is especially significant because of its chronic nature and because of the serious lesions, disabilities, and death resulting from it, as noted earlier.

Medical historians are undecided as to whether syphilis was known in ancient times. During the Middle Ages great epidemics of syphilis broke out in Europe, most notably during the wars of the fifteenth and sixteenth centuries. The name itself was coined in 1521 by an Italian physician Fracastorius in his poem concerning the shepherd Syphilus, who suffered from "the French disease." In 1905 *Treponema pallidum*—the causative spirochaetal organism—was discovered, and in 1906 the Wassermann test for the detection of syphilis was introduced.

Syphilitic infection usually takes place in the genital organs, but not infrequently involves other mucous membranes (such as the mouth, throat, and anus) as well. After an incubation period of about three weeks or so, a chancre sore appears. This primary lesion heals and is succeeded a few weeks later by secondary syphilitic lesions, which also disappear after a few weeks or months. The apparent cure is a tragic illusion, however, because the syphilitic spirochaetes that multiply vigorously during both primary and secondary syphilis continue to damage their victims for the rest of their lives unless they are effectively treated. The result may be serious heart disease, destruction of the spinal cord, paralysis, or death. Pregnant women infected with syphilis are likely to give birth to syphilitic infants suffering from diseases of the heart, skin, bones, and other organs, or else they experience spontaneous abortions or stillbirths.

---

[1]S. W. Becker, 1937, *Ten Million Americans Have It.* Philadelphia: Lippincott.

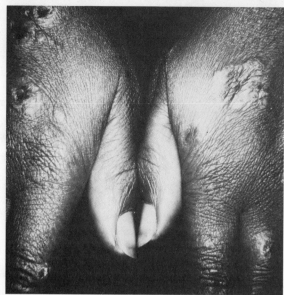

Camera M.D. Studios

During the primary and secondary stages of syphilis, when the spirochaetes are multiplying rapidly in the bloodstream, individuals are highly infectious to others but suffer only the temporary discomfort of genital sores. It is ironical that most of the dreadful complications of syphilis occur when the infected person is no longer harboring active organisms—that is, at a time years later when he or she feels normal and does not suspect the presence of disease.

In 1909 the famous German chemist, Paul Ehrlich, developed the first specific treatment for syphilis, which he named "606," representing the number of compounds tested before success was achieved. Since 1944 penicillin has been the drug of choice in the treatment of this disease. In any event, treatments must be administered during the primary or secondary stages of syphilis. If given later, they have no effect in preventing the irreversible complications.

In contrast with syphilis, gonorrhea primarily affects the mucous membranes of the genital tract and only rarely extends to other organs of the body, such as the heart and brain. It has been estimated that more than 90 percent of women infected with gonorrhea are completely free of symptoms. What are the implications of this in terms of venereal transmission, diagnosis, and prevention?

Two of the more serious chronic complications of gonorrhea are sterility in the male and blindness among infants born of infected mothers. Once recognized, gonorrhea can be effectively treated with antibiotics. There is as yet no blood test for this disease comparable to the Wassermann test or its modifications in syphilis. There is also no acquired immunity, so an individual remains susceptible to reinfection over and over again.

Chancroid, or soft chancre, may be considered a disease of "un-washed" populations. It is caused by a bacillus that is effectively killed by soap and water. Once the disease has established itself, it must be treated vigorously with antibiotics.

Granuloma inguinale is a somewhat unusual venereal disease because only a relatively small proportion of infections develop after venereal exposure. Small nonpainful lesions develop on the genital organs and slowly enlarge and spread out. Antibiotics are quite effective in treatment.

Lymphogranuloma venereum is a venereal infection of the lymph channels and lymph nodes in the genital area. It is the only one of these five venereal diseases to be caused by a virus rather than a bacterium. Swollen and very painful genital glands are usually the first sign of infection. Again, sulfadiazine and other antibiotics are the treatment of choice.

In recent years another venereal disease has come into some prominence. It is caused by the genital herpes virus, and it produces painful pus-filled vesicles on and around the genitalia. Although serious systemic complications have not been attributed to this venereal disease, the patients often suffer from monthly or cyclical recurrences of pain and discomfort as new crops of herpetic vesicles develop. Furthermore, infants born of mothers harboring such infections often have encephalitis of the brain or other life-threatening diseases.

At the time of World War II it was estimated that one in 42 Americans had syphilis, and even more had gonorrhea. If one considers that the risk of venereal diseases is not evenly distributed among all age groups, the statistics become even more impressive. Think about this and calculate some numerical examples, assuming that 28 percent of the 130 million population were under 15 years of age and that 12 percent were 55 years old or more.

The upsurge of cases expected as a consequence of the war was largely contained by a vigorous federal Syphilis Control Program until the early 1950s. By then the medical authorities had become so convinced that venereal diseases no longer posed any serious public health problem that U.S. Government appropriations in this area fell to a mere $3 million in 1955. Hospitals, seeking to save money, dropped their requirement that all patients have a blood test for syphilis. Many states eliminated the mandatory premarital blood test for syphilis as a meaningless gesture. Venereal disease clinics in hundreds of hospitals around the country were phased out. Syphilis and gonorrhea were no longer emphasized in medical school curricula.

Then "the bubble of optimism and smug satisfaction burst."[2] The number of cases of venereal disease reported to health officials began to rise dramatically. Since much venereal disease is still not reported to authorities, the actual number of cases was obviously far higher. By

---

[2]Louis Lasagna, 1975. *The VD Epidemic.* Philadelphia: Temple University Press.

1971 it was estimated that more than a half million Americans suffered from undetected syphilis and were in urgent need of medical attention. By the following year it was estimated that one new case of gonorrhea was being acquired in the United States every 15 seconds 24 hours a day.

What caused the venereal disease epidemic of the past 15 years? There are a number of factors, the most important being the complacency of the public health authorities and the diminishing sums of money made available for operating venereal disease control programs. A somewhat more subtle reason stems from the remarkable ease with which penicillin injections cure early cases of most venereal disease. This contrasts greatly with the prolonged and complicated treatment schedules of earlier days. This easier treatment decreased the fear of venereal disease, both among patients and among physicians. Then the gonorrhea organism began to develop resistance to penicillin as increasing numbers of people received this drug. Finally, sexual habits among young people began to change, if only because of the lessened fear of venereal disease among them. The contraceptive pill was introduced during this time, and it too probably tended to facilitate and therefore increase sexual promiscuity (indiscriminate choice of sexual partners). With promiscuity, of course, the chances of contracting venereal disease increases markedly. Finally, there is the old problem of public attitudes towards syphilis and other venereal diseases. On the one hand, there is the apathy and complacency already referred to. On the other hand, there is the reluctance to teach children in the home and in the public schools about venereal diseases, despite the fact that young people are among the most ignorant about the subject.

Although syphilis and gonorrhea have now attained epidemic proportions again in the United States, there is good reason for optimism. The federal government has recently increased its appropriations for venereal disease control greatly. Active research is under way to develop vaccines that would prevent their occurrence. People have become less reluctant to seek treatment for syphilis, so the long-term complications of the disease are becoming less frequent despite the rising trend of the disease itself. Finally, there is reason to hope that public enlightenment about these diseases, their causes, and their consequences will eventually make possible their control and even eradication.

Present-day venereal disease control programs involve attempts to identify and treat all sexual partners of all detected cases. How would you go about such contact investigations? What would be the problems? How would contemporary mores affect your ability to conduct such activities? Cases can also be detected by means of a Wassermann-type test. Would it be practical to attempt to administer this test to all persons? If not, to whom would you direct the testing? What do you think is the most promising long-term solution to the venereal disease problem in the United States?

1. *Report to class on your conversation with a VD investigator or other VD clinic worker. Consider such subjects as the status of these diseases in the community, techniques and progress in dealing with them, and obstacles to progress.*
2. *For reporting to class, discuss and, if possible, tape record what it means to get VD, using an actual victim of it.*

First introduced to the public in 1960, contraceptive pills are now regularly taken by 8 million or more American women and by several additional millions in other countries. Never before has a drug achieved such widespread use so soon after its introduction. Never before have so many healthy women taken such potent drugs voluntarily over relatively long periods of their lives. Until now, physicians have usually believed that drugs should be used primarily to cure disease or to maintain normal physiological function.

The Pill

How can the phenomenon of "the pill" be explained? There is, first, its extraordinary effectiveness in preventing conception. Depending on the particular compound used and the extent of the woman's cooperation, this varies from 98 to 99.9 percent. Secondly, there is the simplicity and ease of administration, as compared with diaphragms, condoms, and other methods. The latter incidentally, are approximately as effective as the pill when they are properly used. A third possible factor in the rapid acceptance gained by the pill is the enthusiasm it engendered among physicians. A survey taken in 1967 indicated that 95 percent of American gynecologists and obstetricians prescribed the pill, and that 45 percent set no time limits on its use. Whether their enthusiasm infected their patients or vice versa is conjectural. Nevertheless, the end result is that millions of young women are dosing themselves with powerful hormones each day in order to prevent conception.

Because they are so easy to take, contraceptive pills have proved effective in reducing the number of unwanted pregnancies. Since some of these pregnancies and deliveries lead to disease and even death, the pill may be considered to spare some women from such fates. On the other hand, one might argue that the pregnancies could have been avoided by less potentially dangerous mechanical means. Such critics would ask, "What price convenience?"

Religious convictions aside, most physicians would favor the use of the contraceptive pill under specified conditions. These might include honeymoons, the first few months of marriage, and certain illnesses, as well as other limited periods of time in a woman's life when the use of obstructive contraceptive devices might prove inconvenient, impractical, or anxiety-provoking. The key word here is "limited," in contrast to the indefinite periods of time, often running into years, that have become quite common.

435

Why are some physicians concerned with chronic, long-term use of the pill? The reason lies in the fact that these pills contain potent steroid hormones (estrogen and progesterone), the effect of which is to prevent ovulation so that fertilization of the ovum (egg) and pregnancy can be avoided. The hormones accomplish this by affecting the pituitary gland and other parts of the brain that normally secrete a number of other hormones essential for bodily function.

There is an extraordinary delicate balance in the human body between hormones produced by the various ductless glands. For example, when the concentration of hormones secreted by the pituitary gland exceeds a critical level in the blood, further production is shut off by means of a "feedback mechanism" initiated by the other ductless glands. Conversely, when the blood level of a particular pituitary hormone falls, this gland is activated to increase its secretion again. Among the ductless glands involved in this automated system are the ovary, thyroid, and adrenal.

Estrogen is a hormone normally produced by the follicles in the ovary. When you swallow an estrogen pill, you naturally increase the concentration of this hormone in your bloodstream. This activates the feedback mechanism described above to inhibit the pituitary gland from manufacturing and secreting FSH, a hormone that stimulates the ovarian follicles to mature and to secrete estrogen. Because the follicles will not mature, ovulation does not occur, and therefore fertilization is prevented. This is only one example of the complex interplay between the pituitary, the ovary, and the other ductless glands in the body. Can you understand why some physicians are uneasy at the thought of millions of young women swallowing potent estrogen hormone tablets every day over long periods of time?

Some of the side effects and complications of contraceptive pill use are well known. Others are not yet fully understood. Many women taking the pill complain of nausea, breast fullness, depression, apathy, fatigue, fluid retention, migraine headaches, allergic rashes, and so forth. The large majority of pill takers, however, probably suffer only minimally from these reactions.

More important than these symptomatic side effects are the long-term chronic effects. An increase in the size of the thyroid gland is not infrequently seen. Abnormalities in liver function have been detected in 5 to 10 percent of women on the pill. Some changes in function of the adrenal and pituitary glands have been detected. The uterus shows some tissue changes, and, as we have already seen, the ovary fails to develop its follicles.

Laboratory studies in laboratory animals have demonstrated that estrogen and progesterone, the two hormones most commonly used in the pill, can cause cancer under certain conditions. Women taking contraceptive pills manifest changes in the appearance of the cells shed from the uterus during menstruation. Although these changes are not identical to those seen in cancer, some physicians have expressed concern at the possible relationship between these cell changes, long-term pill use, and cancer of the uterine cervix.

The most well-known complication of the contraceptive pill is thromboembolism—that is, the formation of clots and inflammation in the veins of the leg and other parts of the body. As with many of the other side effects, the proportion of women affected is quite small, but when it occurs, the complications can be serious and even life-threatening.

In seeking to give the best possible advice about the pill to young women, the physician is faced with a dilemma. He realizes its convenience and its effectiveness in preventing pregnancy. He feels competent to deal with the relatively mild side effects such as breast enlargement, nausea, and the like. He is less confident in balancing these advantages off against the small but definite risk of serious complications such as thromboembolism.

The crux of the problem arises when a patient says, "I know all about the minor discomforts and the relatively rare case of blood clotting in women taking the pill. I am willing to take my chances. But, doctor, is the pill otherwise really safe?"

To answer this question, one must know about the possible long-term consequences of steroid hormone administration. Most of us can tolerate a little bit of poison, such as radiation from a chest X ray, a few typhoid fever bacteria in a roadside well, the air pollution usually found in our cities, and so on. When the dose of poison is small enough, the immune systems of our bodies can (and usually do) prevent serious disease. However, there are definite limits to what we can tolerate. When the toxic dose exceeds what is called the "threshold" level or when the exposure continues over a long period of time, the results can be deadly. Think about this in terms of Hiroshima, your city's water supply contaminated with typhoid bacilli, and the 809 people who died over a two-week period in New York City because of an episode of intense air pollution in 1963. These examples are appropriate to the contraceptive pill question because in fact there have been very few studies of long-term effects. The women studied have, on the average, taken the pill for about 18 months or so and have been observed for, at most, four or five years. This is not sufficient time to detect risks such as cancer development, which require perhaps 15 or 20 years for their manifestation.

Consider the various reasons for contraception. Are there any besides convenience, medical illness, and the desire to limit one's family size? Consider the various methods of contraception. Is there one method which satisfies all needs best, or might the methods be varied according to the needs? Think about the implications of contraceptive decisions for yourself, your family, your society, other societies, and the world.

TAKING ACTION

1. Discuss use of the pill with such individuals or groups as doctors, girls on the pill, girls who refuse to use it or are advised medically not to take it, and males.

2. Discuss your findings in class with basic reference to the question: Does the convenience justify the risk?

Smoking

A teenager just beginning to smoke said, "Nobody young worries much about some disease they might get 40 or 50 years from now." A few million men and women of 40 or 50 or 60 said, "I'd like to stop but I can't." The former president of one of the largest tobacco companies said, "We are not in the cancer research business." And the tobacco companies, in more than $200 million worth of advertising space and time and in a great variety of ways, said, "Smoke!"

In the area bounded by these four points of view the sales of cigarettes in the United States last year reached the total of one half trillion; this was roughly one hundred billion more than were sold in 1953, the year in which the medical evidence linking cigarette smoking to lung cancer first received widespread attention.

As a statistic for the age of anxiety, as an item for the theater of the absurd, and as a tribute to salesmanship, this figure can only command our respect. On any other ground it must be viewed with real alarm (if we can get past disbelief). And the more than $200 million spent last year for advertising, more than was spent on all but two or three other single products, is hardly less alarming. In 10 years of accumulating evidence indicting cigarette smoking as a major health hazard, the annual advertising expenditure has increased 134 percent. And the number of deaths from lung cancer—a rare disease when cigarette smoking first became popular—last year reached 40,000, about the same as the number of deaths from automobile accidents.[3]

We have already seen that heart disease and cancer are not only the two leading causes of death but that, with the decline in infectious disease, they are accounting for an ever-increasing proportion of total deaths and disabilities. To a significant degree, tobacco smoking accounts for these rising trends.

Consumers Union estimates that there are more than 6 million people in the United States involved to a greater or lesser extent in the tobacco business. This number includes some 300,000 stockholders. Tobacco products are an important United States export, with approximately $500 million worth of cigarettes alone sold abroad each year. What are the implications of these economic statistics? Can you think of other contemporary situations in which society has to make choices between the livelihood of some and the greater good of all?

There are statistics that show that the tremendous increase in

---

[3]Dexter Masters, Director of Consumer's Union in 1963. Excerpted by permission from *The Consumers Union Report on Smoking and the Public Interest—1963.* Copyright © 1963 by Consumers Union of United States, Inc., Mount Vernon, N.Y. 10550.

smoking since the 1930s has been followed by a dramatic increase in the death rate from lung cancer. By itself, can such a correlation *prove* that smoking causes lung cancer? No. Many things have shown an upward trend along with cigarette smoking, such as air pollution, industrialization, consumption of candy, and even telephone poles!

Some skeptics have exploited such meaningless correlations in order to cast doubt on the smoking hypothesis in lung cancer. In the opinion of most experts, however, smoking causes about 90 percent of all lung cancer. There is a substantial body of evidence to support this view. Let us summarize the evidence:

1. Lung cancer is extremely rare among men and women who have never smoked.
2. Nearly all lung cancer patients report heavy smoking habits, whereas this is true for only a small proportion of the general population.
3. There is a "dose-response" relationship between smoking and lung cancer; that is, the more you smoke, the more you significantly increase your risk of developing lung cancer.
4. Smokers who break their habit significantly reduce their subsequent risk of developing lung cancer.
5. At least 15 chemical compounds isolated from tobacco have been shown to cause cancer in laboratory animals.
6. Precancerous changes in the lungs are evident among smokers long before they would be expected to develop cancer. In contrast, the lungs of nonsmokers are usually perfectly normal.

Although nearly all lung cancer patients are heavy smokers, the majority of people who smoke do not in fact ever develop lung cancer.

Although cigarette smoking is the primary cause of lung cancer, it is not the only cause. There is meager evidence that heredity may play a role in some cases. Air pollution is certainly an important factor, especially among coal miners and others exposed to very harsh atmospheric conditions. Finally, viruses may be involved in one way or another in the causation of lung cancer. Here again, however, there is little hard evidence for this, as compared with the evidence for the effect of smoking.

A number of other serious diseases are also associated with smoking. Recent evidence from several countries confirms that cigarette smoking is one of the major risk factors contributing to the development of coronary heart disease. Cigarette smokers also have higher death rates from stroke than nonsmokers. Peripheral vascular disease, an extremely painful condition of the limbs, is also aggravated by smoking. This habit is the most important cause of chronic obstructive bronchopulmonary diseases such as emphysema and chronic bronchitis in the United States. In fact clinical studies of high school students have demonstrated that abnormal lung function and symptoms are more

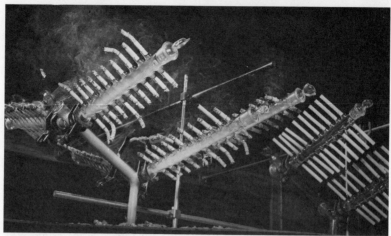

American Cancer Society

common among smokers than nonsmokers even in their youthful years.

Although everyone has probably heard about the association of smoking and lung cancer, the risks of other cancers are not so widely appreciated. Cancers of the larynx, mouth, lips, esophagus, pancreas, and urinary bladder are also significantly increased among smokers.

Smoking is also hazardous to the offspring of pregnant women. Infants of smoking mothers tend to be somewhat retarded in their weight and degree of maturity at birth. Miscarriages may also be increased among such women. Finally, the young person who contemplates smoking should also consider that peptic ulcers, tooth loss, and various allergies are significantly increased among cigarette smokers of all ages.

In 1964 the Surgeon General of the United States and his Advisory Committee on Smoking and Health issued a comprehensive report, the highlights of which we have summarized in this chapter. Since then, the law has required that all cigarette packs be imprinted with a health warning; moreover, cigarette advertising on television has been prohibited. Among adults there has in fact been some decline in the number of individuals smoking. Unfortunately, there has been no significant decrease in the extent of smoking among young adults.

TAKING ACTION

1. Discuss the following possible action programs, and rank them in their potential impact on the national problem:
   a. Prohibition of sales of cigarettes to minors
   b. Increased taxation on cigarette products
   c. Prohibition of cigarette advertising in all media
   d. A program of counteradvertising in the media
   e. Modification of cigarette pack labeling to make the warning more serious.

440

f. Lectures and other health education measures aimed at elementary, high school, and college students

g. Establishment of community clinics to aid smokers in breaking their habit

Design a brief questionnaire based on the foregoing possibilities so as to find out what other groups think. Find out in particular what junior and senior high school pupils think would help.

2. If you're a smoker, get together with some other smokers and discuss: How does all the antismoking propaganda make you feel? The prosmoking? What, if anything, motivates you to want to stop? What keeps you smoking? Under what conditions might you stop?

THE COSTS OF ILLNESS

The nation's medical bill for 1973 exceeded $94 billion, or 7.7 percent of the gross national product. Table 12-4 shows where this money came from and where it went in 1973, 1965, and 1950. Examine the table carefully. Note the three major components of the nation's health bill: medical services (doctor and hospital bills), construction of medical facilities (hospitals, clinics, and laboratories), and medical research.

NATIONAL HEALTH EXPENDITURES BY YEAR AND TYPE (IN BILLIONS OF DOLLARS)*			**Table 12-4**
	YEAR		
Type of Expenditure	1950	1965	1973
Private			
Medical services			
Paid directly	7.11	17.58	28.13
Paid by insurance	1.60	10.45	25.43
Total services	8.71	28.03	53.56
Medical facility construction	0.22	1.17	2.74
Medical research	0.04	0.16	0.22
Total private	8.97	29.36	56.52
Public			
Medical services	2.47	7.64	34.01
Medical facility construction	0.52	0.67	1.49
Medical research	0.07	1.23	2.06
Total public	3.06	9.54	37.56
Both Combined			
Medical services	11.18	35.67	87.57
Medical facility construction	0.74	1.84	4.23
Medical research	0.11	1.39	2.28
Grand total	12.03	38.90	94.08

Source: Adapted from U.S. Department of Commerce, Bureau of the Census, 1974, *Statistical Abstract of the United States.*

What happened to national health expenditures between 1950 and 1973? Inflation alone does not account for much of the rising trend in the nation's medical bill. Consider the following elements in the health establishment, and reflect upon how they might have changed since 1950 as to increase the costs of medical care.

1. Numbers of health professionals and ancillary personnel
2. Types of health professionals and ancillary personnel
3. Medical diagnostic techniques
4. Patterns of medical care
5. Complexity of medical care administration
6. Prepaid medical care (health insurance)

To get a better idea of the impact of rising health costs on the average citizen, estimate per capita health expenditures in the United States for 1950, 1965, and 1973. Does the spending of more money necessarily imply better medical care? What do you think might be a more valid index of the quality of medical care?

The statistics on the declining trends in many of the infectious diseases that we examined earlier offer convincing evidence that our increased national health budget reflects, to some extent, an improved national health profile. The sizable prolongation in average life span of Americans is a similar testimonial. On the other hand, it would be foolish to deny that our present medical care system is in need of much improvement.

Prepaid health insurance has softened the blow of chronic and catastrophic illness for the majority of American families today. Medicare and Medicaid have benefited the elderly and the medically indigent to a significant degree. There are, however, large gaps in the medical care system. Dental services, for example, are not covered by most health insurance plans. Eyeglasses, drugs, and long-term psychiatric care are also excluded in the main. Furthermore, the increasing emphasis on science in medicine has tended to substitute the machine (the automated blood analyzer, the electrocardiogram, and so on) for the human being. These trends, along with the increasing specialization of medical practice, have depersonalized health care significantly.

What do you think can be done about this situation? Can medical students be induced to think about the "whole patient" while at the same time developing expertise in a specific medical specialty? Can health education help citizens to assume greater responsibility for their own health?

Medical Research

Health-related research in the United States is conducted by thousands of investigators in hundreds of medical schools and universities from coast to coast. In addition, large numbers of individuals working in agencies of federal and state governments as well as in commercial establishments are similarly engaged. Who pays for this research?

As you can see in Table 12-4, about 90 percent of the medical research expenses in the United States are paid by government, primarily through the National Institutes of Health and the National Science Foundation. Relatively smaller amounts are spent by such voluntary health foundations as the American Cancer Society and the National Foundation. Drug companies and other business enterprises invest their own funds as well, sometimes for basic research and often for specific applied projects directly related to their commercial interests.

Examine the expenditures listed in Table 12-5. Cancer received the largest amount of money in 1975. Do you think this was justified? How would *you* decide on the allocation of health research funds? Which of the following considerations would you include, and how would you rank their importance?

1. Absolute number of persons dying from the disease per year
2. Number of persons developing the disease per year
3. Number of persons suffering from the disease each year
4. Rate at which the incidence of the disease is increasing or decreasing each year
5. Chronic disability caused by the disease
6. Pain, discomfort, and other acute symptoms caused by the disease
7. Degree of public apprehension concerning the disease
8. Availability of effective therapy for the disease
9. Specific age groups or sex most affected by the disease

NATIONAL INSTITUTES OF HEALTH EXPENDITURES, 1975 (IN MILLIONS OF DOLLARS)	**Table 12-5**

Institute	Amount
Cancer	691.4
Heart and Lung	324.4
Arthritis, Metabolism and Digestive Diseases	173.4
Neurological Disease and Stroke	142.0
Allergy and Infectious Diseases	119.4
General Medical Sciences	187.3
Child Health and Human Development	126.5
Dental Research	50.0
Eye	44.0
Environmental Health Sciences	35.2
Total	2042.9*

*Includes $149.4 million for aging, international studies, and other programs.
Source: Division of Financial Management, National Institutes of Health.

It should be added that administrators of major research institutions would generally agree to allocate relatively more money to areas promising significant scientific advances. For example, if it appeared that a major breakthrough seemed likely in cancer research, cancer would receive extra funding at the expense of other areas. However, the other areas would receive a basic level of funding so as to stimulate new ideas and, hopefully, eventual breakthroughs. What do you think about this policy?

In concluding this section on health expenditures let us attempt to put into perspective the research funds appropriated each year by the federal government for medical research. Consider the following:

1. The National Aeronautics and Space Administration has been spending approximately $4 billion a year to conduct moon orbits and other nonmilitary space ventures.
2. The Department of Defense spends more than $2 billion a year for research and development on missiles each year.
3. The Department of Agriculture spends approximately $250 million for research on plant and animal diseases each year.
4. The Forest Service spends approximately $300 million for forest protection each year.
5. The U.S. Bureau of Outdoor Recreation spends nearly $200 million for the development of public outdoor recreational areas each year.
6. The government allocates well over $100 billion for defense purposes.

Compared with these other expenditures by the federal government, the health research appropriation may not appear to be out of proportion. When it is compared with the spending priorities of private citizens, however, the contrast becomes rather shocking. Each year, Americans spend approximately the following amounts of money:

1. $14 billion on alcoholic beverages
2. $8 billion on tobacco
3. $2.5 billion on cameras and photographic equipment
4. $1 billion on boxed candy
5. $1 billion on greeting cards
6. $300 million on hair sprays

Do these statistics indicate that our budgetary priorities are in order or not? This question is not easily answered. In a free society people make their own decisions on how to spend their money. Through their representatives they influence decisions on national budgets, including health expenditures. Before a patient is operated on, the surgeon discusses with him the rationale as well as the pros and cons of the procedure. Based on this information, the patient then decides whether or not to consent, In quite analogous fashion, it may be advisable for the government to seek the informed consent of the general public when it allocates tax monies for medical research. What is your opinion?

TAKING ACTION

1. *Discuss the question of how our financial priorities might be readjusted so that alcohol, tobacco, candy and perhaps defense would get less of our money and medical research more—that is, if you consider this desirable.*
2. *Discuss with others the medical problems your family has encountered. What would more advanced medical treatment have meant to your family?*
3. *Interview or invite to class an expert on politics to determine just how greater emphasis upon health education and medical research might be achieved.*

DISCUSSION

A major problem of disease is that the etiology of most of the important chronic diseases is unknown. In only a few instances have genetic, microbiological, toxic, or other causal factors been identified. Though direct evidence is lacking, many investigators now believe that it is our environment that holds the key to the pathogenesis of myocardial infarction, cancer, and other serious health problems.

Unfortunately, believing in the effect of environmental factors on disease and proving it are two very different things. Consider the tentative evidence that diets high in cholesterol and fats are responsible for heart disease. How can this theory be proved or, for that matter, disproved? Major efforts are under way to study men whose risk of coronary disease is high. Half of them are given diets low in cholesterol and saturated fats while the remainder maintain their regular eating patterns. By observing the two groups over a period of five years or more, and by documenting whatever heart disease occurs among them, validation of the "cholesterol hypothesis" may be possible. Unfortunately, these clinical trials are very difficult to conduct. Getting people to volunteer, convincing them to maintain their assigned diets, keeping in touch with them to observe developing disease, and so on are all enormous problems. For this and other reasons the riddle of heart disease etiology is still far from solution.

In the meantime, what should we do? The prudent approach would seem to be to maintain a reasonable diet and a reasonable weight. Even if the cholesterol theory proves false, such behavior would offer the benefits of a slimmer and more attractive figure, to say nothing of money saved in the food budget.

We might apply the same argument to another contemporary theory of disease: the "exercise hypothesis." According to this hypothesis, the risk of heart attacks, high blood pressure, and other chronic diseases is increased among excessively sedentary individuals who do not exercise their muscles, blood vessels, and other physiologic functions

445

sufficiently. Although the evidence is still rather meager, the college student of today has a great deal to gain and nothing to lose by accepting this view, at least to the extent of engaging regularly in physical activity.

The cholesterol and exercise hypotheses represent the current "best guesses" by outstanding physicians and medical investigators about important health problems. They are clearly labeled as hypotheses or theories, while research projects are undertaken to test their validity in an objective fashion. Contrasting with them are a number of exotic movements, unsubstantiated by scientific study, which advocate a variety of food fads and "antiestablishment" patterns of behavior. Though many college students are understandably attracted to such nonconformist views, their enthusiasm often wanes as the sense of novelty wears off. The rule of moderation as a guideline to health behavior may seem old fashioned, but it will survive the next generation of health fads as it has the present one.

Despite the dangers and their attendant tensions (which give rise to duodenal ulcers and other psychosomatic diseases), the twentieth and twenty-first centuries offer enormous opportunities for college students and others to make meaningful and rewarding contributions to society. How can this be done? Do we study merely to pass the course? Do we simply go through the motions of getting a job done? All of us can modify our behavior in order to minimize the effects of tension and stress on our ability to enjoy life, to find fulfillment in our work, and to discover that greatest of gifts, peace of mind.

FOR FURTHER READING

Advisory Committee to the Surgeon General, U.S. Public Health Service, 1964. *Smoking and Health.* P.H.S. Publication No. 1103.

This is the famous report that eventually led to such federal actions as labeling cigarettes dangerous and banning their advertisement on television.

Brecher, R., Brecher, E., Herzog, A., et al., 1963. *The Consumers Union Report on Smoking and the Public Interest.* Mount Vernon, N.Y.: Consumers Union.

A year before the Surgeon General's report was issued, Consumers Union commissioned its own study, notable for its frankness and readability.

Facts on the Major Killing and Crippling Diseases in the United States Today, 1971. New York: National Health Education Committee.

Important statistics on all the major diseases are outlined here.

Friedman, G.D., 1974. *Primer of Epidemiology.* New York: McGraw-Hill.

Epidemiology is the medical discipline concerned with the distribution and determinants of disease. This little paperback book provides an excellent introduction to our understanding of causal factors of disease.

Silverberg, E., and Holleb, A.I., 1972. Cancer Statistics, 1972. *Ca—A Cancer Journal for Clinicians* 22:2–20.

Data on cancer are summarized annually in this small journal.

Young, C.G., and Barger, J.D., 1969. *Introduction to Medical Science*. St. Louis: Mosby.

This volume will provide you with a concise introduction to the normal and the abnormal in medicine, from basic principles of pathogenesis to specific disease processes.

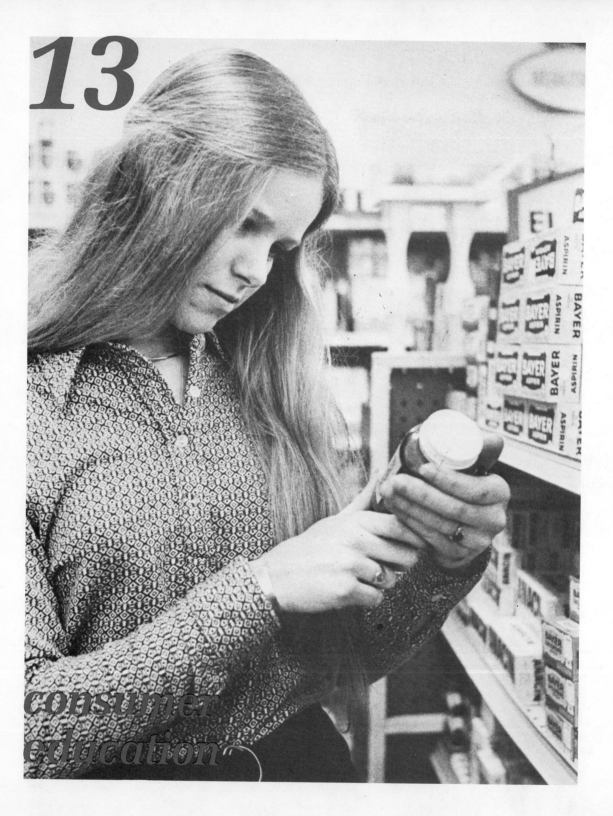

13

*consumer
education*

Consumer education in the field of health places its emphasis on the challenge of prevention. The potential of prevention is highlighted in the marketplace, where choosing the right food and drugs, demanding safer transportation, and refusing harmful goods and services can have a direct impact on producers and, ultimately, on the quality of their products. In the marketplace insistence on comparative information affords the consumer the ability to buy what is safest at the lowest price possible. Where there is little choice but to consume such things as polluted air, contaminated water, and risks of the workplace, prevention measures are effected only through organized action. Ending the compulsory exposure to nuclear power risks and realities, for example, will take persistent citizen action. Finally, the area of professional health care makes special demands on the consumer. Consumers must learn how to shop for doctors and dentists, how to avoid unnecessary surgery, how to choose a hospital, and how to keep medical costs down. As patients, consumers must be aware of their rights, including those to privacy and informed consent. Wherever health and health maintenance are concerned, knowledge is important—as is, supremely, its implementation. To protect their interests consumers must organize not only as consumers but as citizens shaping government policy.

INQUIRY

1. Why is consumer action a necessary part of consumer education?
2. How much can nutrition labeling help in planning a healthy diet?
3. Must America live with 50,000 traffic fatalities every year?
4. What evacuation procedures will you follow in the event of a nuclear accident?
5. How can you be sure that recommended surgery is necessary?
6. What do you do when a dentist wants to pull one of your teeth?

INTRODUCTION

New hazards to health come every day into every home. The shopping bag and even the air and water have become modern-day Trojan horses assaulting human life. Technology and the times require an all-out effort at "defending the home"—that is, education followed by action. In the field of health it means a new emphasis on problem prevention. For the consumer it means learning the connection between health and goods, services and the environment. Finally, it means vigilant citizens organized to lower the cost of living well.

According to the U.S. Department of Health, Education and Welfare (HEW), 10 million Americans have some form of heart disease; over 18 million, arthritis; and over 3 million, ulcers. More than 1 million are under medical care for cancer. There are, in addition, 20 million suffering from some form of mental disorder. Among the many other

449

important health problems are high blood pressure, iron and vitamin A deficiencies, dental diseases, visual and hearing impairments, and drug abuse. Serious health problems, which HEW calls "acute conditions" resulting in medical attention or restricted activity, cannot help but have an effect on personal freedom and the nation's productivity. In 1973 alone 360 million acute conditions caused 1.9 *billion* restricted activity days, averaging more than nine days for each American man, woman, and child.

Attempting to counter the complications of disease and injury, Americans are spending well over $115 billion annually for medical care. Of this, 39 percent goes for hospital care, 18 percent for physicians' services, 6 percent for dentists' services, and 9 percent for drugs. In 1974 spending for medical care amounted to almost 7.7 percent of the gross national product, compared with 7.2 percent in 1970 and 5.2 percent in 1960. In the late 1960s and early 1970s health care costs were rising about 10 percent every year, and no one was predicting a quick leveling off.

Can consumers rationally expect lower medical costs? Of course, they can. There is ample evidence to show many of today's health expenditures are wasted (Table 13-1). Unnecessary hospitalizations alone may cost Americans $10 billion annually by conservative estimates. Hospital beds no one needs cost at least $8 billion more. One estimate puts the total cost of medical waste at $21.5 billion a year, 21 percent of all medical care costs in 1974.[1] Other studies indicate that total waste in the area of health care could amount to 28 percent of all costs or higher.

Well aware of the staggering increases in health care costs and the aggravation of monumental waste, the U.S. Public Health Service in 1974 and 1975 prepared a "Forward Plan for Health." The plan places new emphasis on disease prevention and consumer cost-consciousness. It explains that "In recent years, it has become clear that only by preventing disease from occurring, rather than treating it later, can we hope to achieve any major improvement in the nation's health." Calling attention to a number of preventable health problems, the plan suggests alternatives to overcome them. The proposals include consumer education, legislation, intensified research, and support of improved technology. The plan also anticipates inroads to be made by prevention-oriented health maintenance organizations (HMOs), designed to provide comprehensive and economical health care services.

The need for a national health program of problem prevention is clear, but while the government moves ever so slowly toward implementing new strategies of health improvement, each citizen has a personal responsibility to keep informed on the problems of health and whenever possible to organize, to educate others, and to act. Today defending the home is a full-time job.

---

[1] Sidney Wolfe, HEW Conference on Inflation, September 19–20, 1974.

HEALTH CARE WASTE		Table 13-1
Type of Waste	Magnitude of Waste	Cost per Year (billions)
Unnecessary hospitalizations	10 million per year at $1,000 each	$10
Unnecessary hospital beds	60,000 Construction costs: $50,000 Operating costs: $18,250 per year per bed	$3 $1.1
Unnecessary surgery	2 million operations per year at $1000 each	$2
Drug promotion	Including advertising and retailing	$1
Unnecessary drugs	Overprescribed antibiotics, tranquilizers, noneffective prescription drugs, worthless over-the-counter drugs	$2
Unnecessary X rays	Of $4.8 billion per year spent for diagnostic health and dental X rays, about 30 percent are for "defensive" purposes	$1.4
Profiteering of private insurance industry		$3
Total waste per year (billions)		$21.5

Source: Health Research Group.

Consumers traditionally have best expressed their wants and needs in the marketplace. Theory has it that consumers, ready with the option not to buy, actually restrain the production of products that are harmful, and by exercising their option cause those unsafe products that do appear to disappear. This occurs in practice when consumers are aware of three important facts about each product they consider: (1) what it is supposed to do, (2) what its side effects are, and (3) what alternatives are available. As a quick trip through the marketplace will show, the availability, complexity, and impact of this kind of information varies from product to product—from nothing to little. The consumer is left with the task of finding, understanding, and using enough information to avoid the disease and trauma traps.

Food

Of all products marketed, food has to be the most essential to health maintenance and disease prevention. Yet depending on the way it is consumed, food can hurt as well as help. Obesity, which increases susceptibility to diabetes and other diseases, affects up to 30 percent of all Americans. The increased intake of saturated fats and cholesterol is increasing incidents of coronary heart disease. Sugar ingestion is encouraging tooth decay. Food additives, fortifiers, and artificial colors and flavors are producing side effects of unimaginable proportions. Meanwhile, malnutrition is rife among the poor and the aged.

Almost every problem related to food consumption can also be related to poor consumer information. Unfortunately, little is done that recognizes this reality. Shopping centers have yet to evolve into centers of information. As far as food goes, retailers remain more interested in enlarging their sales volumes than they are in shielding their customers from deceptive marketing practices or from hidden threats to health. In the areas of protection and education the pertinent government agencies, continuing their close relations with food manufacturers, have been almost as neglectful of their duties.

The case of vinyl chloride in food packaging illustrates this state of affairs. Vinyl chloride is used in the production of polyvinyl chloride, a widely used plastic. The National Institute of Occupational Safety and Health (NIOSH) has documented its connection with human cases of angiosarcoma, a very rare and usually fatal cancer of the liver. Animals also have contacted cancer from the inhalation of small amounts of vinyl chloride. While attention was being given the effects on workers exposed to the chemical, it was found that vinyl chloride residues were "migrating" into vegetable oils and other foods packaged in polyvinyl chloride.

One of the vegetable oils was Wesson Oil. When it was shown that a cancer-causing agent was entering the oil, the Food and Drug Administration allowed Wesson (and other food manufacturers) to make a quiet change to glass containers. Consumers were allowed to purchase Wesson in the old polyvinyl chloride containers until the stocks ran out. The FDA obviously put the economic interest of Wesson before the public interest. Not so obvious were the people making the FDA's decisions. One was Virgil Wodicka, then director of the FDA's Bureau of Food. Prior to working with the federal agency, Wodicka had been an executive with Wesson.

Influence like this has a way of circumventing even the most irrefutable evidence of hazards to health. It happens every day in thousands of quiet decisions made without public scrutiny. Time and time again the food industry is found exploiting the disorganization of the citizenry. So what is today's citizen-consumer left with? Practically no means to guarantee that important food information will be made available. In 1973 consumers had no way of knowing that three FDA studies conducted before 1960 had demonstrated that a widely used red food coloring could cause cancer. Since this writing, Red Dye #2 has been banned by the FDA. However, the FDA is allowing all foods manufactured with the dye before the ban to be sold to the public. Now there is still no way a consumer can tell what a hot dog really

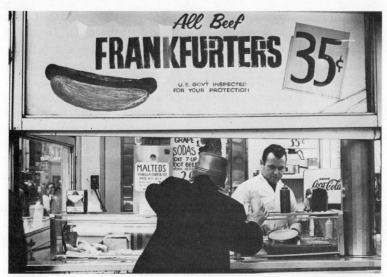

Hugh Rogers/Monkmeyer

holds—no note that even an "all-beef" frankfurter might contain 30 percent fat and 10 percent water. Nor is there any warning about the presence of sodium nitrate in processed meats. There is no indication that the preservative has been implicated in the production of nitrosamines, cancer-causing agents, in the digestive system. The need for new kinds of citizen action becomes clear.

Nutrition Labeling   Of the few handy means for learning something of the food we eat, nutrition labeling is one. Used on food products with nutrients added and others that make nutritional claims, nutrition labels must have three basic parts. The first, at the top, indicates the "serving size" (1 cup, for instance) on which information that follows is based. The second, just under the serving size, shows the number of calories and the amount of protein, carbohydrate, and fat (in grams) in a single serving. The third part lists the percentages of U.S. Recommended Daily Allowances (U.S. RDA) for protein, vitamin A, vitamin C, three of the B vitamins (thiamine, riboflavin, and niacin), calcium, and iron in a serving. Other information, like the types of fat and amount of sodium furnished by a serving, may be added to the labels, but food manufacturers are not known to jump at the chance to tell more than they must.

There are a number of problems with nutrition labels, not the least of which—due to inadequate health education in schools and elsewhere—is the inability of most Americans to understand and use them.

Even to the knowledgeable, nutrition labeling can be confusing. The nutrition information on each label is based on the contents of a single serving, but the manufacturer's serving size can be significantly smaller than what the consumer serves at home; thus the information is easily misinterpreted by anyone not willing to carry a calculator. The amount of protein shown on the label can be further distorted. Because certain kinds of protein are more efficient than others (for example, egg protein is better than wheat protein), simply stating there are x grams of protein in a food product is insufficient.

Similarly, the listed percentages of vitamins can be misleading. Some foods are "fortified" with synthetic vitamins to make them appear as nutritious as other foods that produce like amounts of vitamins naturally. The problem is not that synthetic vitamins are inferior to natural vitamins; rather, it's the fact that natural foods are much more likely to provide a proper balance of vitamins and probably contain important nutrients that scientists have not identified for fortification. By not making a distinction between synthetic and natural nutrients, nutrition labeling actually encourages food manufacturers to overdo their doses of synthetic vitamins like A and D, which are toxic when consumed in excessive quantities.

A wise consumer looks at traditional foods (especially those not touched by chemical toxins) for what they have to offer: the calcium in milk and milk products; the vitamin C and A in fruits and vegetables; the protein in eggs, fish, meat, and poultry; the iron and B vitamins in whole grain or enriched breads and cereals; and so on. After this kind of homework, the daily allowances printed on nutrition labels become particularly valuable.

But the consumer still has to know what a percentage of the U.S. RDA means. One hundred percent of the nutrients listed is more than enough for most people. Table 13-2, prepared by the National Research Council, shows recommended allowances according to age and sex. When properly applied, this information not only helps in planning balanced meals but also serves to restrain unnecessary spending.

Children, Food, and Advertising A balanced diet is especially important for children. Not only are a child's poor eating habits likely to be carried on into adulthood, they are also capable of impairing daily performance including in the classroom. A badly undernourished child is not a child ready to take on new concepts. In spite of this fact, too many parents leave critical dietary decisions to the children themselves. And on what information do children commonly base their decisions? TV commercials.

An estimated $400 million is spent each year for television advertising directed at children. A large part of this is designed to lure children to the kinds of cereals, soft drinks, and snacks they could easily do without. In 1970 a study by the Council on Children, Media and Merchandising (CCMM) in Washington, D.C., revealed the fact that 40 widely advertised dry breakfast cereals were almost entirely without nutritional content. How are children to know their Captain Crunch is more than 40 percent sugar? How are they to know the toll that can take in terms of tooth decay and other health problems? Adults certainly have a responsibility here, but it's too easy for a parent (who might

Table 13-2

ALLOWANCES FOR FOOD ENERGY AND PERCENTAGES OF THE U.S. RECOMMENDED DAILY ALLOWANCES NEEDED TO MEET THE RECOMMENDED DIETARY ALLOWANCES FOR CHILDREN, MEN, AND WOMEN OF DIFFERENT AGES

Age (years)	Food energy (calories) [a]	Protein [b]	Vitamin A	Vitamin C	Thiamin	Riboflavin	Niacin [c]	Calcium	Iron
Child									
1–3	1300	35	40	70	50	50	30	80	85
4–6	1800	50	50	70	60	65	35	80	60
7–10	2400	55	70	70	80	75	50	80	60
Male									
11–14	2800	70	100	75	95	90	55	120	100
15–18	3000	85	100	75	100	110	55	120	100
19–22	3000	85	100	75	100	110	60	80	60
23–50	2700	90	100	75	95	95	45	80	60
51+	2400	90	100	75	80	90	35	80	60
Female									
11–14	2400	70	80	75	80	80	45	120	100
15–18	2100	75	80	75	75	85	30	120	100
19–22	2100	75	80	75	75	85	35	80	100
23–50	2000	75	80	75	70	75	30	80	100
51+	1800	75	80	75	70	65	25	80	60
Pregnant	+300d	+50d	100	100	+20d	+20d	35	120	100+
Nursing	+500d	+35d	120	135	+20d	+30d	35	120	100

[a] Calorie needs differ depending on body composition and size, age, and activity of the person.

[b] U.S. RDA of 65 grams is used for this table. In labeling, a U.S. RDA of 45 grams is used for foods providing high-quality protein, such as milk, meat, and eggs.

[c] The percentage of the U.S. RDA shown for niacin will provide the RDA for niacin if the RDA for protein is met. Some niacin is derived in the body from tryptophan, an amino acid present in protein.

[d] To be added to the percentage for the girl or woman of the appropriate age.

Source: U.S. Recommended Daily Allowance, March 14, 1973, Federal Register 38, no. 49, part II; Recommended Dietary Allowances, 8th ed., National Academy of Sciences, National Research Council, 1974.

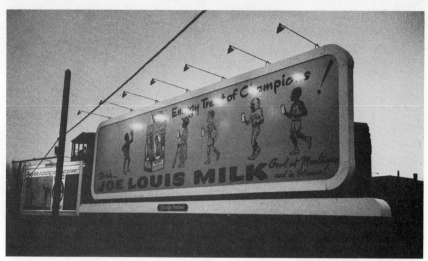

Bruce Davidson/Magnum Photos

think all cereals are the same anyway) to succumb to the pleas of a persuaded child (who remembers only that a cartoon character said the product was good).

An average child (from 3 to 12 years of age) watches some 22,000 commercials each year. The commercials depict another word, a fantasy world of sugar on sugar breakfast, lunches with potato chips that look exactly alike, and dinner dates with Ronald MacDonald. Here sweetness, packaging, and the perception of fun are given priority; health is at best secondary.

Recognizing these distortions to be nothing short of exploitation of children by advertisers, CCMM has asked the Federal Communications Commission (FCC) and the Federal Trade Commission (FTC) to use their authority to protect children against the excesses of advertising. But there has been little federal action. The CCMM suggests action consumers can take on the local level. It notes that a group of only 10 can have a real effect on the programming of an entire city. Documented evidence must be collected. Exact times and wording of questionable programs and commercials are essential.

Compare the number of commercials promoting poor eating habits with the number of public service announcements encouraging proper nutrition and dental health. When a case has been made that a television station has been violating its use of a public trust, get a public interest lawyer to help write a formal letter of complaint to the station. Assuming that the case is a good one, the station should be ready for serious talks at this point. If not, the station's license renewal can be challenged at the FCC. The procedure may seem complicated, but information on it is available at the Office of Communication, United Church of Christ, 289 Park Avenue South, New York, NY 10010.

The consumer typically purchases two kinds of drugs: over-the-counter (nonprescription) drugs and prescription (legally available by medical prescriptions only) drugs. They are a big business. Well over $12 billion are spent on them annually.

Over-the-Counter Drugs These drugs are labeled to help consumers understand what is in each drug, how much of each drug is in its container, and how to use the drug safely. The Federal Food, Drug, and Cosmetic Act requires that each over-the-counter drug label include: (1) the name and address of the manufacturer, packer, or distributor; (2) the net amount of the drug; (3) a list of those ingredients (active ingredients) that will have the intended effect; (4) directions for safe and effective use; and (5) adequate warnings when necessary. A mislabeled drug can be recalled by the Food and Drug Administration.

For both over-the-counter and prescription drugs, manufacturers are required to prove that their drugs are safe and effective before they can be marketed. If, after an over-the-counter drug is marketed, its medical claims are found to be false, legal action may be taken by the FDA or the Federal Trade Commission. The system is far from adequate. The FDA's drug warning system and the FTC's oversight often break down. Complications of even the most popular drugs can go unchecked for years.

For example, in 1973 the FDA found the use of "Alka-Seltzer" for stomach systems alone to be "irrational." All Alka-Seltzer contained aspirin at that time. And aspirin had been implicated as a cause of excess stomach bleeding in people with ulcers and in some normal people. But while it was concluded that use of aspirin in an antacid expected to relieve stomach problems was foolish and possibly harmful, the FDA asked only that Miles Laboratories, the manufacturer, promote Alka-Seltzer for use when a patient has both stomachache and headache.

For obvious reasons, the FDA hadn't gone far enough. Headache or not, the aspirin in Alka-Seltzer wasn't going to help anyone's gastrointestinal symptoms. Public Citizen's Health Research Group surveyed 122 gastroenterologists. The group found that 89 percent of the specialists would not advise use of Alka-Seltzer for stomach upset alone, and 87 percent would not advise it for stomach upset and headache together. Nevertheless, the FDA refused to ban the use of antacid/aspirin combinations for treating stomach ailments. Shortly afterward, Miles placed a new Alka-Seltzer without aspirin on market shelves but continued selling the old Alka-Seltzer too.

As deserving of the consumer's caution is the increasing popularity of the over-the-counter drugs called vitamins. Annual vitamin sales now amount to half a billion dollars. Although there is little information about the safety or efficacy of vitamin doses above Recommended Daily Allowances, few consumers reject the vague statement that "vitamins are good for you." Such confidence has led to outrageously inflated claims (and prices) by vitamin manufacturers. Some declare that massive doses or combinations of vitamins can cure everything from the common cold and baldness to the effects of air pollution. Not only are most of these claims totally unsubstantiated, they tend to distract consumers from dealing with the *causes* of their problems. Such claims can be downright dangerous too.

But no one can argue that the dangers of any over-the-counter drugs are going to be waved away by a warning label, as important as that label can be. It is an undeniable fact that many people don't read labels. And where drugs with potentially damaging side effects are concerned, it is nothing less than criminal to leave consumer awareness to chance. The drug industry spends approximately $300 million each year promoting its over-the-counter drugs on television, but the quality of information leaves much to be desired. Puffery is the order of the day; seldom are Americans given the simple, sober facts.

Prescription Drugs The regulation of prescription drugs presents special problems of consumer education. Practicing physicians prescribe drugs for three-fourths of their patients; they give few of their patients any information they can use as a basis for intelligent questioning. Patients are systematically uninformed of almost every important fact about the drugs they take by prescription. Federal law requires that labels on prescription drugs shipped to pharmacists or physicians include a list of active ingredients and all the information necessary for safe and effective use: when the drug should not be used, possible side effects, and warnings should be indicated. None of this information is required to appear on prescription labels for the consumer.

Neither is the consumer permitted adequate information on drug prices. For years statutory and regulatory restrictions in many states and localities have prohibited advertising the retail prices of prescription drugs. In other regions peer pressure among pharmacists has had the same effect on advertising. Although this system caused price discrepancies of up to 300 percent and had nothing beneficial to offer consumers, as of 1975 the federal government had only initiated action to remove the anticompetitive checks on disclosure of prescription drug prices.

In the early 1970s consumer groups in 11 states and the District of Columbia surveyed the pricing of prescription drugs and found more than an unfair and arbitrary price structure. Student-funded Public Interest Research Groups (PRGs) found that in many drugstores pharmacists were filling generic prescriptions with expensive brand-name drugs, effectively nullifying doctors' attempts to give their patients a price break. The groups also discovered the curious fact that drugstores offering free delivery and 24-hour emergency services did not necessarily charge the highest prices. They had discovered the value of comparison shopping.

Every year automobile accidents are responsible for about 50,000 fatalities, 4.5 million injuries, and $30 billion of economic waste. For Americans between 5 and 25 years of age, car accidents are the leading cause of death.

The sad fact is that carnage on the highway is among America's most preventable problems. Indeed, technology already promises significant progress in car safety. But as long as the automobile manufacturers are able to obstruct efforts to establish government safety standards, avoidable auto casualties will continue to occur in the millions annually.

Auto manufacturers will have their first readings of the demand for safety when consumers receive comparative information. Federal regulations, to be enforced by the National Highway Traffic Safety Administration (NHTSA), will soon require all car dealers to provide data on vehicle damageability and crashworthiness. Once a safety rating system is developed, the consumer will be able to compare such information as brake stopping distance and the likelihood a driver will live through an accident. If the NHTSA comes around to requiring passive restraint systems, consumers would be able to compare them too.

With facts on hand, consumers would soon see the advantages of the "air bag," one form of passive restraint system. During a car crash the air bag automatically inflates in front of the passenger, distributes the force of the crash, and effectively prevents serious injury. It also deflates in a fraction of a second. Making use of space-age technology, each air bag can be calibrated to inflate only at certain crash speeds. Its reliability has been proved so convincingly in sample cars on the highway that the Allstate Insurance Company actively promotes its uniform use for all automobiles.

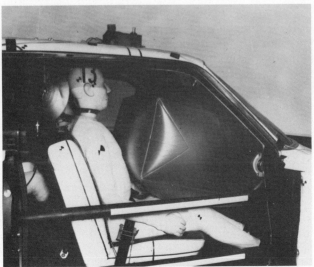

A crash resistant bag, designed to protect a car's occupant, shown here in fully inflated condition.

Wide World Photos

459

Requiring the installation of air bags or similar passive restraint systems will add less than $100 to the cost of a car (less than the cost of a vinyl roof cover), but the requirement will also prevent tens of thousands of fatalities and serious injuries a year.

In the absence of more meaningful data and higher safety standards, consumers can use their own good judgment in choosing a car. They have to look behind the romance. They have to ask questions. After cars are purchased, they can use existing safety devices. (The properly designed shoulder harness-lap belt combination, though seldom used, is a most effective restraint.) And when auto safety problems arise, consumers should report them to the dealer, the manufacturer, and the NHTSA. Consumers have to exhibit and transmit a concern for safety right back to the auto companies.

Cigarettes

The smoking epidemic tests the nation's concern for its health. Forty-five million Americans smoke 600 billion cigarettes annually. Since the Surgeon General's 1964 report on the hazards of smoking, there has been a decline in smoking in the population 25 and older, but teenage smoking, especially by women, has increased. By the time they are 18 years old, 42 percent of men and 28 percent of women are regular smokers.

The practice has created a slew of preventable health problems. As we have noted elsewhere, lung cancer, a rare disease at the turn of the century, now kills 81,000 Americans annually. Between 80 and 90 percent of these deaths are caused by smoking. Heart disease, chronic bronchitis, emphysema, unsuccessful pregnancies, and cancers of the larynx, lip, oral cavity, esophagus, and bladder have also been linked to smoking. The President's Science Advisory Committee estimated that 16 percent of total mortality was related to smoking in 1967.

By ending televised cigarette commercials in 1971, Congress did little to alleviate the problem. In fact the ban led to a reduction of antismoking television spots, thus impeding the national effort to educate the public. Today almost every American adult knows something about the effects of smoking, but too many remain unpersuaded.

And just how can the nation fully sense the urgency of the problem when at the same time the government advises people to stop smoking it continues multimillion-dollar subsidies to the tobacco industry? The Health Research Group asked this question in 1975. In a letter to President Gerald Ford, it noted that while $900,000 was being spent each year on the government's campaign against smoking, approximately $60 million in federal funds was going to support programs keeping tobacco growers in business. Recommended was an end to tobacco supports, a transfer of the $60 million to a full-scale antismoking program, and federal aid to assist tobacco growers in a transition to other crops.

Cigarette smoking has to be discouraged whenever it can be, particularly in public transportation vehicles, public buildings, and hospitals. Nonsmokers have rights they are starting to assert against being exposed to smokers. Consumer education is only part of this problem's solution, but it is the part every citizen can promote.

Consumer Products

For the purposes of the U.S. Consumer Product Safety Commission, consumer products are articles used in or around households, schools, or in recreation. Specifically excluded from the commission's authority are food, drugs, cars, tobacco, alcohol, boats, and aircraft. But the number of products under its purview is large enough that, with adequate consumer input, its actions can prevent literally millions of injuries every year. Toys, flammable fabrics, household chemicals, bicycles, and aerosol sprays are a few of the products for which the commission issues and enforces standards of safety.

Currently 30,000 people die and 110,000 are permanently disabled each year as a result of injuries suffered in and around the home. To monitor the causes of these injuries, the staff of the Consumer Product Safety Commission examines injury reports from 119 hospital emergency rooms across the land. Complaints directly from consumers are equally as important in the commission's efforts.

By writing the commission,[2] consumers can have their names placed on a "roster" that indicates their areas of expertise and a willingness to share their knowledge in the development of certain product safety standards. Consumers can testify at information-gathering hearings. They can take part in meetings between the commission and industry. They can comment on proposed standards. And they can petition the commission to begin proceedings to issue, amend, or revoke a consumer product safety rule. Petitions may be handwritten or typed; the commission has to consider them either way. If a request is granted, proceedings begin; if not, the commission must publish reasons for the denial.

The activities of the Consumer Product Safety Commission, of other government agencies, and of the business community highlight an already conspicuous reality. In every phase of life in the marketplace—in shopping for food or a means of transportation, for toys or shaving cream—the consumer much more than ever needs to learn the fine art of self-defense. Shrewd consumerism is no longer a simple matter of knowing how to buy; where health is concerned, it is the more involved matter of knowing how to act.

TAKING ACTION

1. Use the chart of Recommended Daily Allowance, and perhaps Nutrition Labeling *(see For Further Reading) to help you plan a meal that is both*

---

[2]The commission can be telephoned free of charge anywhere in the continental United States. Dial 800-638-2660 in most states. Dial 800-492-2937 in Maryland. In Alaska and Hawaii write the Consumer Product Safety Commission, Washington, D.C. 20207.

nutritious and inexpensive. Defend your selections in group discussions.

2. Form a family drug study committee. Look at the drugs in homes. How much did they cost? Find out what they do. If you can, get opinions on each of the drugs from two different physicians. How much money could be saved by living without unnecessary drugs and by purchasing drugs under their generic, rather than brand, names?

3. Visit the people at the nearest regional offices of the Consumer Product Safety Commission. Ask them about one area of product safety. Toys would be a good one. In that case, ask them what kinds of hazards toys present. Ask to see their file of complaints on toys. Ask how the regulations are enforced. Ask them how they inform communities as to their location and functions. Later, study the regulations, and go toy shopping. Note whether all the toys you see appear safe to you and whether they meet Consumer Product Safety Commission regulations. Then do something with what you learn.

4. Organize a Public Interest Research Group. The book Action for a Change (Nader and Ross, 1971) and the booklet A PIRG Organizer's Notebook (Nader and Ross, 1974) will help.

COMPULSORY CONSUMPTION

By buying and refusing to buy, consumers in the marketplace have at least the opportunity to use information in the interest of their health. Consumers are deprived of this choice outside the marketplace, where the most ferocious threats to health are bred. Although no one purchases these threats through a monetary expression of want or need, everyone pays for them. The results are shorter lives, special medical treatment, property damage, and a diseased environment.

Pollution

Pollution is a prime example of compulsory consumption. Only a fool would ask to breathe poisoned air or drink contaminated water, but

Smoke pollution from a Texan factory.

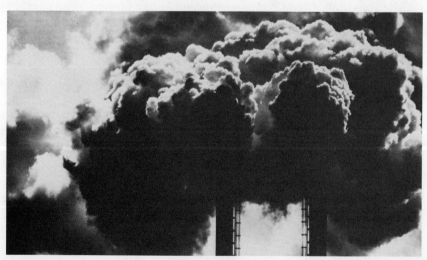

Wide World Photos

millions of Americans have no choice but to be victimized in these ways. And millions are beginning to feel the impact of their sullied world. Each citizen knows that an individual refusal to purchase the products of chronic polluters like the steel and auto industries is not likely to change the direction of industry decision makers. It's going to take the action of united consumers to (1) expose the polluters and the cost of pollution, (2) monitor the enforcement of existing state and federal pollution control laws, (3) fund court action against businesses and government agencies derelict in their compliance with the law, and (4) pressure U.S. senators and representatives for new and improved legislation.

Risks of the Workplace

Citizen groups can take the same approach to counter the occupational hazards over which the worker has little control. The U.S. Department of Health, Education and Welfare estimates that each year 100,000 workers die and more than 2 million are disabled by injuries and illness related to adverse working conditions. Even so, the Occupational Safety and Health Administration (OSHA), the federal agency that is supposed to protect workers by setting and enforcing good safety and health standards, has treated its responsibilities with apathy. Just four and a half years after its establishment, OSHA's review commission was taking an average of eight months to hear each case before it. Its case backlog was in the hundreds. And penalties for violations of safety regulations were averaging $25, hardly enough to encourage compliance.

No worker wants to consume carcenogenic gas or be exposed to deafening noise or any of the many dangers of the workplace. But unless adequate standards are adequately enforced, workers can live each day with risks beyond their power to control or avoid. As a partial

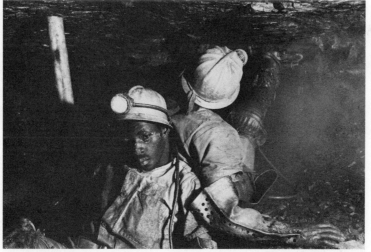

Underground fumes and dust are common hazards to the health of mineworkers.

Rene Burri/Magnum Photos

463

response to the problem, Public Citizen's Health Research Group in 1975 published the *Workers Handbook on Enforcing Safety and Health Standards* to guide worker involvement in enforcement proceedings. The handbook points up the importance of employees' participating in OSHA workplace inspections, checking OSHA violation citations for accuracy, and challenging any unreasonably long time period ("abatement period") OSHA proposes for correcting a hazard. Use of the book's suggestions can balance employers' testimony with that of well-prepared employees, speed up the review commission's proceedings, and in the process save workers from disease, injury, and death.

Any further action (through collective bargaining, petitioning for new standards, and other means) in the field of occupational safety and health is contingent upon information made public. Until recently neither industry nor government considered it the right of workers to have access to detailed information on their working conditions. Industry still does its best to keep hidden hazards hidden. Government is looking for guidance. And workers remain defenseless against many threats they do not know exist. It will be a giant step toward a safe and healthy workplace when workers, consumer groups, and the scientific community cooperate with government to give workers the means to evaluate for themselves the gravity of the risks that surround them.

Nuclear Power

Beyond all risks is the risk presented by the use of nuclear power plants and the associated technology, containing awesome amounts of radioactive materials. It is a test of credulity to watch the mad rush to build nuclear power plants, which are widely considered to be unsafe, uneconomical, and unnecessary. The energy industry, relentless in its attempt to perpetuate its blundering and overreaching, continues to portray nuclear power as the clean, efficient answer to our energy needs. Americans who have learned about nuclear energy from the industry's slick television commercials aren't likely to have many doubts about the "peaceful use of the atom." But the plain fact is that the billions of dollars spent on developing nuclear power have been wasted.

A 1965 study sponsored by the Atomic Energy Commission estimated that one big nuclear plant accident would cause $17 billion worth of property damage, 45,000 deaths, and hundreds of thousands of injuries throughout a contaminated area the size of Pennsylvania. One way this colossal calamity could occur would be through a failure of a plant's emergency core cooling system (ECCS) to back up normal cooling systems that fail. The reactor core would overheat, everything around it would melt, and enormous quantities of radioactive waste would be spewn into the atmosphere.

It is not paranoia, then, that makes one flinch at the less than perfect construction and operation of nuclear power plants. In March 1975 a serious fire at the world's largest nuclear plant, the Browns Ferry plant in Alabama, caused at least $50 million worth of direct damage and disabled all components of the ECCS in one reactor unit. How did it happen? Workmen were inspecting electric cable penetrations into the Browns Ferry Reactor Building. A technician using a 4-inch candle to check for air leakage accidentally ignited the foam used as sealant around the penetrations. The fire spread quickly and burned for seven hours before it was extinguished. For good reason, the accident frightened even the staunchest proponents of nuclear power. When nuclear power plants lack the competence to handle their small problems, their ability to deal with such massive problems as deadly nuclear wastes, sabotage, and fuel reprocessing has to be called into question.

Trying to prepare for the worst, the Nuclear Regulatory Commission (NRC) requires all operators of nuclear plants to prepare contingency plans for the evacuation of populations around their facilities. As of 1975 these planning efforts were inadequate at best. Except in Oregon there was no effort anywhere to let the public know even that evacuation plans existed. The omission could be catastrophic. In New York, for instance, 66,000 people live within 5 miles of the three Indian Point reactors, and 900,000 live within 20 miles. If a serious accident occurs there, these people (and more) are subject to lethal contamination.

In August 1975, 30 citizen groups in 19 states, with the assistance of the National Public Interest Research Group in Washington, D.C., took this message to the NRC. They petitioned the commission to require

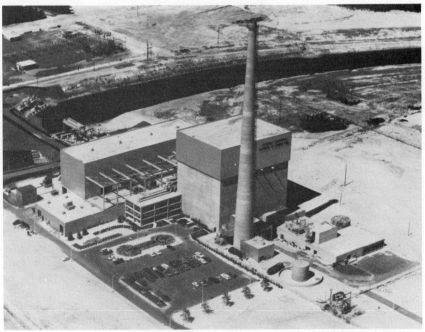

A nuclear station in New Jersey.

Wide World Photos

each utility company seeking a nuclear license to disseminate emergency plans to all those living within a 40-mile radius of a nuclear plant, and they asked that evacuation drills be conducted annually. Emergency evacuation plans are the least consumers can demand. However, they do not prevent accidents, nor do they approach the other problems of nuclear power.

The nuclear industry has yet to decide what to do about the waste produced by nuclear power plants. Each atomic reactor produces radioactive materials that are capable of causing cancer, death, and, in future generations, genetic disorder. With an efficient dispersal, less than 20 pounds of one product, plutonium 239, could give lung cancer to every man, woman, and child on earth.

It is difficult to sense the urgency of this menace, as it is unseen, silent, and slow. According to John Gofman at the University of California, plutonium fallout produced by past atmospheric weapons testing is just beginning to show its effects. He calculates the fallout has already condemned 116,000 people to die of lung cancer over the next 30 to 40 years. His data also show that even if the nuclear industry were to contain 99.99 percent of its reactor-produced plutonium, by the year 2020 it will cause an additional 500,000 lung cancer deaths a year.

Plutonium 239 remains lethal for over 250,000 years, which means it must be stored and guarded for just as long. An educated maniac managing to pirate 30 pounds of the material would have the wherewithal to construct a small atomic bomb. If government and industry projections are correct, by 1990 there will be 55 tons of plutonium used each year in the reactor industry. Citizens need to inform themselves about the full meaning of nuclear plant exports to lesser developed countries, where governments can easily divert weapons-grade materials from their atomic power plants to produce their own nuclear weapons. Citizens critical of nuclear power point to the sharply increasing costs of the energy source, its unresolved safety problems, and its lack of reliability. They believe that the superior availability of energy conservation and faster application of clean and truly safe solar power is the future.

TAKING ACTION

1. *Interview an inspector at one of the regional offices of the Occupational Safety and Health Administration. Ask which local workplaces OSHA has inspected and which (or how many) the agency has not. Ask about the common hazards of the workplace. And find out what is given the most careful scrutiny during a workplace inspection. Then ask to be present during an OSHA inspection. If that cannot be arranged, check a local workplace on your own. Try to get permission from management or through a labor union to look at the premises firsthand. If that is impossible, interview workers. Ask them pointed questions based on the information you obtained during your interview with the OSHA inspector.*

If you find violations of OSHA regulations, ask both OSHA and the management of the firm what will be done about them and how.

2. *If you live near a nuclear power plant in operation or under construction, find out what's going on at the plant. There are several ways to do this. First, you might contact the power plant coordinator with your local utility company. This coordinator might be able to arrange a tour of the plant or a workshop on nuclear power. If you get involved in either of these projects, prepare yourself before you go. Be ready with questions on the efficiency of nuclear power compared with other energy sources. Ask about the plant's safety features, area evacuation plans, and the kind of insurance policies held by the utility. Ask where the waste goes. In other words, arrange for a productive dialogue.*

3. *Another way of learning about your neighbor, the nuclear risk, is to visit the local power plant's Public Documents Room. Each of these is to be found in the library closest to each of the nuclear plants. Ask the librarian for help, and sort through the mountain of material on file. The "Emergency Planning" section of the preliminary or final "Safety Analysis Report" should be of particular interest—for what it shows and for what it fails to show. The section is supposed to outline plans for the emergency evacuation of the surrounding area. If the plan is typical, it is woefully inadequate. If you know your region well, you should be able to catch the inadequacies. To complement your study, look at the "Environmental Impact Report" and any "Abnormal Occurrence Reports" in the same file. If information is not easily available at the local Public Documents Room, contact Public Documents Room, Nuclear Regulatory Commission, Washington, D.C. 20555.*

PROFESSIONAL HEALTH CARE

Sooner or later almost everyone receives professional medical care. In the doctor's office, in the hospital, in the dentist's office, or wherever it is dispensed, today's professional medical care, in all its bewildering forms, demands of the consumer a new kind of skepticism that breaks through the mist of professional secrecy. Where their most intimate problems are concerned, consumers cannot afford blind faith in anyone, regardless of his credentials. Consumers have to know what they are paying for, understand any risks they face, and learn what their alternatives are. Active consumer participation in the choice of professional care is a necessity.

Doctors

How do you make an informed choice of a doctor? How do you compare one physician with another? It isn't easy. If you really want to be conscientious about picking a doctor, you've got a lot of digging to do. The medical profession does not make public ascertainable information on the quality or skill of each doctor. There is, however, information available with which consumers can evaluate their area physicians in terms of availability, services offered, and fees. The information is in the Yellow Pages, in professional medical directories, in files of local medical societies, and even in doctors' offices. The problem is putting it all together. In January 1974 the Public Citizen's

Figure 13-1
What a directory for doctors holds. This is the kind of information a consumer will want to have before choosing a physician. (Original format by Consumers Union, revised by the Health Research Group.)

DOE, JOHN

Introductory Information

101 First Avenue
Medville, New York 10022
212-111-2222

Internist
Fee-for-service, solo practice
Office personnel: one RN, one secretary, one X ray technician

Education, Appointments, and Affiliation

Doctors Medical College, Centreville, N.Y. 1954
Internship: Good Hope Hospital, Centreville, N.Y. 1954–55
Residency: Vista General Hospital, Chester City, N.Y. 1956–59
Fellowship in Cardiology: Doctors Medical College, Chester City, N.Y. 1959–60
Board Certified, intern
Sub-specialty, Cardiology
Chairman of Medical Education, Medville Hospital
Assistant Professor of Medicine, Westside Medical School
Chief, Department of Cardiology, Urban Medical Center, Chester City, N.Y.

Admits patients to: Medville Hospital—accredited, voluntary, affiliated with Westside Medical School; Urban Medical Center—accredited, municipal, nurses' training program.

Availability

Office hours: 8 A.M.–noon, Mon.–Thurs. and Sat.; 2–5 P.M., Wed.
After-hours coverage: answering service; can be reached at home; if out of town, other doctors cover.
Make house calls. Standard fee—$15.00.
Accepts new patients.
Required advance notice for routine visit—1–3 days; for complete physical examination—3 months.
Schedules 30 minutes for each patient if not seeing patient for first time or doing complete physical.
Sees walk-in patients without appointment if patient is known.

Languages: English only

Figure 13-1
(Continued)

Fees and Billing

Accepts Medicaid and Medicare patients; does accept Medicare patients on assignment. Sometimes accepts Medicare fee schedule as payment in full, depending on patient's economic status.

Standard fee for initial office visit: $30.00
Routine office visit: $10.00
Routine hospital visit: $15.00

Does not request fees prior to seeing the patient or at the time of service. Bills monthly.

Practice Information

Sometimes prescribes drugs by generic name. Does so if patient requests.
Usually advises patients of possible drug side effects.
Allows patients to view their medical records upon request.

Office equipped for: Chest X ray — Fee: $10.00
Urinalysis — 4.00
Complete blood count — 6.00
Throat culture — 8.00
Electrocardiogram — 10.00
Prescribes contraception.

Health Research Group compiled the first consumer's directory for doctors (Figure 13-1). The directory covered the physicians of Prince Georges County, Maryland. Since then, public interest groups in over a dozen states have published directories for their own communities.

The publications are milestones of consumer education. Medical societies have made it a matter of tradition to resist the public disclosure of any useful data on doctors. Many state doctor antiadvertising laws, originally enacted to protect the public from quacks, still are interpreted by some medical societies as prohibiting doctors from publishing their fees or their educational backgrounds. Consumers preparing directories are not subject to these restrictions inasmuch as it will be the consumers, not the doctors, who publish the information. When the doctor directory phenomena was making its first appearances, some physicians claimed medical ethics forbade their participation in the surveys. For these doctors the American Medical Association amended its *Principles of Medical Ethics* in December 1974 to permit doctor cooperation with consumers.

There are four steps in the preparation of a doctor directory: (1) *preliminary research*, (2) *contacting the doctors*, (3) *verification*, and

(4) *publication.* Depending on its scope and the number of people who work on it, a directory should take between two and four months to complete. Access to a medical library would be essential. To cover stationery and duplicating and mailing costs, funding of $200 to $300 would also be required. For details, a guide for compiling a consumers director for doctors is available from the Health Research Group (see For Further Reading).

Surgery The consumer's job does not end with the selection of a doctor. A number of critical decisions have to be made by the consumer in the doctor's office. One very difficult decision is whether or not to have surgery, once the need has been suggested. Few people are competent to decide on their own; so the decision is usually left to the doctor, who is often a surgeon. The problem with this is simple: the greater the number of operations performed the greater the economic reward to the surgeon. A good physician genuinely committed to quality care will insist on the participation of the patient in any choice of medical treatment and will help with the necessary information. On the other hand, a doctor preoccupied with keeping hospital beds filled is likely to exploit the confusion of the patient in recommending surgery that is not only expensive and dangerous but unnecessary.

Needless surgery in the United States results in at least 10,000 deaths each year. It is conservatively estimated that of the 18 million surgical operations performed annually, more than 3 million, or one-sixth, are unnecessary. Unwarranted hysterectomies, hemorrhoidectomies, and tonsillectomies are common. In the belief that a little consumer education could prevent a lot of pain and save a lot of money, a "Shopper's Guide to Surgery" was issued in 1972 by Herbert Denenberg, then Pennsylvania Commissioner of Insurance. It lists 14 rules for avoiding unnecessary surgery. Here is a brief summary in checklist form:

1. Don't go directly to the surgeon for medical treatment. Go to a general practitioner or internist, who tend to be more conservative.
2. Make sure that any surgeon who is to perform surgery on you is qualified by one of the American specialty boards.
3. Be sure your surgeon is a Fellow of the American College of Surgeons or the American College of Osteopathic Surgeons.
4. Consider getting an independent consultation or opinion before surgery, even if your family doctor and surgeon agree that surgery is necessary.
5. Make sure that surgery is performed in a hospital accredited by the Joint Commission on Accreditation of Hospitals or the American Osteopathic Association.
6. If you insist on surgery, even if it is unnecessary, you are likely to find a surgeon willing to perform it. Don't push.

7. Make sure that your doctor and surgeon explain both the alternatives to surgery and the possible benefits and complications of surgery.

8. Forget the mistaken notion that it's somehow improper to inquire about all the cost of surgery. If the surgeon seems unwilling to discuss fees, then he doesn't know much of his obligation to the patient.

9. Check out the surgeon with those who know him or have used him.

10. Be sure that the surgeon knows and is willing to work with your personal doctor. If they can't work as a team, you may be the loser.

11. You are more likely to have a doctor available at all times who is familiar with your case if your physician is part of a group practice.

12. Surgeons who handle too many cases are bad news for the patient. Select one who isn't too busy to give you enough time and attention.

13. Watch out with special care for those operations that are most often unnecessarily performed: hysterectomies, hemorrhoidectomies, and tonsillectomies.

14. The patient, and not the doctor or surgeon, is supposed to and is entitled to make the decision on surgery. This is your life.

Mimi Forsyth/Monkmeyer

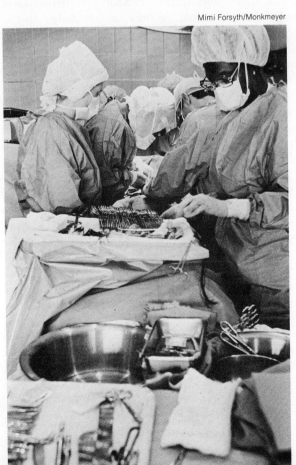

Surgery is more complicated—and expensive—than ever before.

A word about item 11 of the surgery checklist. A growing form of group practice is the Health Maintenance Organization (HMO). Doctors working in an HMO get paid as much for keeping a patient well as they do for giving a patient treatment when he is sick. Unlike standard health insurance plans, which pay doctors on a per-case basis, the HMO provides no economic incentive to perform unnecessary surgery. It's a program worth considering. If you don't belong to an HMO, however, always seek a second independent opinion as to whether an operation is really necessary. When you are employed, urge your employer to get a health insurance policy that pays for this second opinion.

Hospitals

Of all categories of health care, hospitalization is by far the most taxing of the consumer's budget. Over $40 billion is spent each year on hospital care in America. This is about $190 for each man, woman, and child. In 1975 the Health Research Group reported that at least $8 billion of this money was wasted on excess hospital beds. Of that $8 billion, $2 billion was spent just for the upkeep of 100,000 unused beds, and another $6 billion was wasted on 250,000 more beds filled by patients who should not have been hospitalized in the first place or who stayed in the hospital too long. Today this "hospital bed overrun" continues to encourage unnecessary surgery, diverts badly needed funds from other, less costly health facilities like outpatient clinics and ambulatory surgical centers, and inflates the cost of going to the hospital.

With charges as high as they are, the consumer must do everything possible to see that any recommended hospital care is (1) necessary, (2) safe, and (3) as economical as reason will allow. *Before hospitalization* a patient should talk to his physician about alternatives to hospital care, such as outpatient treatment or home care programs. If hospital care is deemed necessary, the patient should work with his physician in choosing a hospital. If, for no apparent reason, the physician will not admit the patient to the hospital of his choice, the patient should go to another physician. When a hospital is chosen, financial arrangements have to be made. The patient should review his health insurance with his employer or insurance advisor. Next, the patient should find out more about his hospital, including what it charges and what these charges include.

During hospitalization the patient should let his physician and the hospital staff know when there is anything about which he has questions or complaints. The doctor should be willing to discuss anything about the patient's care and should be ready to show the patient any part of his medical record he asks to see. The patient should ask his doctor how the hospital safeguards the confidentiality of this record. The patient should also be aware that his doctor may not force him to take part in any research projects; if the patient agrees to such participation, he should be able to withdraw from the experiment at any time.

As the patient leaves the hospital, and he has the right to do this any time he wishes, he should make sure his bills are correct. It does not matter whether Medicare, Medicaid, an insurance company, an employer, or the patient himself paid the bill; the patient has a right and a responsibility to check the hospital bill. Finally, the patient should give the hospital his opinion of its service. This can be done by talking to a "patient advocate" or another hospital contact person.

Through the entire process of hospitalization, the patient should have in mind the "Patient's Bill of Rights," adopted in 1973 by the American Hospital Association. Although they have not become legal rights, they do review standards of good practice. A patient should ask if his hospital has adopted such a policy. The "Bill of Rights," in abbreviated form, states that the patient has:

1. The right to considerate and respectful care
2. The right to obtain from his physician complete current information concerning his diagnosis, treatment, and prognosis in terms the patient can be reasonably expected to understand
3. The right to receive from his physician information necessary to give informed consent prior to the start of any procedure or treatment
4. The right to refuse treatment to the extent permitted by law and to be informed of the medical consequences of his action
5. The right to every consideration of his privacy concerning his own medical care program
6. The right to expect that all communications and records pertaining to his care should be treated as confidential
7. The right to expect that within its capacity a hospital must make a reasonable response to the request of a patient for services
8. The right to obtain information as to any relationship of his hospital to other health care and educational institutions insofar as his care is concerned
9. The right to be advised if the hospital proposes to engage in or perform human experimentation affecting his care or treatment
10. The right to expect reasonable continuity of care
11. The right to examine and receive an explanation of his bill regardless of source of payment
12. The right to know what hospital rules and regulations apply to his conduct as a patient

The right repeated throughout is the consumer's right to be informed. It was the right addressed by the Connecticut Citizen Action Group, the Connecticut Citizen Research Group, and the New Haven Health Care, Inc., in their 1974 publication of the first statewide guide to general hospitals.

Dentists Tooth decay is America's most common chronic disease, afflicting 95 percent of the population. Some 90 million Americans have at least 18 missing, decayed, or filled teeth, and 25 million Americans, middle-aged and older, have lost all their teeth. About 90 percent of those over 65 have gum disease, as do 80 percent of the middle-aged and 60 percent of young adults. American dentists are kept busy. Extractions alone amount to 56 million teeth a year.

And yet dentistry is about as familiar to the American consumer as the other forms of professional health care—the consumer in the dentist's chair has no idea of what the dentist should be doing. Government does very little to regulate dentistry, and local professional societies do even less. In fact until 1973 the code of the American Dental Association deemed it unethical for one dentist to criticize the poor work of another. So the modern dentist is very much on his own, often to make his own rules.

Evidence now suggests that too many dentists are taking unfair advantage of this independence. Faulty diagnosis, faulty dental work, and outright deception by dentists are not uncommon. In a study of 11,000 Medicaid patients in New York State, 11 percent of their dental work was found deficient or in need of review; 8 percent was found to involve fraud. More than a waste of money, these mistakes and misdeeds are likely to be the cause of new, more painful dental problems in the future. The victims failed to carry with them the best defense against the swindler—that is, information.

There are a few basic rules you can follow in selecting a dentist. If you can contact dental specialists for advice, you should certainly do that first. Look for a specialist likely to be prevention-oriented. Orthodontists (specializing in straightening teeth), periodontists (gums), endodontists (root canal work), and pedodontists (children's teeth) ought to have valuable information on dentists. When you find a dentist, evaluate him for yourself, remembering your rights.

The Right to Quality Dentistry The best dentist is one primarily interested in the prevention of dental disease. At your first appointment this dentist will obtain from you your medical and dental history. You should advise the dentist of any of your drug allergies and about any medication you might be taking. He will ask for a record of your past dental treatment, including X rays. During your examination, note whether your dentist checks (1) your lips, tongue, and throat (soft tissue) for any abnormalities that might indicate cancer of the oral cavity, (2) your gums for bleeding, unusual coloring, tooth mobility, and other signs of disease, and, of course, (3) your teeth (hard tissue). Throughout your examination and then your treatment, consider how well organized your dentist is. One who is constantly interrupted or has to rush to meet a fast-paced schedule can be dangerous.

The Right to the Knowledge of Preventive Techniques You should not feel uneasy about asking questions, and your dentist should not be unhappy to provide answers you can understand. You should have some idea of the risks involved with any treatment. When the dentist decides to give you an anesthetic, ask him about it. Ask him what specialized training he has had. Ask him how he is prepared for an emergency. And if you have even the slightest doubt about your dentist's judgment, ask the advice of another dentist or a dental specialist.

The Right to Minimize X-Ray Exposures Whenever a dentist says he needs X rays of your teeth, ask him why. X rays are capable of causing cancer and genetic damage and should be used sparingly. Nevertheless, it is estimated that over half of all diagnostic X rays taken are unnecessary. Slipshod practice and poorly functioning equipment compound the problem. To guard against excessive exposure to radiation, a dentist taking X rays should cover his patient with a lead apron. A good dentist will not have to be asked to do this. To shorten X-ray exposures, he should also use ultraspeed dental film. The patient should request older X rays from any previous dentists. Under normal circumstances, this will reduce the need for new X rays, particularly full-mouth sets, which are necessary only every three to five years.

The Right to the Most Conservative Therapy   An extraction is the last thing you want from your dentist. If he advises a removal, ask him why he has rejected periodontic treatment or root canal therapy. Then, if you are still hesitant, go to a specialist who does not know your dentist. Losing a tooth may appear more economical than saving it, but consequent dental problems can turn an extraction into a financial disaster. Be wary too of dentists who suggest capping before a more conservative therapy, or who without good explanation want to remove your wisdom teeth.

The Right to a Written Estimate of Costs in Advance of Treatment After your examination and before any dental treatment, your dentist should present you with a treatment plan, with a written itemization of costs and fees. After the treatment, you should be given an itemized bill, breaking down the charges.

The Right to Your Own Dental X Rays and Records When a dentist X-rays your mouth or records your treatment, you pay him to do it. You then have a right to the records. Before you move or change dentists, you should ask your last dentist for a copy of all your X rays and records to give your next dentist. This saves needless expense and exposure to radiation and provides your newest dentist with information he will require.

To explain these rights, a "Consumer's Guide to Dentistry" was released in 1974 by the Connecticut Citizen Action Group, in concert with the Connecticut State Dental Association (CSDA). It was the first time a professional dental society had joined with a citizen group to advise consumers on avoiding low-quality dentistry. The CSDA was, in effect, conceding the fact that some dentists are flunkies—a good first step toward better dental care.

In 1975 another group went even further. That year, the Health Research Group published a "Dentist Directory" for the citizens of Washington, D.C. In addition to office hours, practice patterns and fee schedules, the directory spells out insurance programs (Blue Cross, Medicaid, Medicare, and so on) in which each dentist participates (see Figure 13-2). The information was first collected over the telephone, then sent to each dentist for confirmation. Only 127 of the 430 D.C. dentists provided the information during the phone interviews, and only 68 ultimately confirmed in writing what was collected. However, the data that were collected, outlining the practices of 15 percent of the city's dentists, go far beyond anything Washingtonians had previously had to work with. It's the kind of information the consumers of any city could use.

High Cost of Dental Care   As experience or a "Dentist Directory" will show, going to a dentist is expensive. The costs of dental care might not be so high as those of hospital care or physicians' services, but they can be just as traumatic. About 90 percent of all hospital bills and over 60 percent of all physicians' bills are covered by "third-party payments" from private insurance, government, and philanthropy. In contrast, these payments cover only 14 percent of bills for dental care. The rest comes directly from the patient's pocket. Thus in 1974 direct payments for hospital and physicians' services amounted to only $12 billion of the astounding $60 billion total, but nearly all the $6.2 billion for dental care was paid directly.

Dental costs have an impact that encourages consumers to put off sorely needed tooth care, only to wind up with more pain, more expense, and tooth loss in the long run. Most affected by the reluctance to see a dentist are the children of the disadvantaged. This is what the Vermont Public Interest Research Group (VPIRG) was thinking in 1972, when it decided to study the dental health of Vermont's children. The student-run group found that only half the school children in that state had seen a dentist by their fifteenth firthday, that over two-fifths of the children were in urgent need of dental care, and that the majority of Vermont families could not afford dental care for their children. In January 1973 VPIRG released their report on the dental health of Vermont's children. The report led to the passage that year of the "Tooth Fairy Bill," cutting by 50 percent the cost of children's dental care to Vermont families with adjusted gross incomes under $8750 and cutting by 75 percent the cost to families with incomes under $5750.

The action in Vermont, the work in the District of Columbia and in Connecticut, and the rules for finding a dentist: all manifest the fact that good dental care need not be a luxury, nor need it be left to dentists alone. Consumers can find out what their teeth need and don't need.

Figure 13-2

Sample data on one dentist listed in "D.C. Dentist Directory."

General Practice

N———, EDWARD D.,   Graduated: 1966   Office Phone: 000-0000

Office Address: _____ Avenue N.W.   Home Phone: Listed
              Washington, D.C.

Office Hours: Mon., Tues., Thurs., Fri., Sat. Group practice
                                            of 2 dentists

2-3 day interval between request and date of appointment.

Emergencies: Will take emergency calls without an appointment
             for anyone during office hours.

Practice Patterns
   INITIAL EXAMINATION includes the following, cost varies:
      1) medical and dental history, 2) full set of X rays
   X RAY: New unit. Lead apron routinely used. Fast film and long cone
      technique. Full mouth series taken every 2-3 years.
   PERFORMS ROUTINELY: Pericsurgery; oral surgery (simple third mo-
      lars, impacted third molars); endodontics (anterior, posterior).
   PLAQUE CONTROL PROGRAM: Sessions last from 15–30 minutes and
      are as frequent as necessary. Patient is seen by both dentist and
      hygienist. Cost of program varies depending on number of sessions.
   HANDICAPPED: Mentally retarded.
   GENERAL: Uses steam autoclave. Has an emergency kit which con-
      tains epinephrine, glucose, nitroglycerin, ephedrine, oxygen, endo-
      tracheal equipment.

Fee Schedule
   STANDARD FEES:
      Full mouth series - $25; 2 bitewing films - $8; minimum charge for
      emergency treatment - $10; Class II surface fillings - $15; prophylaxis
      - $20; complete denture maxillary and mandibular - $500; anterior
      ceramco crown - $180; extraction of simple third molar - $20; extrac-
      tion of impacted third molar $25 up; anterior endodontics - $95; pos-
      terior endodontics - $125-$150.

General Information
   Participates in Blue Cross insurance program. Records are released to
      patient upon request. Has a faculty or hospital appointment at Chil-
      dren's Hospital and Georgetown University. Attended a continuing
      education course in pedodontics in the last six months. Willing to
      undergo Peer Review.

Consumers can save their teeth, even without dentists. Good diet and
proper home care do more for teeth than fillings. Dentists might have
your teeth a couple hours a year; if you do your part, you'll have them
all your life.

TAKING ACTION

1. *Visit and evaluate your family doctor.*
2. *Visit and evaluate your local hospital.*
3. *Go through the process of a dental examination and treatment.*
4. *If you think you can raise the required funds, get the material from Public
   Citizen's Health Research Group to compile a local directory of doctors,
   dentists, or hospitals.*

EDUCATION AND THE STUDENT: A DISCUSSION

Methods of counteraction are gradually emerging from the manifold
threats to health. Again and again consumers are proving the value of
information applied to defense of the home. They have discovered that
even large-scale problems, once the sacred domain of private interests
working with government, can be taken on in the public interest. The
new vigor of the "public citizen" is manifested in expert testimony
before Congress and state legislatures, the petitioning of governmental
agencies, the publication of consumer guides to health care, and the
preparation of data for coverage in the press. Consumers are beginning
to meet a basic need: organization.

Students have a major role to play in meeting this need. Today 24
Public Interest Research Groups (PIRGs) in 24 states are run by college
students. The groups are funded each semester by student fees paid at
registration. Students exercise control over each PIRG by electing a
board of directors. Each board, working within its budget, hires lawyers
and other staff (scientists, doctors, and others) who together have the
expertise to act on problems an individual would find impossible to
approach. Through student financing they also have the resources to
gather and publish information, such as that necessary to proper and
economical health care.

In addition to organization, students have another role to play in the
implementation of consumer information. This they accomplish by
making the personal transition from knowledge to action. For too long
some students, many who know better, have turned abuse of alcohol,
tobacco, and drugs into a way of life. There is no longer an excuse for it.
It's bad enough that companies often conceal important facts; it's a
disgrace that life-saving information is ignored.

For the multitudes of students who are actively concerned about
health, there is the job of supplying and maintaining the vital link
between self-care and self-respect. Students can make it clear to other
students that there is nothing "cool" about debasing life, by whatever

means. Like everybody else, students must come to grips with the real world. Campuses should be living examples of a better way. Institutions of learning must demonstrate their commitment to one basic tenet: that only with the rational *use* of information is there a completion of education.

FOR FURTHER READING

Choate, Robert, 1973. *The Selling of the Child.* Washington, D.C.: Council on Children, Media and Merchandising.

Congressional testimony on the role of motivational research houses and television advertising in manipulating the wants of children.

A Consumer's Guide to Connecticut Hospitals, 1974. Hartford: Connecticut Citizen Action Group.

An excellent model for future consumer guides. Available from CCAG, Box 6465, Hartford, Conn. 06106.

Cottine, Bert, Birrel, Linda, and Jennings, Robert, 1975. *Winning at the Occupational Safety and Health Review Commission: Workers Handbook.* Washington, D.C.: Health Research Group.

A citizen's guide to claiming the right to a safe workplace. Available for $5 from the Health Research Group, 2000 P Street, N.W., Washington, D.C. 20036.

A Guide for Compiling a Consumers Directory of Doctors, 1975. Washington, D.C.: Health Research Group.

A detailed plan for breaking through the secrecy of the medical profession. Available for $1 from the Health Research Group.

Lanoue, Ron, 1975. *Evacuation Plans: The Achilles' Heel of the Nuclear Industry.* Washington, D.C.: Citizen Action Group.

Suggestions and facts on how to be sure public officials have done their job in preparing for the possibility of an accident at a nuclear power plant. Available for $1.50 from the Citizen Action Group, 2000 P Street, N.W., Washington, D.C. 20036.

Nader, Ralph, and Ross, Donald, 1974. *A PIRG Organizer's Notebook.* Washington, D.C.: Citizen Action Group.

Information for establishing a local student-funded, student-run Public Interest Research Group. Available for $1.

Nader, Ralph, and Ross, Donald, 1971. *Action for a Change.* New York: Grossman Publishers.

This 118-page book also presents useful information for campus organizers.

our health and society

Nash, Greg, and Wolfe, Sidney, 1975. *Taking the Pain Out of Finding a Good Dentist.* Washington, D.C.: Health Research Group.

A guide for publishing a consumer's directory of dentists, with a model D.C. dentist directory. Available for $2 from the Health Research Group.

U.S. Department of Agriculture, 1975. *Nutrition Labeling: Tools for Its Use.* Washington, D.C.: U.S. Government Printing Office.

A 57-page government publication, discussing not only the use of nutrition labeling but also the nutrients provided by foods that have no labels. Available from the GPO for $1.15.

INDEX